NEUROBEHAVIOR OF LANGUAGE AND COGNITION
Studies of Normal Aging and Brain Damage

Honoring Martin L. Albert

NEUROBEHAVIOR OF LANGUAGE AND COGNITION
Studies of Normal Aging and Brain Damage

Honoring Martin L. Albert

edited by

Lisa Tabor Connor
Boston University School of Medicine

Loraine K. Obler
City University of New York Graduate Center

KLUWER ACADEMIC PUBLISHERS
Boston / Dordrecht / London

Distributors for North, Central and South America:
Kluwer Academic Publishers
101 Philip Drive
Assinippi Park
Norwell, Massachusetts 02061 USA
Telephone (781) 871-6600
Fax (781) 681-9045
E-Mail <kluwer@wkap.com>

Distributors for all other countries:
Kluwer Academic Publishers Group
Distribution Centre
Post Office Box 322
3300 AH Dordrecht, THE NETHERLANDS
Telephone 31 78 6392 392
Fax 31 78 6546 474
E-Mail <services@wkap.nl>

 Electronic Services <http://www.wkap.nl>

Library of Congress Cataloging-in-Publication Data
Neurobehavior of language and cognition: studies of normal aging and brain damage: honoring Martin L. Albert / edited by Lisa Tabor Connor, Loraine K. Obler.
  p. ; cm.
  Includes bibliographical references and index.
  ISBN 0-7923-7877-6 (alk. paper)
  1. Language disorders. 2. Cognition disorders. 3. Aphasia. 4. Neurolinguistics. 5. Cognition. 6. Brain damage. 7. Albert, Martin L., 1939- I. Albert, Martin L., 1939- II. Connor, Lisa Tabor. III. Obler, Loraine K.
  [DNLM: 1. Language Disorders. 2. Aging—physiology. 3. Aphasia. 4. Brain Damage, Chronic. 5. Cognition—physiology. 6. Dementia. 7. Neuropsychology—methods. WL 340.2 N4934 2000]
  RC423 .N36 2000
  616.85'5—dc21

00-033103

Copyright © 2000 by Kluwer Academic Publishers

All rights reserved. No part of this publication may be reproduced, stored in a retrieval system or transmitted in any form or by any means, mechanical, photocopying, recording, or otherwise, without the prior written permission of the publisher, Kluwer Academic Publishers, 101 Philip Drive, Assinippi Park, Norwell, Massachusetts 02061
Printed on acid-free paper. Printed in the United States of America

The Publisher offers discounts on this book for course use and bulk purchases. For further information, send email to <michael.williams@wkap.com>.

TABLE OF CONTENTS

CONTRIBUTORS — ix

PREFACE — xiii

ACKNOWLEDGMENTS — xvii

LANGUAGE IN HEALTHY ADULTS

Neural Change, Cognitive Reserve and Behavioral Compensation in Rapid Encoding and Memory for Spoken Language in Adult Aging
Arthur Wingfield, Kristen Prentice, Christine K. Koh, and Deborah Little — 3

Factors Underlying Comprehension of Accented English
Mira Goral, Loraine K. Obler, and Elizabeth Galletta — 23

LANGUAGE IN BRAIN DAMAGE: DEMENTIA

Word and Pseudoword Repetition in Alzheimer's Disease
Marie-Claire Goldblum, Catherine Tzortzis, Thérèse Jahchan, and François Boller — 45

Sentence Comprehension in Alzheimer's Disease
David Caplan and Gloria Waters — 61

Writing Impairments in Alzheimer's Disease
Guila Glosser and Victor W. Henderson — 77

LANGUAGE IN BRAIN DAMAGE: APHASIA

Neurobehavioral Models for Aphasia Rehabilitation
Nancy Helm-Estabrooks — 95

Self-Determination and Self–Advocacy: New Concepts for Aphasic Individuals and Their Partners
Audrey L. Holland — 109

Neuroimaging in Severe Aphasia and Outcome Following Treatment with the Nonverbal, Computer-Assisted Visual Communication Program, C-ViC
Margaret A. Naeser, Errol H. Baker, Carole L. Palumbo, Marjorie Nicholas, Michael P. Alexander, Ranji Samaraweera, Malee N. Prete, Steven M. Hodge, and Tamily Weissman — 117

Combinatorial Operations in Sentence Comprehension
Edgar Zurif and Maria Piñango — 141

Primary Progressive Aphasia: Dissociation of the Loss of Syntax and Semantics in a Biologically Determined Brain Degeneration
Andrew Kertesz — 149

Pharmacotherapy of Aphasia
Yutaka Tanaka and David L. Bachman — 159

UNDERSTANDING COGNITIVE FUNCTIONING THROUGH BRAIN DAMAGE

The Neural Basis of Working Memory: Evidence from Neuropsychological, Pharmacological and Neuroimaging Studies
Mark D'Esposito — 179

Language Functions in Parkinson's Disease: Evidence for a Neurochemistry of Language
Patrick McNamara and Raymon Durso — 201

Asymmetries of Brain Function in Alcoholism: Relationship to Aging
Marlene Oscar-Berman and Haline E. Schendan — 213

Cognitive Perspectives on Humor Comprehension after Brain Injury
Hiram Brownell and Andrew Stringfellow — 241

Anosognosia
Kenneth M. Heilman, Anna M. Barrett, and John C. Adair — 259

Doctor François: A Case-Study of Deep Dyslexia
André Roch Lecours, Marie-Josèphe Tainturier, and Sonia Lupien — 269

Dissociating Speed from Automaticity in the Stroop Task: Evidence from a Case of Progressive Posterior Cortical Atrophy
Kimberly C. Lindfield, Harold Goodglass, and Arthur Wingfield — 299

The Role of Memory in Estimating Time: A Neuropsychological Analysis
Marcel Kinsbourne — 315

NEUROBEHAVIORAL ASSESSMENT

Neuropsychiatric Symptoms in Alzheimer's Disease:
Assessment and Management
Susan McPherson and Jeffrey Cummings   327

Cross-Cultural Neuropsychology of Aging and Dementia:
An Update
Nicola Wolfe   347

Validation of the Neurobehavioral Evaluation System (NES) in
Patients with Focal Brain Damage
Rhea Diamond, Roberta F. White, Maxine Krengel, Karen Lindem,
Robert G. Feldman, Carole Palumbo, Richard Letz, Ellen Eisen, and
David Wegman   359

Neurology of Aging
Janice E. Knoefel and John C. Adair   381

INDEX   391

Contributors

John C. Adair
Department of Neurology, University of New Mexico; Department of Veterans Affairs Medical Center, Albuquerque, NM

Michael P. Alexander
Department of Neurology and Harold Goodglass Aphasia Research Center, Boston University School of Medicine; Medical Research Service, Veterans Affairs Boston Healthcare System, MA

David L. Bachman
Department of Neurology, Medical University of South Carolina, Charleston, SC

Errol H. Baker
Department of Neurology and Harold Goodglass Aphasia Research Center, Boston University School of Medicine; Medical Research Service, Veterans Affairs Boston Healthcare System, MA

Anna M. Barrett
Department of Neurology, Pennsylvania State University College of Medicine, Hershey, PA

François Boller
Centre Paul Broca, Paris, France

Hiram Brownell
Department of Psychology, Boston College, Chestnut Hill, MA; Department of Neurology and Harold Goodglass Aphasia Research Center, Boston University School of Medicine; Medical Research Service, Veterans Affairs Boston Healthcare System, MA

David Caplan
Department of Neurology, Harvard Medical School; Neuropsychology Lab, Massachusetts General Hospital, Boston, MA

Jeffrey L. Cummings
Department of Neurology, UCLA School of Medicine, Los Angeles, CA

Mark D'Esposito
Department of Neurology, University of Pennsylvania, Philadelphia, PA

Rhea Diamond
Department of Neurology, Boston University School of Medicine; Department of Environmental Health, Veterans Affairs Boston Healthcare System, MA

Raymon Durso
Department of Neurology, Boston University School of Medicine and Veterans Affairs Boston Healthcare System, MA

Ellen Eisen
Department of Work Environment, University of Massachusetts, Lowell, MA

Robert G. Feldman
Department of Neurology, Boston University School of Medicine, Boston, MA

Elizabeth Galletta
Program in Speech and Hearing Sciences, City University of New York Graduate Center, New York, NY

Guila Glosser
Department of Neurology, University of Pennsylvania School of Medicine, Philadelphia, PA

Marie-Claire Goldblum
Centre Paul Broca, Paris, France

Harold Goodglass
Department of Neurology and Harold Goodglass Aphasia Research Center, Boston University School of Medicine; Medical Research Service, Veterans Affairs Boston Healthcare System, MA; Volen National Center for Complex Systems, Brandeis University, Waltham, MA

Mira Goral
Program in Speech and Hearing Sciences, City University of New York Graduate Center, New York, NY

Kenneth M. Heilman
Department of Neurology, University of Florida College of Medicine; University Hospital Medical Center; Department of Veterans Affairs Medical Center, Gainesville, FL

Nancy Helm-Estabrooks
Department of Neurology and Harold Goodglass Aphasia Research Center, Boston University School of Medicine; Medical Research Service, Veterans Affairs Boston Healthcare System, MA; National Center for Neurogenic Communication Disorders, University of Arizona, Tucson, AZ

Victor W. Henderson
Department of Neurology, University of Southern California School of Medicine, Los Angeles, CA

Steven M. Hodge
Department of Neurology and Harold Goodglass Aphasia Research Center, Boston University School of Medicine; Medical Research Service, Veterans Affairs Boston Healthcare System, MA

Audrey Holland
Department of Speech and Hearing Sciences, University of Arizona, Tucson, AZ

Thérèse Jahchan
Centre Paul Broca, Paris, France

Andrew Kertesz
Department of Clinical Neurological Sciences, University of Western Ontario, London ON, Canada

Marcel Kinsbourne
Department of Psychology, New School University, New York, NY; Center for Cognitive Studies, Tufts University, Medford, MA

Janice Knoefel
University of New Mexico, Albuquerque, NM; Geriatrics/Extended Care Section, Veterans Affairs Medical Center, Albuquerque, NM

Christine K. Koh
Acoustics Laboratory, Department of Psychology, Queen's University, Kingston, Canada

Maxine Krengel
Department of Environmental Health, Veterans Affairs Boston Healthcare System; Department of Neurology, Boston University School of Medicine; Department of Psychiatry, Harvard Medical School, Boston, MA

André Roch Lecours
Centre de Recherche en Sciences Neurologiques, Faculté de Médecine, Université de Montréal; Centre de Recherche de l'Institut de Geriatrie, Université de Montréal, Québec, Canada

Richard Letz
Department of Behavioral Science and Health Education, Rollins School of Public Health, Emory University, Atlanta, GA

Karen Lindem
Department of Neurology, Boston University School of Medicine; Veterans Affairs Boston Healthcare System, MA

Kimberly C. Lindfield
Department of Neurology and Harold Goodglass Aphasia Research Center, Boston University School of Medicine; Medical Research Service, Veterans Affairs Boston Healthcare System, MA; Volen National Center for Complex Systems, Brandeis Univ., Waltham, MA

Deborah M. Little
Volen National Center for Complex Systems and Department of Psychology, Brandeis University, Waltham, MA

Sonia Lupien
Department of Psychiatry, McGill University; Douglas Hospital & Geriatric Institute of Montreal, Montreal, Canada

Patrick McNamara
Department of Psychiatry and Program in Behavioral Neuroscience, Boston University School of Medicine, Boston, MA

Susan McPherson
Department of Neurology, UCLA, School of Medicine, Los Angeles, CA

Margaret A. Naeser
Department of Neurology and Harold Goodglass Aphasia Research Center, Boston University School of Medicine; Veterans Affairs Boston Healthcare System, MA

Marjorie Nicholas
Speech Pathology and Audiology Service, Veterans Affairs Boston Healthcare System; Harold Goodglass Aphasia Research Center, Department of Neurology, Boston University School of Medicine; Medical Research Service, Veterans Affairs Boston Healthcare System, MA

Loraine K. Obler
City University of New York Graduate Center, Program in Speech and Hearing Sciences, New York, NY; Department of Neurology and Harold Goodglass Aphasia Research Center, Boston University School of Medicine; Medical Research Service, Veterans Affairs Boston Healthcare System, MA

Marlene Oscar Berman
Department of Psychiatry, Boston University School of Medicine; Veterans Affairs Boston Healthcare System, MA

Carole L. Palumbo
Boston Environmental Hazards Center, Veterans Affairs Boston Healthcare System; Department of Neurology and Harold Goodglass Aphasia Research Center, Boston University School of Medicine; Medical Research Service, Veterans Affairs Boston Healthcare System, MA

Maria M. Piñango
Department of Linguistics, Yale University, New Haven, CT

Kristen J. Prentice
Volen National Center for Complex Systems and Department of Psychology, Brandeis University, Waltham, MA

Malee N. Prete
Department of Neurology and Harold Goodglass Aphasia Research Center, Boston University School of Medicine; Medical Research Service, Veterans Affairs Boston Healthcare System, MA

Ranji Samaraweera
Department of Radiology, Boston University School of Medicine; Veterans Affairs Boston Healthcare System, MA

Haline Schendan
Department of Psychiatry, Boston University School of Medicine, Boston, MA

Andrew Stringfellow
Harold Goodglass Aphasia Research Center, Department of Neurology, Boston University School of Medicine; Medical Research Service, Veterans Affairs Boston Healthcare System, MA

Marie-Josèphe Tainturier
Université Pierre-Mendès-France, Grenoble, France

Yutaka Tanaka
Mie University, Nara, Japan

Catherine Tzortzis
Centre Paul Broca, Paris, France

Gloria Waters
Department of Communication Disorders, Boston University, Boston, MA

David Wegman
Department of Work Environment, University of Massachusetts at Lowell, Lowell, MA

Tamily Weissman
Department of Neurology and Harold Goodglass Aphasia Research Center, Boston University School of Medicine; Medical Research Service, Veterans Affairs Boston Healthcare System, MA

Roberta F. White
Departments of Neurology, Psychology, and Environmental & Occupational Health, Boston University School of Medicine; Boston Environmental Hazards Center, Veterans Affairs Boston Healthcare System, MA

Arthur Wingfield
Volen National Center for Complex Systems and Department of Psychology, Brandeis University, Waltham, MA; Department of Neurology and Harold Goodglass Aphasia Research Center, Boston University School of Medicine; Medical Research Service, Veterans Affairs Boston Healthcare System, MA

Nicola Wolfe
Psychopharmacology Program, California School of Professional Psychology, Alameda, CA

Edgar Zurif
Volen National Center for Complex Systems, Brandeis University, Waltham, MA; Harold Goodglass Aphasia Research Center, Department of Neurology, Boston University School of Medicine and Medical Research Service, Veterans Affairs Boston Healthcare System, MA

PREFACE

This volume has been composed as an appreciation of Martin L. Albert in the year of his 60th birthday. At least one contributor to each paper in this volume has been touched by Marty in some way; he has mentored some, been a fellow student with some, and been a colleague to most. These contributors, as well as many others, view Marty as a gifted scientist and a wonderful human being. The breadth of his interests and intellectual pursuits is truly impressive; this breadth is reflected, only in part, by the diversity of the papers in this volume. His interests have ranged from psychopharmacology to cross-cultural understanding of dementia, through the aphasias, to the history of the fields that touch on behavioral neurology, especially neurology *per se*, cognitive psychology, speech-language pathology, and linguistics. Throughout his scholarly work, Martha Taylor Sarno notes, Marty never loses the human perspective, e.g., the "powerfully disabling effect on the individual person" with aphasia or other neurological disorder.

For those readers who only know a portion of his work, we thought that we should describe him here. Many of the people whom Marty has influenced have been able to contribute to this volume. We have invited some others who were unable to contribute to express their appreciation for him, as well. We have attempted to weave in the sentiments of all (attributed when the quotation was unique, unattributed when more than one person made reference to a particularly appreciated characteristic) with our own, in what follows.

Marty's predilection is, most certainly, for interdisciplinary work and he is able to plumb a number of fields to stimulate thinking. Terms used to characterize his thinking are "synthetic, comprehensive, ecumenical, and international" (David Bachman); he has the ability to "see important connections among disparate elements, that otherwise, on first glance, would seem absurd" (Marlene Oscar Berman). He takes risks in making connections, going beyond the conventional understanding that, Janice Knoefel reminds us, he's mastered, to ask new questions and/or give new answers. Marty's characteristic breadth extends to his appreciation of the counter-intuitive, reminiscent of Normal Geschwind's, as David Bachman pointed out. Marty's intellectual style and openness to ideas (Marney Naeser cites the idea of using acupuncture for treating the consequences of stroke, and, more recently, laser acupuncture) is appreciated by many.

Marty's approach to intellectual endeavors is serious and thoughtful, leavened by a certain humor and whimsy and imagination. His style of thinking, as well as of interacting, is always questioning. His insights are profound. He is a creative thinker who makes certain to mark what is known and what is speculation. Marty is not afraid to go out on an intellectual "limb." He enjoys making provocative statements to challenge thinking beyond current boundaries of an issue, to push envelopes, to expand our horizons.

Short- and long-term visitors from around the world, Yutaka Tanaka indicates, are proud to have studied with Marty. Marty teaches in many contexts – certainly not just the formal classroom: bedside rounds, grand rounds, over lunch, and at meetings from the laboratory-level to the international, synthesizing and sharing knowledge from a broad array of disciplines. As a teacher, Marty is known for his eloquent and well-organized discourse. He is willing to find time to discuss any topic, and to share all his knowledge. He teaches, too, through his stimulating writings across a wide range of topics.

As a mentor, Marty can be counted on to be supportive. Many wrote us that they owe him a lot, professionally, but personally as well, for what he has done, and continues to do, in discussing their lives and careers with them. Not only is he "there for one" as necessary, as Edgar Zurif observes, he is invariably available for counsel and suggestions. Lise Menn and others have appreciated Marty's important advice and guidance that have gotten them to their current positions. Howard Gardner and Nancy Helm-Estabrooks credit him with being influential in their introduction to the field and the Aphasia Research Center, respectively. Nikki Wolfe remembers the importance of his enthusiastic encouragement. Hiram Brownell concludes that Marty "wants people to succeed in their carecrs." Moreover, Marty often develops a friendship with those he has mentored that continues on as they move to more advanced stages of their careers. Few can count as many colleagues as friends as Marty can.

As a leader, Marty has been appreciated by many in the roles he has taken at what is now named the Harold Goodglass Aphasia Research Center where he is currently Director. He is appreciated for his ability to collaborate with and support a group of independent thinkers with different perspectives. Sheila Blumstein terms this latter the ability to be patient with "challenges, debates and disagreement, and the refusal to take anything at face value, leading this group being like herding cats!" Many mention his cheerful, optimistic attitude (even when it is not warranted by reality, Marlene Oscar Berman points out), and the fact that he actually seems happy to see his colleagues. That he takes on his administrative function with a sense of humor, never hurting others, but including himself as a target, has been important. His willingness to share his knowledge and resources is appreciated by many. Also, his ability to contribute content as well as administrative structure is valued in part for its rarity in someone with an administrative role.

In sum, Marty is appreciated for his superb human interactional abilities that extend beyond his life with family and friends to his colleagues at every level. His ability to get the larger picture in any intellectual realm he approaches, and to convey this larger picture to those he works with, advises, teaches, and leads in various ways stand out to all who have worked with him in this, the early part of his career.

The papers in this volume are united by the fact that they represent neurobehavioral approaches to unraveling the diversity of human behavior. What constitutes a neurobehavioral approach is, of course, wide-ranging itself, as many methodologies can be deployed and many subject populations studied. Research on neurobehavior includes study of the behavior of individuals with a particular brain disorder or lesion, as well as examination of ways in which individuals adapt to the aging process or alteration of incoming information.

This volume is organized by the cognitive functions that are examined in the individual papers and the populations in which these functions are disordered. The first section, *Language in Healthy Adults*, includes two papers, one by Wingfield, Prentice, Koh, and Little on the role of compensation in speech recognition and memory for speech in old age, and the other by Goral, Obler, and Galleta on accommodation to accented speech. The second section, *Language in Brain Damage: Dementia*, also details language changes, but in individuals with Alzheimer's disease. Three papers, the first by Goldblum, Boller, Jahchan, and Tsortzis on word repetition, the second by Caplan and Waters on sentence comprehension, and the third by Glosser and Henderson on writing abilities, each demonstrate that individuals with Alzheimer's disease have impairment of many of the components of communication but that these abilities degrade in a predictable way along the lines of extant psycholinguistic theory of language functioning.

Chapters in the third section, *Language in Brain Damage: Aphasia*, examine language in aphasia, the intellectual domain with which Marty Albert is most strongly associated. The first two chapters, by Helm-Estabrooks and by Holland, are focused on aspects of aphasia treatment. Helm-Estabrooks synthesizes work on aphasia treatment arising from a neurobehavioral approach, while Holland discusses focusing treatment on aphasic individuals' functional communication. Naeser et al. report on brain-behavior correlates of recovery of propositional language following treatment with an alternative computerized communication system (C-ViC). The last three chapters in this section, by Zurif and Piñango, Kertesz, and Tanaka and Bachman, focus on theories of language representation and show how aphasic language disorders may be interpreted in terms of theories from linguistic, neuropsychological, and psychopharmacological perspectives.

Section four, *Understanding Cognitive Functioning through Brain Damage*, contains eight chapters that each discuss cognitive processes and their neural substrates: D'Esposito discusses the role of prefrontal cortex; McNamara and Durso examine language changes during Parkinson's Disease; Oscar-Berman and Schendan report on cognitive changes associated with aging and alcoholism; Brownell and Stringfellow examine evidence for a neuropsychological model of humor appreciation; Heilman, Barrett, and Adair develop a neuropsychological model of anosagnosia; Lecours, Lupien, and Tainturier discuss aphasic alexia; Lindfield, Goodglass, and Wingfield discuss the nature of automaticity as it interacts with speed of responding; and Kinsbourne hypothesizes that disorders of time estimation emanate from memory dysfunction in specific subsystems.

The final section, *Neurobehavioral Assessment*, is devoted to current advances in assessment of neurobehavioral functioning either in particular populations such as older adults, Knoefel and Adair, the dementing, McPherson and Cummings, or in cultures other than our own, Wolfe, or with new computerized instruments, Diamond et al.

ACKNOWLEDGMENTS

We have a sincere debt of gratitude to pay to our research assistant, Kristal Nevarez, for her careful and patient work on this volume. Kristal was responsible for turning all of the authors' words of wisdom into works of art. She dedicated countless hours to dotting our *i*s and crossing our *t*s. Without Kristal we would not be paying tribute to Marty. Thank you. We would also like to express our thanks to people at the Language in the Aging Brain Laboratory who served supporting roles in this endeavor, Rachel Albert, Eunice Yang, Anthony J. Velez, and Anna J. MacKay. Our colleagues at the Harold Goodglass Aphasia Research Center, especially Marjorie Nicholas, have stimulated our thinking and have challenged us over the years; we appreciate your engaging us intellectually. And, of course, we thank Marty Albert for his being and all of his work that made this festschrift necessary.

Lisa Tabor Connor and Loraine K. Obler

LANGUAGE IN HEALTHY ADULTS

NEURAL CHANGE, COGNITIVE RESERVE AND BEHAVIORAL COMPENSATION IN RAPID ENCODING AND MEMORY FOR SPOKEN LANGUAGE IN ADULT AGING

Arthur Wingfield, Kristen Prentice,
Christine K. Koh, and Deborah Little

INTRODUCTION

The aging nervous system is marked by gradual but progressive changes in gross brain anatomy, metabolic activity, and cell function that have been increasingly well-described in the literature (Ivy, MacLeod, Petit, & Markus, 1992; Raz, Gunning-Dixon, Head, Dupuis, & Acker, 1998). We begin by reviewing these changes and their implications for rapid encoding, comprehension, and memory for spoken language. Finally, we present experimental evidence bearing on the ability to use linguistic knowledge to compensate for what might otherwise be a more serious loss.

NEURAL CHANGE, LANGUAGE, AND COGNITIVE RESERVE

Reviews of the anatomical changes in the nervous system in adult aging describe a 10% decrease in brain surface area between the third and ninth decades (Brody & Vijayashankar, 1977), with the largest increases in cell loss occurring in most cases in the sixth decade and after. Such loss is not evenly distributed. Cortical areas showing substantial neuronal loss in elderly populations include the superior temporal gyrus (Brody & Vijayashankar, 1977; Kohn, 1971) and the superior frontal gyrus, both of which have been estimated to decrease by as much as 45% by the ninth decade (Brody & Vijayashankar, 1977). Additionally, the frontal polar region has shown cell loss of up to 28% in adults aged 77 and older (Brody & Vijayashankar, 1977). Subcortical regions showing age-related cell loss include the hippocampal formation (Strong & Garruto, 1994; Simic, Kostovic, Winblad, & Bogdanovic, 1997), where the CA1 region has shown up to a 3.6% drop in cell count per annum between the ages of 15 and 96, as well as the amygdala (Strong & Garruto, 1994). Anderson and Rutledge (1996) have reported an age-related decline in dendritic structure (e.g., number of dendritic branches and spines) for select neurons in the temporal gyrus of both hemispheres, and Kohn (1971) observed a 15% decline in the conduction velocity of nerve cells between the third and ninth decades.

A recent study by Raz et al. (1998) of 95 healthy adults between the ages of 18 and 77 employed structural magnetic resonance imaging (MRI) to assess age-related changes in the volume of particular regions of interest (ROIs). The results confirmed data from earlier studies outlined above. An ROI referred to as prefrontal cortex (PFC) was a composite area encompassing the dorsolateral prefrontal cortex and the orbitofrontal cortex. The volume of this ROI was found to have a significant negative correlation with age ($r = -0.46$, $p < 0.001$). The fusiform gyrus (FG), a second ROI under investigation, also correlated negatively with age ($r = -0.30$, $p < 0.01$), as did the hippocampal formation (HF) ($r = -0.24$, $p < 0.01$) and the visual (pericalcarine) cortex (VC) ($r = -0.26$, $p < 0.01$). Although all of these ROIs showed significant negative correlations with age, the PFC showed a significantly greater negative correlation than any of the other regions.

Age is also associated with declines in brain tissue's production and responsiveness to hormones and neurotransmitters including dopamine (Bannon & Whitty, 1997; Hess & Roth, 1984; Norlen & Allard, 1996; Wong, Young, Wilson, Meltzer, & Gjedde, 1997), which has been implicated in the regulation of the circuitry underlying working memory function (Goldman-Rakic, 1996). Regional cerebral blood flow is also reported to be negatively correlated with age in many areas of the brain (London, 1984).

The behavioral consequences of the age-related neural changes sampled here include a general slowing of perceptual and cognitive operations and memory limitations that begin to appear in middle age and increase to more noticeable proportions in subsequent decades. Among the most noticeable are occasional memory lapses and an increase in tip-of-the tongue (TOT) experiences, especially for proper names (Burke, MacKay, Worthley, & Wade, 1991; Nicholas, Barth, Obler, Au, & Albert, 1997).

Language comprehension is not totally spared from such declines. Studies of healthy elderly adults show increased difficulty comprehending long and syntactically complex sentences (Kemper, Kynette, & Norman, 1992; Obler, Fein, Nicholas, & Albert, 1991) and in handling sentences and discourse when anaphoric distances are especially great, as when a pronoun and its referent are separated by several sentences in a text (Light & Capps, 1986). This distance factor appears to hold even for referent trace activation in on-line sentence comprehension (Zurif, Swinney, Prather, Wingfield, & Brownell, 1995). By contrast with these performance deficits, linguistic knowledge per se remains quite stable in normal aging (Light, 1990) (see Kempler & Zelinski, 1994, for a comparison of these factors in normal aging and dementia).

Rather than reflecting a loss of linguistic knowledge, the comprehension deficits one sees are thought to result from age-related declines in rapid encoding of the linguistic input (Gordon-Salant & Fitzgibbons, 1993; Wingfield & Lindfield, 1995; Wingfield, Poon, Lombardi, & Lowe, 1985) and declines in the working memory resources needed to support language comprehension (Carpenter, Miyaki,

& Just, 1994). Perhaps the most interesting feature of language processing in the aging brain is the finding that the supporting processes (sensory acuity, speed of processing, and memory) typically decline at a faster rate than the performance levels for language processing would suggest. This mis-match between the magnitude of the changes in language comprehension and the more marked changes in neural structure, sensory acuity, and working memory defines the notion of *cognitive reserve*: in this case, the utilization of spared linguistic knowledge to compensate for biological loss. As we shall see, age differences in language comprehension and recall of what has been heard are relatively small when the listening task is an easy one, appearing only to a notable degree as the task approaches the limits of compensation. Such overload conditions may thus serve to more accurately define the limits of compensation or cognitive reserve than typical performance levels in low-demand situations.

Our focus in this paper is on behavioral changes in the perception, comprehension, and memory for spoken language. Our goal is to see what this may tell us about compensatory operations that occur in healthy elderly adults and how these operations may ameliorate what might otherwise be far more dramatic declines in everyday language processing.

SENSORY CHANGE AND SPEECH PERCEPTION IN ADULT AGING

Because our focus is on spoken language, we will concentrate on sensory change in elderly audition. It should not be forgotten, however, that equally important age-related changes occur in other sensory domains as well. In the case of vision, changes include a yellowing of the lens that reduces transmission of light, especially in the shorter (blue) wavelengths and losses in spatial resolution and contrast sensitivity (Fozard, 1990). Although changes are less dramatic with olfaction, tactile perception, and taste, such changes do occur, most especially in olfaction, with the loss more marked for some odors than others. These deficits in high-level visual processing and olfaction, present in normal aging, are further amplified in Alzheimer's disease. (A good review of the physiological basis of these changes can be found in Ivy, MacLeod, Petit, & Markus, 1992.)

The change in auditory sensitivity and auditory perception in aging is referred to as *presbycusis*. The most obvious change is a loss of sensitivity to pure tones, especially in the higher frequency ranges. Although such declines may be a natural part of the aging process, there are wide individual differences in the occurrence and rates of such declines. In the left panel of Figure 1 we have plotted data taken from a large scale study conducted some years ago by the National Center for Health Statistics (U.S. Congress, Office of Technology Assessment, 1986). Our plot of these data shows the incidence of pure tone hearing loss at various frequencies across five different age groups. (Hearing loss was defined by subjects' ability to hear tones varying from 500 to 4000 Hz at an intensity level of 31 dB at least 50% of the time.) The range of 500 to 2,000 Hz covers the general range of speech frequencies (Sekuler & Blake, 1994).

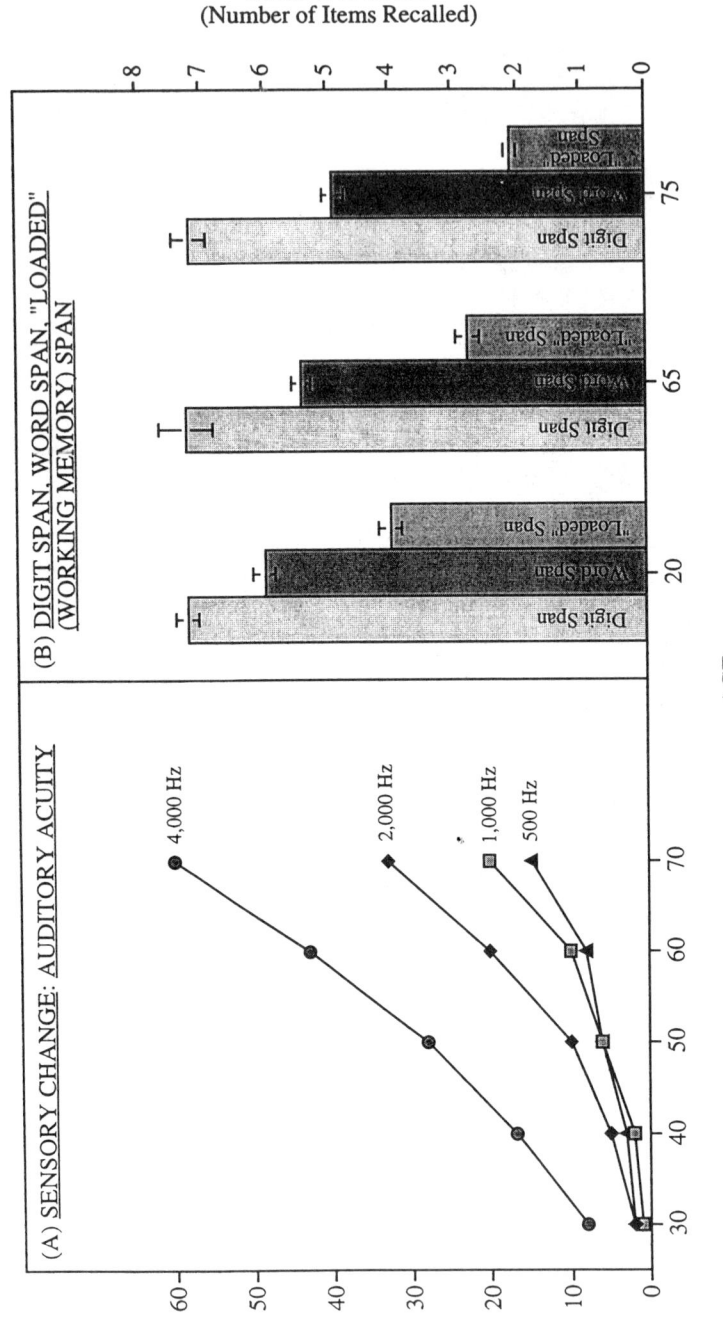

Figure 1. Left panel shows the incidence of hearing loss for five age groups for pure tones varying in frequency from 500 to 4,000 Hz (U.S. Congress, Office of Technology Assessment, 1986). Right panel shows three memory test scores (digit span, word span, and loaded word span) for young adults and two groups of older adults (based on data from Wingfield, Stine, Lahar, & Aberdeen, 1988).

Although it can be seen that a large number of elderly adults in this study did not have clinically significant hearing losses even for the higher frequencies, pure-tone audiograms do not directly measure age-related phonemic regression in which the perception of speech sounds (hence *phonemic*) is especially difficult, even when the amplitude of the speech is increased. These age-related deficits in audition arise from selective loss of hair cells at the high frequency (basal end) of the organ of Corti, atrophy of cochlear nerve fibers, and presumed neural change at higher auditory processing centers. Thus, while it is the case that many people overestimate the incidence of clinically significant hearing loss in elderly adults, it is certainly true that its incidence statistically increases with older populations.

Before leaving this topic, it is important to note that data derived from hearing in a quiet environment can overlook special difficulties elderly listeners may have in real-world environments such as the perception of speech in noisy environments or in rooms with poor acoustics (e.g., rooms with poor reverberation characteristics; Gordon-Salant & Fitzgibbons, 1993). A combination of rapid speech rate s and a noisy background can be especially devastating for the older listener (Tun, 1998). Of special concern is that the extra effort elderly listeners may need to allocate to the perception of the speech signal itself may draw resources from higher-level interpretive operations and working memory (Pichora-Fuller, Schneider, & Daneman, 1995). Indeed, we are just now beginning to understand the complexity of the interaction between sensory change in auditory and visual modalities and downstream cognitive performance (Baltes & Lindenberger, 1997).

WORKING MEMORY, PROCESSING SPEED, AND PROCESSING RESOURCES

In the cognitive science literature a distinction is made between short-term memory, as the ability to temporarily hold spoken or written items in a verbatim form, and working memory, which represents the ability to hold material while engaging in some other cognitive activity such as manipulating material in memory or engaging in a concurrent task that draws on the same cognitive resources (Baddeley, 1986). The question of whether language comprehension is constrained by limitations in the capacity of working memory is currently a matter of controversy between those who say that it does (Carpenter, Miyaki, & Just, 1994; Daneman & Merikle, 1996) and those who claim that language comprehension may rely on brief memory representations, but that these representations are not measured by standard span tests usually associated with working memory capacity (Waters & Caplan, 1996; Wingfield & Lindfield, 1995; Wingfield, Waters, & Tun, 1998).

This question is an important one because working memory capacity unarguably does change with age. We have illustrated this change in the right panel of Figure 1 with data from our own laboratory that compares three common types of span tests. In the original report of this study, we contrasted performance levels for a group of 34 young ($M = 19$ years) and 34 elderly ($M = 70$ years) adults (Wingfield, Stine, Lahar, & Aberdeen, 1988). In Figure 1 we show the elderly subjects from that study separated into two groups based on a median-split at age

70. The resulting two groups consisted of 17 *young-old* subjects: ages ranging from 59 to 69 years ($M = 65$ years), and 17 *old-old* subjects: ages ranging from 70 to 84 years ($M = 75$). All of the elderly subjects were healthy, community-dwelling, well-educated volunteers with high vocabulary scores. The two elderly subject groups did not differ significantly from each other in mean WAIS vocabulary scores or years of formal education, and both sets of scores were higher than those of the young adults who were university undergraduates. Thus, any differences observed among the three groups would not be due to inadvertent differences in education or verbal ability. The three span tests were presented auditorily over earphones. All subjects had received audiometric testing to insure age-normal hearing.

The first vertical bar on the left (right panel, Figure 1) shows the young subjects' mean digit spans, measured as the number of digits they could correctly repeat back immediately after one hearing. The second bar shows the mean memory span for these same subjects for lists of unrelated words. The final bar shows the same subjects' scores on an auditory version of Daneman and Carpenter's (1980) well-known working memory span test in which subjects had to listen to and comprehend the meaning of sets of sentences while holding in memory the last word of each sentence. We refer to this as the loaded span test. To the right of the young subjects' data, we have plotted the scores on the same three span tests for the two groups of elderly subjects.

The first feature to be noted in the figure is that there are no age differences in simple digit spans, with all three groups showing a mean digit span score of 7.2 items. This is a common finding in aging research where forward digit spans for healthy adults typically show minimal or no age differences (Craik, 1977). A significant difference does appear for word list recall, with a small but significant difference appearing between the young and the young-old subjects ($p < 0.05$) and a further drop in performance for the old-old group relative to the young-old group ($p < 0.05$).

By far, the greatest difference, however, appears for the loaded span test, demonstrating the usual findings in the literature of substantial age differences in working memory span. On this test of working memory scores, there was a significant difference between the young and the young-old subjects ($p < 0.001$) and the young-old subjects versus the old-old ($p < 0.01$).

An Analysis of Variance (ANOVA) comparing simple word spans versus the loaded spans for the young and the young-old showed a significant age interaction, $p < 0.05$. Interestingly, the analogous interaction for the young-old versus the old-old was not significant, $p > 0.05$. That is, although there was a significant main effect of age on the loaded span scores for the old-old versus the young-old subjects, the reduction in the loaded span scores was not differentially greater than the reduction in simple word spans. One should treat this finding with caution for two reasons. First, the number of subjects in these two groups was small which means that the likelihood of detecting an interaction could be limited by statistical power. It is also important to recall when examining these data that the elderly subjects in this study were especially healthy, high-functioning, and intellectually active adults. This is a group that typically shows smaller age effects in memory and other cognitive tasks than elderly subjects not sharing these characteristics

(Stine, Wingfield, & Poon, 1989). Thus, these results may be marking the lower end of expected age differences in working memory in the more general aging population.

It should be noted that the expression *working memory* has acquired a rather elastic meaning in the cognitive literature, ranging from the three-part structure described by Baddeley (1986) (a phonological or articulatory loop, a visuo-scratchpad, and an executive control), to the more abstract notion of an age-sensitive computational space (Carpenter, Miyaki, & Just, 1994). The frequency with which the term has been used in the human and animal literature in the past decade has not been matched by a uniformity in its definition, with some studies emphasizing the holding feature of working memory and others emphasizing its computational limits. In the human cognitive aging literature, characterizations of age-related resource limitations have taken the form of a general resource-deficit hypothesis (see Hartley, 1993, for evidence and an excellent critique), as the consequences of generalized slowing (Salthouse, 1991) or as an inability to inhibit off-target stimuli (Zacks & Hasher, 1994). The decline in processing resources with age is not at issue. We have seen, for example, that working memory spans decline significantly, even with healthy and active adults with good verbal abilities. The question currently engaging the cognitive aging literature is only how best to characterize this cognitive change.

WORKING MEMORY RESOURCES AND SINGLE CHANNEL MODELS

Salthouse (1991) has characterized the theories of cognitive aging in terms of the metaphors of time (perceptual and cognitive slowing), space (reductions in working memory capacity), and energy (reductions in available attentional resources). To this list one might also add age differences in allocation, or the way in which the limited resources are distributed (Hartley, 1993). From whichever metaphor current theories spring, most accounts would find little disagreement with the empirical reality of the complexity hypothesis: the notion that cognitive or perceptual operations that the young find hard, or more time-consuming to accomplish, will be differentially more difficult or time-consuming for the elderly (Cerella, 1994).

Probably no area of research in cognitive psychology has received as much attention as the question of whether individuals, regardless of age, must draw on a single pool of processing resources for all cognitive functions (Kahneman, 1973) or whether different cognitive operations draw on different resource pools (McLeod, 1977). Indeed, the origins of limited channel capacity models can be traced to early Information Theory, with its proposition that one should be able to measure information flow in terms of the amount of information contained in a message and the rate at which this information is delivered (Attneave, 1959). A counterpart to the *single* versus *multiple resource pool* argument appears in two debates in the current literature. One of these debates is whether aging can best be described in terms of a single slowing function (Cerella, 1994) or whether different perceptual and cognitive operations may slow at different rates (Fisher & Glaser, 1996). The second debate is over whether a single working memory system underlies all levels of language processing from syntactic parsing to interpretive processes (Carpenter, Miyaki, & Just, 1994) or whether a number of memory systems with different kinds of representations and different decay rates may operate in language comprehension (Waters & Caplan, 1996; Wingfield, Waters, & Tun, 1998).

These debates focus on the internal structure of the capacity and the rate of processing limitations observed in normal aging. In his review of the literature on attention and aging, Hartley (1992) has noted the increase in studies over the years that have involved a dual-task method to study capacity limitations in cognitive aging. In such studies, subjects first perform one task alone (e.g., listening to speech for later recall), a second task alone (e.g., pressing a key when a particular stimulus is flashed on a computer screen), and then performance on the two tasks is measured by having the subjects perform them concurrently. The change in performance when the two tasks are performed together (e.g., lowered recall accuracy or longer reaction times in the visual detection task), relative to single-task performance, is then taken as a measure of the subjects' limits in resource capacity and the cost of having to divide these resources.

Such dual-task studies reliably show that concurrent activities drain resources from each other, with the relative draw on resources defined by which task the subject considers to be the primary one. Careful reviews of the literature, however, document somewhat mixed findings on whether elderly adults are differentially impaired in dual-task studies relative to young adults (Hartley, 1992; Tun & Wingfield, 1993). Because elderly adults typically start at a lower baseline level than the young, even when differential interference effects do not appear in the performance of the elderly, they may still drop to a level below that which might be necessary for effective processing. The same point may be made about working memory performance levels as discussed previously.

Given the rapid speed at which speech arrives even in ordinary conversation and the multiple operations that must be performed on this rapid signal, language comprehension and the recall of linguistic materials are far better preserved in normal aging than would be predicted from the age-related declines in working memory and general processing speed. That is, the sensory and working memory deficits observable in normal aging should predict significantly poorer performance in comprehension and memory for spoken language than actually occurs. The answer to this apparent paradox lies in the ability of the intact systems to compensate for the measurable neurologic and sensory loss. Word recognition offers an excellent model of how this compensation operates.

TOP-DOWN COMPENSATION IN WORD RECOGNITION

The *gating* paradigm in its present form was introduced some years ago by Grosjean, who tested subjects' ability to identify spoken words simply from their opening sounds. (See Grosjean, 1996, for a review of the gating paradigm and its development.) In this technique, the subject first hears the first 50 milliseconds (ms) of a word and is asked to attempt to identify the word. If the subject is unable to do so, he or she then hears the first 100 ms of the word then the first 150 ms of the word and so on, until the word is correctly identified. (The technique was called *gating* because, in the early experiments, an electronic gate was opened and closed to control the amount of speech a subject would be allowed to hear.) Grosjean demonstrated that words in context can be recognized with as little as the first 175 to 200 ms of their onsets. Words heard alone without a linguistic context can be recognized with an average of only 333 ms of their onsets, or when half or less than half of their full acoustic duration has been heard. (Depending on the speech rate, typical one-, two-, and three-syllable words may average between 550 to 830 ms in full duration.)

The reason words can be recognized with so little of their full acoustic duration is because there is only a limited number of words that share the same onsets (the word-initial cohort), and this number decreases rapidly as more and more of a word's onset is heard. This fact underlies the so-called *cohort theory* of word recognition (Marslen-Wilson, 1987). Theoretical disagreement centers on whether, in natural speech, context limits the size of the word-initial cohort even before the word is heard or whether context operates only after the word has been accessed in the lexicon and whether word-onsets have any special priority over a general goodness-of-fit in driving word recognition (Connine, Blasko, & Titone, 1993; Wingfield, Goodglass, & Lindfield, 1997). It is clear, however, that the more probable the word is in a linguistic context, the more rapidly it will be recognized and that natural word-stress is an important variable in the reduction of cohort size (Wingfield, Goodglass, & Lindfield, 1997).

In the case of aging, we and others have shown that in order to correctly identify a word heard in isolation elderly adults need to hear more of the word's onset than do young adults (Craig, 1992; Perry & Wingfield, 1994; Wingfield, Aberdeen, & Stine, 1991). This difference is most probably due to the perceptually driven (*bottom-up*) stages of processing rather than to age differences in the use of the phonological information, once encoded, to access the lexical entries that share the word onset phonology (Marshall, Duke, & Walley, 1996). As Marshall et al. suggest, however, difficulties with both factors may operate in cognitively impaired patients with Alzheimer's disease when tested with this paradigm. The potency of an intact linguistic system in normal aging to compensate for perceptual encoding deficits can be illustrated by contrasting the amount of word onset information necessary for word identification when a word such as *book* is presented in a neutral context ("The word is...."), when it is presented with a moderately constraining sentence ("John found a note in his...."), or in a high context sentence frame ("John wrote a chapter in the...."). Studies such as these make use of the so-called *cloze* procedure in which large numbers of subjects are given sentence contexts such as these and are asked to say what they think the most likely final word of the sentence might be. Based on cloze norms, for example, the probability of *book* in the above moderate and high context sentence frames are $p = 0.06$ and $p = 0.86$, respectively (Perry & Wingfield, 1994).

To conduct an experiment on the effects of context on word recognition, one would need to make sure that the recording of the target word (e.g., *book*), is exactly the same in all three sentence contexts. This would be done by making a single recording of the target word and splicing that same recording onto each of the different sentence frames. This method also controls for possible coarticulation cues: the fact that phonemes take on different acoustic coloring depending on the adjacent speech sounds, a subtle cue listeners can use to facilitate word perception. By taking such care, one can insure that any differences in perceptual accuracy are a result of the linguistic context in which the word is presented rather than any differences in the physical clarity of the word.

Figure 2 shows data from three experiments that compared the effects of linguistic context on word identification for young and elderly adults (Perry & Wingfield, 1994; Experiments 1 and 2, Single-Task conditions; Wingfield et al., 1991). In all cases, the probabilities of occurrence of the target words in the various linguistic contexts were determined using a cloze procedure, as described above, in which separate groups of subjects were given the sentence contexts and simply asked to say what they thought was the most likely word to complete that sentence. (As is typical in such studies, the pairings of the target words and their possible sentence contexts were counterbalanced across subjects such that, by the end of the experiment, one has equal amounts of data for each target word heard in each of its sentence contexts.)

All three experiments used three conditions: a Neutral Context condition, a Low Context condition, and a High Context condition. In Wingfield et al. (1991) the Low Context sentence frames had an average probability of 0.05 (*range* = 0.02 to 0.14) of predicting the target word, and the High Context frames had an average probability of 0.33 (*range* = 0.16 to 0.89) of predicting the target word. In Experiments 1 and 2 of Perry and Wingfield (1994) the Low Context frames had an average probability of .11 (*range* = 0.02 to 0.25) of predicting the target word, and the High Context frames had an average probability of 0.82 (*range* = 0.75 to 0.98) of predicting the target word. In all three experiments, the young subjects were university undergraduates, and the elderly adults were healthy community-dwelling volunteers with levels of education and verbal ability at least equal to the young adults. In the Wingfield et al. (1991) study, the mean age of the elderly group was 69 years. In Experiments 1 and 2 of Perry and Wingfield (1994), the mean ages of the elderly subjects were 71 and 72 years, respectively. In all three experiments, subjects received audiometric testing to insure age-normal hearing.

We have used different symbols in Figure 2 to indicate the mean gate sizes needed for correct word identification for the young and elderly subjects in each of the three experiments. The mean word probabilities for the three conditions (Neutral Context, Low Context, and High Context) are plotted on the abscissa on a logarithmic scale. Best fitting straight lines are shown for the young and the elderly subjects averaged across the three sets of data. It can be seen from the age difference in the Neutral Context condition that the elderly subjects in all three experiments required a longer gate duration to recognize the target words than the young subjects, reflecting an expected age difference in auditory processing efficiency. We also can see, however, that when a High Context sentence frame was used (strong top-down context) the age difference disappears.

It is important to note in these studies that subjects were not consciously guessing the identity of the words based on the context. Rather, in the High Context conditions, the word onset fragments seemed to the subjects to be clearer or more informative as to the full word identity than when the words were presented in a neutral context or in the Low Context conditions. This result is a consequence of the fact that speech perception is heavily context dependent for both young and elderly subjects. When context is present, as it usually is under natural circumstances, word recognition represents the product of the summed information from both bottom-up and top-down sources (Wingfield & Stine, 1991).

LIMITS TO TOP-DOWN CONTEXT UTILIZATION

There are many examples in the literature that show how age differences can be reduced in perceptual and memory tasks for written and spoken materials when the materials are presented in the context of structured sentences (e.g., Madden, 1988; Stine & Wingfield, 1987; Wingfield, Poon, Lombardi, & Lowe, 1985). Indeed, so strong is this evidence that one might be tempted to conclude that the more structure linguistic materials contain, the smaller will be the age differences. We and others have drawn exactly this conclusion. On reflection, however, one realizes that this will be true only to the extent that the listener is able to detect this structure.

Imagine, for example, that one were to present young and elderly subjects with prose passages that varied in their difficulty with instructions to recall as much of the content of the passages as possible. One way to do this is to use passages that are made up of normal English prose but that vary in their average inter-word probabilities based on a cloze procedure. In this case the cloze probabilities had been obtained by giving subjects the full passages with words periodically deleted and asking them to guess the identities of the missing words (Miller & Coleman, 1967). These average inter-word probability levels can be taken as reflecting the combined effects of linguistic structure and the strength of linguistic context across the passages.

Based on a simple context-use principle and the previously cited complexity hypothesis, one could make several predictions. First, to the extent that elderly adults can make good use of linguistic knowledge to compensate for a poorer memory capacity, one would expect age differences in recall of passage content to be smaller for high inter-word probability passages than for low inter-word probability passages. This would be so to the extent that elderly subjects can use the linguistic context to help organize the material when hearing it and to guide recall in the memory phase of the experiment. Second, one would expect that if one increased the rate of presentation, the elderly should show differentially poorer recall for the passage content than the young subjects. This prediction would be based on the presumption that elderly listeners require more time to encode the incoming prose so as to lay down a more effective memory representation. There is considerable support for this latter prediction in the form of many experiments that show elderly adults to have more difficulty with artificially accelerated (time-compressed) speech than do young adults (Gordon-Salant & Fitzgibbons, 1993; Wingfield, Poon, Lombardi, & Lowe, 1985). This vulnerability to rapid speech input in adult aging is a robust finding that appears even when young and elderly adults are carefully matched for hearing acuity (Gordon-Salant & Fitzgibbons, 1993).

14 Neurobehavior of Language and Cognition

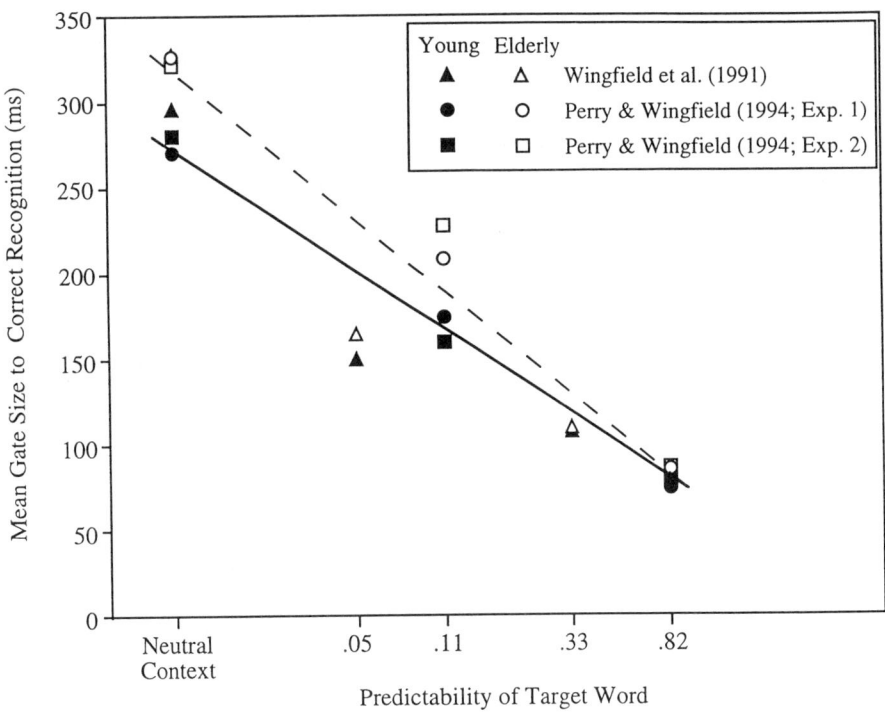

Figure 2. Data taken from three experiments showing mean word-onset gate sizes necessary for correct word identification for words presented either in a neutral context ("The word is....") or with words varying in their degree of predictability based on a preceding sentence context. (Note that predictability levels are plotted on a logarithmic scale.)

When we conducted such an experiment with young and elderly adults screened for age-normal hearing and good levels of education and verbal ability (Riggs, Wingfield, & Tun, 1993), only part of these predicted results appeared. (The young subjects were university undergraduates and the elderly were healthy, community-dwelling volunteers with a mean age of 70 years. The elderly subjects' WAIS vocabulary scores and years of education equaled or exceeded that of the young subjects.)

In Figure 3 we have plotted data for two of the three speech rate s that were used in that experiment: a normal speech rate of 170 words per minute (wpm) and the same passages time-compressed to produce speech delivered at twice the normal rate (340 wpm). The compression was accomplished using a speech-editing computer program that reduced both speech and silent durations to an equal degree, thus maintaining the relative temporal patterning of the original sample as well as maintaining normal pitch and intonation. The result is speech that continues to sound normal, although arriving at an unnaturally rapid rate. The passages, which averaged 150 words in length, varied from an average inter-word predictability of just above 0.30 (low predictability) to just under 0.70 (high predictably). These values are plotted on the abscissa. The dependent measure was the average percentage of propositions (idea units) correctly recalled from each passage after it had been heard. For each set of data we have plotted least-squares lines of best fit. (Comprehension and recall were also tested with multiple choice questions and a cued recall test, with similar although more attenuated results.)

We can see by comparing the left and right panels of Figure 3 that time-compression reduces recall performance and differentially so for the elderly adults. An ANOVA showed significant main effects of age ($p < 0.001$), of speech rate ($p < 0.001$), and a significant age by speech rate interaction ($p < 0.0001$). We also see that for both subject groups, the higher the average inter-word predictability of the passages, the better was their recall performance ($p < 0.001$). Most interestingly, however, we can see by comparing the left and right panels of the figure that although both the young and the elderly subjects gained equivalent value from increases in passage predictability for passages heard at the normal speech rate of 170 wpm (left panel), as evidenced by the approximately parallel slopes of the recall functions, the rate of gain in performance with increasing passage predictability is much less for the elderly than the young subjects for the speech heard at 340 wpm (right panel).

One can assume that the predictability levels of the passages facilitated the recall at several levels. On the perceptual side, high inter-word predictability would be expected to facilitate the rapid perception of the individual words, much as we illustrated in the previous section. Also, high predictability passages would be expected to facilitate detection of the linguistic structure of the incoming speech, as well as aiding development of a meaningful coherence structure for the passage as a whole. Finally, high predictability passages would offer structure to aid recall of the passage content, both by providing rich retrieval cues and by allowing reasonable reconstruction of missing elements (Alba & Hasher, 1983; Wingfield, Tun, & Rosen, 1995).

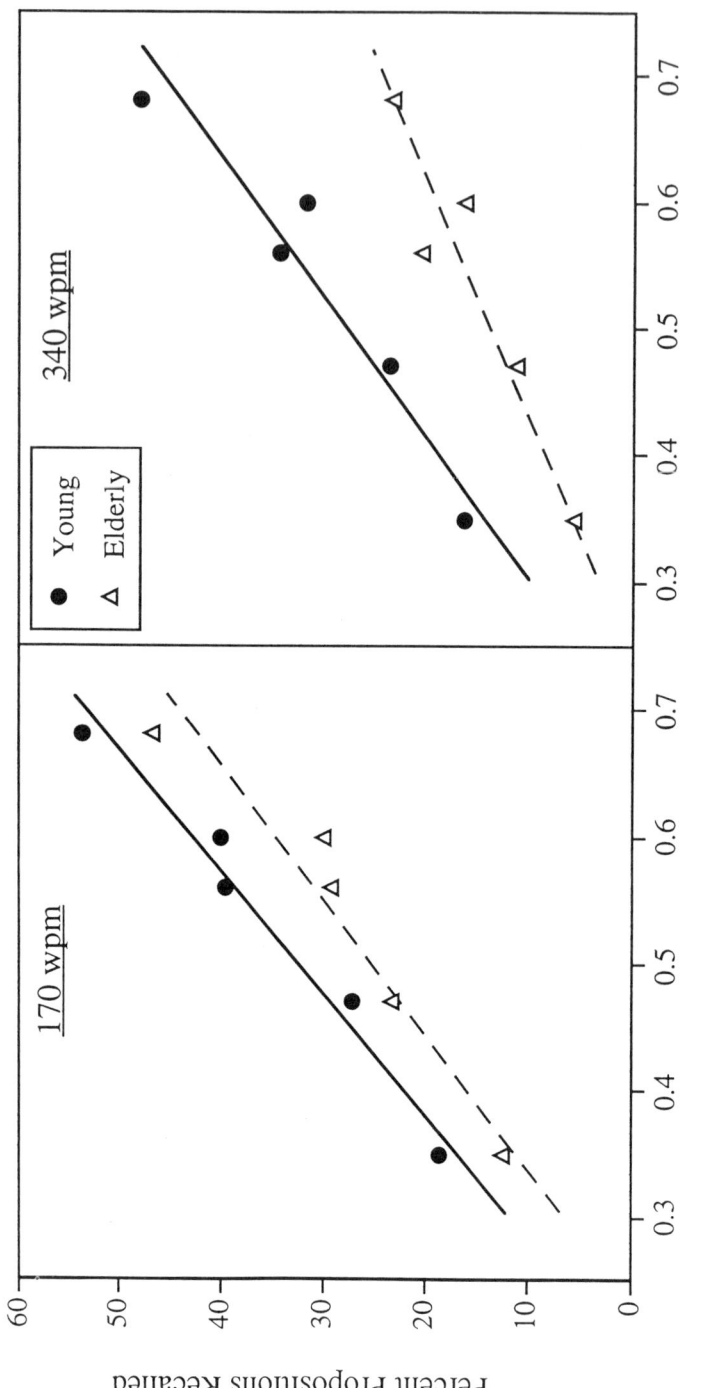

Figure 3. Percentage of propositions (idea units) correctly recalled by young and elderly adults as a function of passage difficulty based on mean inter-word predictability levels of the test passages for passages presented at 170 words per minute (wpm; left panel) and 340 wpm (right panel) (Riggs, Wingfield, & Tun, 1993).

In order to exploit the high predictability levels of the passages, however, the listener must rapidly gain an understanding of both the theme of the story and the linguistic structure of what is being heard. The fact that the elderly adults' recall performance increased for passages with increasing inter-word predictability levels at the fast speech rate (340 wpm) shows that they were able to extract meaning from the passages as they were hearing them. The shallower slope to their function, however, shows that they were less able to do this than were the young adults at this very rapid speech rate. This would suggest that, for the elderly subjects, there was a rate overload at the fast speech rate that impaired extraction of high-level passage structure. For this reason, the greater predictability of the high probability passages could not be as effectively exploited at the faster speech rate by the elderly subjects as it could be at the slower speech rate.

The implications of the Riggs et al. study represent an important qualification to the usual picture of compensatory operations in language processing in normal aging. Elderly subjects can utilize their spared linguistic knowledge to facilitate language comprehension and accurate recall of what they have heard. There is now a large body of evidence showing that this is so (Wingfield & Stine, 1991). The above results show that they can do so, however, only to the extent that the speech materials do not so overload the system that this structure cannot be detected.

CONCLUSIONS

Kliegl, Smith, and Baltes (1989) have argued that there exists, for both young and elderly adults, a sizable reserve capacity for cognitive performance. The extent of this cognitive reserve can be demonstrated to the degree that training or experience can raise performance level from a pre-training baseline or from a baseline condition in which training and experience cannot be brought to bear on performance. In the case of language, such a contrast is illustrated by age differences observed in the perception of single words in isolation, or recall of lists of unrelated words, versus the smaller age differences that are observed for perception of words in context or recall of meaningful sentences and prose. As Kliegl et al. have pointed out, however, the extent of this capability will have upper-bound limits constrained by the neurophysiological limits in the aging brain. We showed one example of this in the Riggs et al. study in which elderly adults' ordinarily excellent use of linguistic context in comprehension and recall was limited by inducing a processing overload through presentation of the stimulus materials at a high speech rate.

The source of the cognitive reserve in language processing in the aging adult must come from several sources, some of which we have illustrated here. The most potent of these is the way a preserved procedural knowledge of linguistic rules can be used to compensate for weakened bottom-up processing attributable to sensory declines and lowered efficiency in auditory processing. As we have argued, speech perception in both young and elderly adults represents a dynamic mix of bottom-up (perceptual input) and top-down (context driven) sources of input. What emerges with age and the accompanying reduction in efficiency of bottom-up processing is a spontaneous shift in the ratio of top-down to bottom-up input used in the task performance (Wingfield & Stine, 1991).

There are numerous examples across a number of domains of how expertise can ameliorate age differences, such as the way in which significant age differencesin speed of visual search can be eliminated when the search targets are visual forms with which the subject is familiar (Clancy & Hoyer, 1994). In the case of language, we have seen how elderly adults can compensate for sensory and processing declines by utilizing the natural redundancy of language supplied by the syntactic and semantic structure that carries the speech message. Other features that systematically accompany normal language production can also serve comprehension in both young and elderly adults, but they may take on special importance in the elderly listener. These may include the use of visible speech (visible articulatory movements of the speaker) to aid perception (Thompson, 1995), as well as the use of naturally occurring prosodic structure (intonation, stress, and timing) to help guide rapid detection of syntactic structure in sentence comprehension (Wingfield, Wayland, & Stine, 1992).

The key to behavioral plasticity in a variety of domains is represented by the spontaneous utilization of intact processing architectures to compensate for degraded ones. We believe that language processing in healthy aging serves as an excellent model of how this can be accomplished.

ACKNOWLEDGMENTS

Our work is supported by NIH Grant R37-AG04517 from the National Institute on Aging. We also acknowledge support from Training Grant T32-AG00204 to Brandeis University and support from the W.M. Keck Foundation.

REFERENCES

Alba, J. W. & Hasher, L. (1983). Is memory schematic? *Psychological Bulletin*, *93*, 203-231.
Anderson, B. & Rutledge, V. (1996). Age and hemisphere effects on dendritic structure. *Brain*, *119*, 1983-1990.
Attneave, F. (1959). *Applications of information theory to psychology*. New York: Holt-Dryden.
Baddeley, A. D. (1986). *Working memory*. Oxford: Oxford University Press.
Baltes, P. B. & Lindenberger, U. (1997). Emergence of a powerful connection between sensory and cognitive function across the adult life span: A new window to the study of cognitive aging? *Psychology and Aging*, *12*, 12-21.
Bannon, M. J. & Whitty, C. J. (1997). Age-related and regional differences in dopamine transporter mRNA expression in human midbrain. *Neurology*, *48*, 969-977.
Brody, H. & Vijayashankar, N. (1977). Anatomical changes in the nervous system. In C. Finch & L. Hayflick (Eds.), *Handbook of the biology of aging* (pp. 241-261). New York: Von Nostrand Reinhold.
Burke, D. M., MacKay, D. G., Worthley, J. S., & Wade, E. (1991). On the tip of the tongue: What causes word finding failures in young and older adults? *Journal of Memory and Language*, *30*, 542-579.
Carpenter, P. A., Miyaki, A., & Just, M. A. (1994). Working memory constraints in comprehension: Evidence from individual differences, aphasia, and aging. In M. Gernsbacher (Ed.), *Handbook of psycholinguistics* (pp. 1075-1122). San Diego, CA: Academic Press.
Cerella, J. (1994). Generalized slowing and Brinley plots. *Journal of Gerontology: Psychological Sciences*, *49*, P65-P71.
Clancy, S. M. & Hoyer, W. J. (1994). Age and skill in visual search. *Developmental Psychology*, *30*, 545-552.

Connine, C. M., Blasko, D. G., & Titone, D. (1993). Do the beginnings of spoken words have a special status in auditory word recognition? *Journal of Memory and Language, 32*, 193-210.

Craig, C. H. (1992). Effects of aging on time-gated isolated word-recognition performance. *Journal of Speech and Hearing Research, 35*, 234-238.

Craik, F. I. M. (1977). Age differences in human memory. In J. E. Birren & K. W. Schaie (Eds.), *Handbook of the psychology of aging* (pp. 384-420). New York: Van Nostrand Reinhold.

Daneman, M. & Carpenter, P. A. (1980). Individual differences in working memory and reading. *Journal of Verbal Learning and Verbal Behavior, 19*, 450-466.

Daneman, M. & Merikle, P. M. (1996). Working memory and language comprehension: A meta-analysis. *Psychonomic Bulletin and Review, 3*, 422-433.

Fisher, D. L. & Glaser, R. A. (1996). Molar and latent models of cognitive slowing: Implications for aging, dementia, depression, development, and intelligence. *Psychonomic Bulletin and Review, 3*, 458-480.

Fozard, J. L. (1990). Vision and hearing in aging. In J. E. Birren & K. W. Schaie (Eds.), *Handbook of the psychology of aging* (pp. 50-83). San Diego: Academic Press.

Goldman-Rakic, P. S. (1996). Regional and cellular fractionation of working memory. *Proceedings of the National Academy of Sciences USA, 93*, 13473-13480.

Gordon-Salant, S. & Fitzgibbons, P. J. (1993). Temporal factors and speech recognition performance in young and elderly listeners. *Journal of Speech and Hearing Research, 36*, 1276-1285.

Grosjean, F. (1996). Gating. *Language and Cognitive Processes, 11*, 597-604.

Hartley, A. A. (1992). Attention. In F. I. M. Craik & T. A. Salthouse (Eds.), *The handbook of aging and cognition* (pp. 3-49). Hillsdale, NJ: Erlbaum.

Hartley, J. T. (1993). Aging and prose memory: Tests of the resource-deficit hypothesis. *Psychology and Aging, 8*, 538-551.

Hess, G. D. & Roth, G. S. (1984). Receptors and aging. In J. E. Johnson (Ed.), *Aging and cell function* (pp. 187-210). New York: Plenum Press.

Ivy, G. O., MacLeod, C. M., Petit, T. L., & Markus, E. J. (1992). A physiological framework for perception and cognitive changes in aging. In F. I. M. Craik & T. A. Salthouse (Eds.), *The handbook of aging and cognition* (pp. 273-314). Hillsdale, NJ: Erlbaum.

Kahneman, D. (1973). *Attention and effort*. Englewood Cliffs, NJ: Prentice-Hall.

Kemper, S., Kynette, D., & Norman, S. (1992). Age differences in spoken language. In R. West & J. Sinnott (Eds.), *Everyday memory and aging: Current research and methodology* (pp. 138-152). New York: Springer-Verlag.

Kempler, D. & Zelinski, E. M. (1994). Language in dementia and normal aging. In F. A. Huppert, C. Brayne, & D. W. O'Connor (Eds.), *Dementia and normal aging* (pp. 331-365). New York: Cambridge University Press.

Kliegl, R., Smith, J., & Baltes, P. B. (1989). Testing-the-limits and the study of adult age differences in cognitive plasticity of a mnemonic skill. *Developmental Psychology, 25*, 247-256.

Kohn, R. R. (1971). *Principles of mammalian aging*. New Jersey: Prentice-Hall.

Light, L. L. (1990). Interactions between memory and language in old age. In J. E. Birren & K. W. Schaie (Eds.), *Handbook of the psychology of aging* (pp. 275-290). San Diego, CA: Academic Press.

Light, L. L. & Capps, J. L. (1986). Comprehension of pronouns in young and older adults. *Developmental Psychology, 22*, 580-585.

London, E. D. (1984). Metabolism of the brain: A measure of cellular function in aging. In J. E. Johnson (Ed.), *Aging and cell function* (pp. 187-210). New York: Plenum Press.

Madden, D. J. (1988). Adult age differences in the effects of sentence context and stimulus degradation during visual word recognition. *Psychology and Aging, 3*, 167-172.

Marslen-Wilson, W. D. (1987). Parallel processing in spoken word recognition. *Cognition, 25*, 71-102.

Marshall, N. B., Duke, L. W., & Walley, A. C. (1996). Effects of age and Alzheimer's disease on recognition of gated spoken words. *Journal of Speech and Hearing Research, 39*, 724-733.

McLeod, P. (1977). A dual task response modality effect: Support for multiprocessor models of attention. *Quarterly Journal of Experimental Psychology, 29*, 651-667.

Miller, G. R. & Coleman, E. B. (1967). A set of thirty-six prose passages calibrated for complexity. *Journal of Verbal Learning and Verbal Behavior, 6*, 851-854.

Nicholas, M., Barth, C., Obler, L. K., Au, R., & Albert, M. L. (1997). Naming in normal aging and dementia of the Alzheimer's type. In H. Goodglass & A. Wingfield (Eds.), *Anomia: Neuroanatomical and cognitive correlates* (pp. 166-188). San Diego, CA: Academic Press.

Norlen, M. & Allard, P. (1996). Reduction in number of dopamine uptake sites but unchanged number of piperazine-acceptor/CYP450IID6 binding sites in the human caudate nucleus in aging. *Neuroscience Letters, 209*, 161-164.

Obler, L. K., Fein, D., Nicholas, M., & Albert, M. L. (1991). Auditory comprehension and aging: Decline in syntactic processing. *Applied Psycholinguistics, 12*, 433-252.

Perry, A. R. & Wingfield, A. (1994). Contextual encoding by young and elderly adults as revealed by cued and free recall. *Aging and Cognition, 1*, 120-139.

Pichora-Fuller, M. K., Schneider, B. A., & Daneman, M. (1995). How young and old adults listen to and remember speech in noise. *Journal of the Acoustical Society of America, 97*, 593-607.

Raz, N., Gunning-Dixon, F. M., Head, D., Dupuis, J. H., & Acker, J. D. (1998). Neuroanatomical correlates of cognitive aging: Evidence from structural MRI. *Neuropsychology, 12*, 95-114.

Riggs, K. M., Wingfield, A., & Tun, P. A. (1993). Passage difficulty, speech rate, and age differences in memory for spoken text: Speech recall and the complexity hypothesis. *Experimental Aging Research, 19*, 111-128.

Salthouse, T. A. (1991). *Theoretical perspectives on cognitive aging*. Hillsdale, NJ: Erlbaum.

Sekuler, R. & Blake, R. (1994). *Perception* (3rd ed.). New York: McGraw-Hill.

Simic, G., Kostovic, I., Winblad, B., & Bogdanovic, N. (1997). Volume and number of neurons of the human hippocampal formation in normal aging and Alzheimer's disease. *Journal of Comparative Neurology, 379*, 482-494.

Stine, E. A. L. & Wingfield, A. (1987). Process and strategy in memory for speech among younger and older adults. *Psychology and Aging, 2*, 272-279.

Stine, E. A. L., Wingfield, A., & Poon, L. W. (1989). Speech comprehension and memory through adulthood: The roles of time and strategy. In L. W. Poon, D. C. Rubin, & B. A. Wilson (Eds.), *Everyday cognition in adulthood and late life* (pp. 195-229). New York: Cambridge University Press.

Strong, M. J. & Garruto, R. M. (1994). Neuronal aging and age-related disorders of the human nervous system. In D. E. Crews & R. M. Garruto (Eds.), *Biological anthropology and aging* (pp. 214-231). New York: Oxford University Press.

Thompson, L. A. (1995). Encoding and memory for visible speech and gestures: A comparison between young and older adults. *Psychology and Aging, 10*, 215-227.

Tun, P. A. (1998). Fast noisy speech: Age differences in processing rapid speech with background noise. *Psychology and Aging, 13*, 424-434.

Tun, P. A. & Wingfield, A. (1993). Is speech special? Perception and recall of spoken language in complex environments. In J. Cerella, J. Rybash, W. Hoyer, & M. L. Commons (Eds.), *Adult information processing: Limits on loss* (pp. 425-457). San Diego, CA: Academic Press.

U.S. Congress, Office of Technology Assessment (1986, May). Hearing impairment and elderly people - A background paper (OTA-BP-BA-30). Washington, DC: U.S. Government Printing Office.

Waters, G. S. & Caplan, D. (1996). The capacity theory of sentence comprehension: Critique of Just and Carpenter (1992). *Psychological Review, 103*, 761-772.

Wingfield, A., Aberdeen, J. S., & Stine, E. A. L. (1991). Word onset gating and linguistic context in spoken word recognition by young and elderly adults. *Journal of Gerontology: Psychological Sciences, 46*, P127-P129.

Wingfield, A., Goodglass, H., & Lindfield, K. C. (1997). Word recognition from acoustic onsets and acoustic offsets: Effects of cohort size and syllabic stress. *Applied Psycholinguistics, 18*, 85-100.

Wingfield, A. & Lindfield, K. C. (1995). Multiple memory systems in the processing of speech: Evidence from aging. *Experimental Aging Research, 21*, 101-121.

Wingfield, A., Poon, L. W., Lombardi, L., & Lowe, D. (1985). Speed of processing in normal aging: Effects of speech rate, linguistic structure, and processing time. *Journal of Gerontology, 40*, 579-585.

Wingfield, A. & Stine, E. A. L. (1991). Expert systems in nature: Spoken language processing and adult aging. In J. D. Sinnott & J. C. Cavanaugh (Eds.), *Bridging paradigms: Positive development in adulthood and cognitive aging* (pp. 237-258). New York: Praeger.

Wingfield, A., Stine, E. A. L., Lahar, C. J., & Aberdeen, J. S. (1988). Does the capacity of working memory change with age? *Experimental Aging Research, 14*, 103-107.

Wingfield, A., Tun, P. A., & Rosen, M. J. (1995). Age differences in veridical and reconstructive recall of syntactically and randomly segmented speech. *Journal of Gerontology: Psychological Sciences, 50*, P257-P266.

Wingfield, A., Waters, G. S., & Tun, P. A. (1998). Does working memory work in language comprehension?: Evidence from behavioral neuroscience. In N. Raz (Ed.), *The other side of the error term: Aging and development as model systems in cognitive neuroscience* (pp. 319-393). Amsterdam: Elsevier.

Wingfield, A., Wayland, S. C., & Stine, E. A. L. (1992). Adult age differences in the use of prosody for syntactic parsing and recall of spoken sentences. *Journal of Gerontology: Psychological Sciences, 47,* P350-P356.

Wong, D. F., Young, D., Wilson, P. D., Meltzer, C. C., & Gjedde, A. (1997). Quantification of neuroreceptors in the living human brain: III. D2-like dopamine receptors: Theory, validation, and changes during normal aging. *Journal of Cerebral Blood Flow and Metabolism, 17,* 316-330.

Zacks, R. T. & Hasher, L. (1994). Directed ignoring: Inhibitory regulation of working memory. In D. Dagenbach & T. H. Carr (Eds.), *Inhibitory mechanisms in attention, memory, and language* (pp. 241-264). New York: Academic Press.

Zurif, E. B., Swinney, D., Prather, P., Wingfield, A., & Brownell, H. (1995). The allocation of memory resources during sentence comprehension: Evidence from the elderly. *Journal of Psycholinguistic Research, 24,* 165-182.

FACTORS UNDERLYING COMPREHENSION OF ACCENTED ENGLISH

Mira Goral,
Loraine K. Obler,
and Elizabeth Galletta

INTRODUCTION

In recent years, attention has been given to the apparent increase in the proportion of college instructors and teaching assistants in the United States who are nonnative speakers of English. In response to various concerns about the language proficiency among foreign teaching assistants and the status of higher education, several studies have addressed aspects of the communication problems that may be associated with *nonnative speaking teaching assistants* (NNSTAs) (Hofstede, 1986; Norris, 1991). Shifting the attention from the linguistic competence of nonnative teaching assistants to their perceived proficiency by their students, researchers such as Rubin (1992) and Brown (1992) investigated undergraduate students' evaluation of NNSTAs who spoke English with various degrees of accents and found that variables other than the actual degree of accentedness of the NNSTAs' speech influenced undergraduates' evaluation of their teaching abilities.

Rubin and Smith (1990), for example, used a matched-guise procedure to investigate undergraduates' comprehension and attitude toward NNSTAs. The authors varied three instructors' variables: ethnicity, level of accentedness, and topic of lecture. The relations between comprehension performance of 92 undergraduate students, as measured by their scores on a cloze test of listening comprehension (following their listening to a tape-recorded lecture), their evaluation of the instructors as measured by a questionnaire (including a general impression scale, level of accentedness, level of teaching proficiency), and their self-reported previous experience with NNSTAs, were studied. While comprehension scores were not found to be affected by level of instructors' accentedness, a significant correlation was found between the level of perceived accentedness and the teaching rating. Moreover, a positive correlation was found between comprehension scores and the number of courses previously taken with NNSTAs. Based on this correlation, however, it cannot be determined whether exposure to other NNSTAs' accents facilitated comprehension or whether students who are more talented at understanding accented English are more likely to choose courses taught by NNSTAs.

Brown (1992) studied the effect of speakers' perceived country of origin, educational status, and native language on students' evaluation of the speakers' personal qualities, language competence, and teaching competence. Using a matched-guise paradigm and collecting evaluation data from 438 students, Brown found that perceived country of origin correlated with judgment of language competence, and perceived educational status correlated with judgments about personal qualities. The findings of these studies indicate that factors such as students' stereotypical attitudes toward other cultures and their exposure to NNSTAs interact with their evaluation of instructors.

Relevant to the compromised communication that may be associated with the accented speech of NNSTAs is the fact that attitude factors were found to be related not only to undergraduate students' evaluation of the NNSTAs, but also to the students' academic performance in their classes. However, while a relation between students' comprehension performance and attitude toward foreign teaching assistants was found in a number of studies (Rubin & Smith, 1990; Rubin, 1992; Mettler, 1991), such a relation is not sufficient to determine that differences in attitude account for the differences in performance. To summarize, both students' attitudes toward and their evaluation of nonnative-English speaking instructors are closely related to the students' varied ability to comprehend English spoken with a nonnative accent. Evidently, students who confront the task of comprehending accented English vary in their ability to adjust to the accented speech. Intriguing yet under-investigated questions arise with respect to possible accounts for this variability.

Varying ability to tolerate, adjust to, and understand English spoken with nonnative accents may be related to several factors. One such factor may be the overall attitude toward foreigners, as described above (e.g., Rubin, 1992). Secondly, listening comprehension scores among undergraduates may be related to their experience with NNSTAs, as suggested by Rubin and Smith (1990). More broadly, greater exposure to foreign accents in general may enhance overall ability to adjust to a new accent. Enhanced ability to adjust to accented speech following previous exposure to accents may be expected particularly in view of the effect that previous exposure to a nonnative language has been reported to have on the ability to learn an additional foreign language. Although evidence is not conclusive, several studies found differences between monolinguals and multilinguals learning a foreign language (Klein, 1995; Nayak, Hansen, Krueger, & McLaughlin, 1990; Eisenstein, 1980). For example, Nayak et al. (1990) reported differences found in the strategies used by monolinguals and multilinguals learning a foreign language. They compared monolingual and multilingual speakers learning a new, artificial language. Learners were instructed to use either a memorizing strategy or a rule-discovering strategy. While no differences were found between the monolingual and multilingual groups in the memorizing task, significant differences were obtained between the two groups in the rule-discovering task. Namely, the multilinguals outperformed the monolinguals. The authors concluded that previous experience with learning a foreign language facilitated the process of learning an additional linguistic system.

Similarly, Eisenstein (1980) compared monolinguals, childhood bilinguals, and childhood multilinguals on measures of language-learning ability, including language aptitude. The author found that bilinguals scored higher than monolinguals, and multilinguals scored higher than both other groups. In a more recent study, Klein (1995) found support for enhanced nonnative-language acquisition by multilinguals as compared to monolinguals. Based on a *Universal Grammar* (UG) model of parameter setting, Klein predicted that when learning a new language, monolinguals and multilinguals will not differ with respect to the process of parameter setting per se. This prediction follows from the assumption that UG and the whole range of parameter setting is available to all language learners, not only in the course of acquiring one's native language. On the other hand, Klein predicted that multilinguals will demonstrate a better lexical knowledge (of verb subcategorization) and thus enhanced knowledge of the relevant syntactic rule (preposition stranding). Klein compared monolingual and multilingual speakers learning English as a nonnative language on a grammaticality judgment and correction task. Her findings demonstrated that the multilinguals performed better than the monolinguals and that there was a relation between students' level of lexical learning and their ability to set and apply the corresponding parameter. These findings provide further evidence that experience with learning a nonnative language enhances ability to learn an additional language.

This facilitation for foreign-language learning can be explained in terms of overall greater flexibility in the representation and processing of various linguistic systems resulting from previous experience with more than one language. It may be associated with generally superior linguistic skills, and therefore can be expected to be manifested in tasks that require linguistic and metalinguistic flexibility (for example, in tasks that involve application of linguistic rules to unknown words or recognition of various interpretations of a given linguistic unit).

The notion of flexibility of representation and processing plays a role in theories concerning special talent. Indeed, a third factor that may account for variability in comprehension skills concerns varying degrees of special talent in adjusting to and comprehending accented English. Neuropsychological research in special talents includes studies concerning special talent in learning a foreign language. For example, Schneiderman and Desmarais (1988a; 1988b) hypothesized that neurocognitive flexibility may distinguish talented second-language learners from most second-language learners. Underlying this hypothesis was the assumption that the mechanisms responsible for nonnative-language learning and their underlying neural networks may vary among learners. In the course of first language acquisition, certain pathways and strategies are established as the linguistic system is being set. While most learners apply these existent mechanisms when learning a second language, talented learners may be able to avoid the fixed pathways when acquiring a new linguistic system. Instead, it is assumed, they establish new pathways for the purpose of processing the new language. This may contribute to their superior ability in adjusting to the features of a second language and modifying their linguistic system to accommodate the new language.

Similarly, general cognitive flexibility can be hypothesized to underlie the ability to adjust to a foreign accent. Presumably, listening to a foreign accent requires a decoding process and then a matching process. Encountering an unintelligible word but assuming that it was nevertheless spoken in English, the listener may undertake a process of matching the heard word to a known word. For many listeners, after a brief period of listening to the accented speech, it becomes more transparent and the matching process is facilitated. Some transforming system has presumably been established so that listeners can hear the speech as English. The extent to which such adjustment takes place and the length of the period of exposure needed are assumed to vary across listeners.

Ability to adjust to foreign accents may thus be related to superior performance on tasks of general cognitive flexibility. Skills associated with cognitive flexibility, such as ability to switch sets, are measured by neuropsychological tasks such as the Wisconsin Card Sorting Test. In this test, subjects are asked to match cards according to one of three possible visual criteria (color, shape, and number). The target criterion is altered periodically by the examiner without explicitly telling the subject (e.g., suddenly a subject's choice based on a criterion that got a *right* response previously now gets a *wrong* response). Performing this task successfully requires cognitive flexibility. We set out to test whether such general cognitive flexibility or explicitly language-related cognitive flexibility might be linked to the ability to adjust to English spoken with a foreign accent.

A unique theory concerning special talents is the neurological theory of talent developed by Geschwind and Galaburda (1985). Geschwind and Galaburda hypothesized that there is a neurological basis for talent, attributing certain types of talent such as mathematical or musical talent to superior functioning of the right hemisphere. Based on this view, special talents are related to neural development and certain neuroimmunoendocrinological features. More specifically, both talents and certain disabilities can be explained by hormonal activity that takes place in early-mid stages of fetal life at the time when the immunological system is developing and the right hemisphere is developing faster than the left. Unusual amounts of hormones result in a delay in cellular organization in the left hemisphere. Thus, superior skills may be related to the right hemisphere as well as to unaffected areas surrounding the affected area in the left hemisphere (Geschwind & Galaburda, 1985, discussed in Fein & Obler, 1988). Geschwind developed a questionnaire designed to reveal neurological, immunological, and endocrinological characteristics associated with this theory. A number of studies (e.g., in Obler & Fein, 1988: Benbow, Novoa, Fein, & Obler; Schneiderman & Desmarais) have explored the application of the theory to specific areas of talent.

Obler has been particularly interested in talent and lack of it in the language realms. Novoa et al. (1988) studied talent in acquiring a foreign language. The case they reported showed slow overall development, mild difficulty in learning to read, and an exceptionally good ability in acquiring native-like proficiency in foreign languages. We hypothesized that neuroimmunoendocrinological characteristics associated with talent in foreign language acquisition are also associated with talent in understanding and adjusting to new accents.

The purpose of the present study was to explore the factors discussed above as they may relate to undergraduate students' varying abilities to comprehend accented English. In particular, the study was designed to evaluate subjects' ability to adjust to English spoken by a nonnative speaker of English with respect to each of the following factors: linguistic and cognitive flexibility; talent and the neuroimmunoendocrinological characteristics that have been hypothesized to be linked to it; exposure to foreign languages and accents; and attitude toward foreign languages and foreign speakers.

The study involved two stages. The purpose of the first stage was to assess the ability of a large sample of native English speakers to comprehend accented English. The second stage was designed to explore four possible accounts for good adjustment to accented English. First, good adjusters and matched nonadjusters' performance on cognitive and linguistic flexibility measures was evaluated. Next, their self-reported neuroimmunoendocrinological profiles were analyzed. Additionally, all subjects' scores on a questionnaire concerning exposure to and attitude toward foreign accents and foreigners were considered.

SELECTING THE GOOD ADJUSTERS: DISCRIMINATION SCORES

Method

Subjects

One hundred and twelve undergraduate students from the New York metropolitan area participated in the study. Students' ages ranged from 18 to 43 with a *mean* of 21.8. Number of years of education ranged from 13 to 18 with a *mean* of 15.1. Each student agreed to participate and signed an informed consent form.

Materials

Listening Task A two-page segment of an article about the life of monkeys in Peru (*Natural History*, May, 1994) was used for the listening task. This text was chosen assuming its topic would be universally unfamiliar.

A nonnative English speaker was tape-recorded reading the two-page segment. The speaker's heavy accent served our purpose, creating a passage of reduced intelligibility. The speaker's accent was characterized by a number of phonological deviations from standard American English production such as consonant reduction, consonants collapsing, vowel substitutions, and vowel collapsing, as well as by a different lexical and sentential stress pattern.

The speaker read the article to herself before the audio recording. She was then asked to read it aloud, speaking at an average rate. Recordings were made using a Marantz PMD 201 portable cassette recorder and an Electro-Voice 635A Dynamic omni-directional microphone.

Discrimination and Comprehension Tasks A review of the speaker's tape-recorded passage enabled identification of three phoneme pairs spoken differently from standard American English production. The following phoneme pairs were judged by the researchers to be minimally distinguishable: /l/ and /r/, /I/ and /i/, and /s/ and /z/ in word-final position. Five minimal pairs were chosen to contrast each pair of minimally distinguishable phonemes, thus creating a list of 30 monosyllabic CVC experimental words (15 minimal pairs). Word frequencies (based on Francis & Kucera, 1982) were matched within each group of words containing the same phoneme. An additional 20 words (ten minimal pairs, monosyllabic CVC) that did not contain the experimental phonemes served as fillers. This list of 50 words (30 experimental words and 20 fillers) was pseudo-randomized so that no more than two consecutive words included phonemes of the same minimal pair. The list was read by the same speaker and was tape-recorded using the system described above. The 50 words were digitized using waveform editing software for waveform display, segmentation, and subsequent playback (*WAVEXAM*) via a P5-90 computer system. Three lists were created using three different pseudo-randomized orders of the 50 words. The lists were recorded onto an analog tape using a Marantz PMD 430 cassette recorder.

Ten multiple-choice questions based on the content of the recorded passage were used to motivate the students' attention throughout the listening tasks. We deliberately created difficult questions to avoid ceiling effects or students' answering based on general knowledge.

Questionnaires A questionnaire was created to elicit information regarding students' attitude toward and exposure to foreigners, foreign languages, and accented English. The questionnaire consisted of 46 statements. Twenty-three items were included to determine the degree of exposure to languages other than English and to foreign accents and to determine whether English was the student's native language. The remaining 23 items were included to elicit information regarding attitude toward foreigners and foreign languages. The students indicated whether they agreed or disagreed with each item using a five-point scale. For example, presented with the following items, the students indicated whether they agreed or disagreed: "It is better to live in a place where everybody has the same culture" or "I enjoy socializing with people from different countries." The attitude items were worded such that opportunity to both agree and disagree with items denoting both positive and negative attitudes was provided. For instance, in the examples above, agreeing to the first statement would indicate a more negative attitude toward foreigners, while agreeing to the second statement would indicate a positive attitude.

A modified Geschwind-Galaburda Questionnaire was given to obtain information about neuroimmunoendocrinological factors involved in talent (Geschwind & Galaburda, 1985). The questionnaire included items inquiring about history of handedness and familial handedness, history of hearing problems, history of hereditary and immune diseases, and history of special talents, language delay, and learning disability. The modification consisted of eliminating from the original questionnaire items that were inappropriate for this college-student population (e.g., questions concerning fertility) and adding a question concerning hearing status.

Procedure

Groups of 15 to 30 students were tested in their classrooms. The testing procedure was explained to the students. They then listened to the tape-recorded passage, to the three word-lists (one after 2 minutes, one after 7 minutes, and one at the end of the 12-minute passage), then answered the comprehension questions and filled out the questionnaires. Each testing session lasted about 45 minutes and consisted of the following steps:

> Students listened to an explanation of the procedures and then signed the informed consent forms.

Students listened to the first two minutes of the tape-recorded passage.

Students listened to the first order of the word list and indicated, on an answer sheet in front of them, the word they heard given a binary choice (for example, when the speaker said *lake* the choices on the answer sheet were *lake* and *rake*).

Students listened to the next five minutes of the tape-recorded passage.

Students listened to the second order of the word list and again indicated on an answer sheet the word they heard.

Students listened to the last five minutes of the passage.

Students listened to the third order of the word list and indicated on the third answer sheet the word they heard.

Students answered the ten multiple-choice comprehension questions.

Students completed the two questionnaires.

Scoring

Comprehension Tasks For each student, a total number of correctly identified experimental words was calculated for each list. The maximum possible score for each list was 30. The students' overall mean improvement (i.e., the mean increase in scores from list 1 to list 3) was calculated. An increase of at least one and a half standard deviations above the overall mean increase was considered an excellent improvement in comprehension of accented English, taken as evidence for subjects' adjustment to the speaker's accent in particular and for their talent in adjusting to a new accent more generally.

A total number of correct answers for the ten multiple-choice comprehension questions was also calculated for each subject. As this score reflects factors beyond mere adjustment to accented speech, it was not incorporated into the selection criteria for particularly good adjusters.

Exposure and Attitude Questionnaire Total exposure scores were calculated for each student by adding up the scores of 21^1 exposure items. Recall that possible scores on each item ranged from 0 to 4. Thus, possible overall exposure scores ranged from 0 to 84 (such that lower scores denoted native English speakers with minimal exposure to other languages). Similarly, for the attitude component of the questionnaire, total attitude scores were calculated from 22^1 attitude items. Here too, possible scores for each item ranged from 0 to 4 and possible overall scores ranged from 0 (most negative attitude toward foreigners and foreign languages) to

---

[1] Three questionnaire items were excluded from the analysis due to their ambiguity with respect to providing exposure or attitude information exclusively. In addition to total scores for each student and across students, individual scores on each item followed by mean scores for each item, collapsed across students, were also calculated. Mean scores on clusters of items reflecting specific areas of exposure and attitude (for example, exposure to foreign languages, exposure to English spoken with a foreign accent, etc.) were also calculated, as described below.

88 (most positive attitude). Scores were calculated after adjusting for directionality of items. Recall that some items were presented such that choosing *0* (*strongly agree*) would reflect positive attitude, while for others a choice of *0* reflected negative attitude. This was reflected in the calculation such that for all items lower adjusted scores denoted a more negative attitude and higher adjusted scores denoted a more positive attitude.

Results

Out of the 112 undergraduate students tested, 104 were identified as native speakers of English. Data from the eight nonnative English-speaking subjects were excluded from analysis in the current study.

Discrimination Task

Based on students' performance on the three word lists, 7 (out of the 104, 7%) students were identified as particularly good adjusters by virtue of their ability to adjust to the new accent. Specifically, those students who improved from list 1 to list 3 by more than one and a half standard deviations above the overall mean improvement, were defined as good adjusters. Students who did not improve from list 1 to list 3 (e.g., improved by the overall mean improvement or less) were defined as nonadjusters. Mean improvement scores of the seven good adjusters and the group of 97 remaining students are shown in Table 1.

In addition, 7 students were selected from the group of 97 nonadjusters. These 7 were matched to the seven good adjusters on age, education, and exposure and attitude scores (see Table 2).

Comprehension Task

The scores of the comprehension questions of the 7 adjusters (*mean* = 3.9; *SD* = 2.4) did not differ from those of the 97 remaining students (*mean* = 3.9; *SD* = 1.9). Comparing the good adjusters, the matched nonadjusters, and the remaining subjects (*n* = 90) using a one-way ANOVA revealed no significant differences among the three groups ($p = 0.76$).

The exposure and attitude scores as well as the data from the Geschwind-Galaburda questionnaire served initially for the purpose of matching the group of seven nonadjusters to the seven good adjusters. These measures were then used to investigate whether exposure, attitude, and special talent can account for the good adjustment, as will be discussed below.

Table 1. Mean Improvement of the Seven Good Adjusters and the 97 Remaining Students

Students	Mean (SD)		
	List 1	List 3	Improvement from List 1 to List 3
Good Adjusters ($n = 7$)	19.3 (2.2)	25.4 (1.6)	6.1 (1.1)
Remaining Students ($n = 97$)	22.6 (1.8)	22.3 (1.9)	−0.3 (2.3)
All Students ($n = 104$)	22.4 (2.0)	22.5 (2.1)	0.1 (2.8)

Table 2. Good Adjusters and Nonadjusters Students' Characteristics

	Adjusters			Nonadjusters		
	Mean	SD	Range	Mean	SD	Range
Age	23	3.2	19-29	23	6.2	20-37
Education (yrs.)	15.6	1.4	13.5-18	14.7	0.8	14-16
GPA	3.2	0.5	2.25-3.75	3.4	0.4	2.25-3.75
Exposure Score	32.1	18.9	12-59	34.9	13.6	15-53
Attitude Score	63	12.1	41-79	60.9	10.1	44-73

FACTORS UNDERLYING GOOD ADJUSTMENT TO ACCENTED ENGLISH: TALENT, EXPOSURE, AND ATTITUDE SCORES

A second set of analyses was carried out to answer the following questions: (a) whether cognitive and linguistic flexibility can distinguish good adjusters and nonadjusters to accented English; (b) whether adjusters and nonadjusters differ in their neuroimmunoendocrinological profiles; (c) whether exposure to foreign languages, foreign accents, and NNSTAs can distinguish good adjusters from nonadjusters; and (d) whether attitude toward foreign languages, foreign accents, and NNSTAs can distinguish good adjusters from nonadjusters to accented English.

Method

Subjects

Recall that seven particularly good adjusters to accented English and seven matched nonadjusters were selected based on their discrimination scores (see above and Table 2). To answer the first question, (a), the seven good adjusters were tested in a second session on a battery of cognitive and linguistic flexibility tasks and were compared to the seven matched nonadjusters on these tasks. For the purpose of answering questions (b), (c), and (d), the 7 good adjusters were compared to the remaining 97 students on the questionnaires data.

Procedure

Each of the 14 students described above (7 good adjusters and 7 matched nonadjusters) was tested individually on the following tests:
Cognitive Flexibility Tasks
The *Wisconsin Card Sorting Test* (WCST) (Heaton, 1993): Participants' ability to shift sets is measured by variables such as overall number of trials and number of errors (i.e., failure to shift to the new criterion).
Trails B (timed; Halstead and Reitan Battery): participants are asked to connect numbers and letters according to a certain pattern as quickly as they can. This task measures participants' ability to rapidly alternate between sets.
Breskin's Rigidity Test (Breskin, 1968): in this test, participants are asked to indicate which shape of each pair of shapes they prefer. The test measures preference for symmetry or asymmetry.
Linguistic Flexibility Tasks The following subtests are from the Gjerlow-Johnson Metalinguistic Battery (1991):
Phonology subtest (based on Scholes & Willis, 1988b): for each word presented to the participants they are asked to provide a target word by omitting or adding a sound (for example, spit - /p/ => sit; ocean + /n/ => notion). Instructions are given to complete the task based on the way the words sound rather than how they are spelled. This test measures phonological awareness.
Quick Answers (coreference) subtest (based on Scholes & Willis, 1988a): participants are presented with short sentences that include more than one potential agent and are asked to identify the correct one (identifying within-sentence

coreference), for example: "If a young man watching a pretty girl talking to a tall boy rides a bicycle, who rides a bicycle?" (MAN, GIRL, or BOY).

Morphology subtest: in this test participants are asked to use derivational and inflectional suffixes with nonwords. For example: "...[We] call this kind of stripe a *zar*. If a cat has more than one zar it has many _____. A cat with many of these stripes is a very _____ cat." This task measures ability to use morphological patterns productively.

Ambiguity Detection subtest (based on Brooks, 1980): participants' ability to detect ambiguities is measured by asking them to read a list of sentences and identify those that are ambiguous.

Stress Interpretation subtest (Gleitman & Gleitman, 1971): in this task, participants are asked to listen to three-word novel compounds and paraphrase them. The meaning of the novel compounds is to be determined based on their stressed components (for example, *old bird-house* versus *old-bird house*). Thus, this test measures ability to use stress patterns in interpreting novel compounds.

Results

Results for each of the four measures used in our second set of analyses are detailed below. While comparisons on three variables (namely, linguistic and cognitive flexibility, special talent, and previous exposure to foreign languages) did not differ between good adjusters and nonadjusters, attitude scores were found to significantly distinguish between the two groups.

Cognitive and Linguistic Flexibility

Accuracy scores for each task were obtained for each of the seven good adjusters and seven matched nonadjusters (see Table 3). Mean scores of the good adjusters on each task were compared to those of the nonadjusters. Statistical analysis using a repeated-measure ANOVA revealed no significant differences between the two groups ($F = 0.14$; $p = 0.71$).

Neuroimmunoendocrinological Characteristics Associated with Talent

Next, the adjusters and nonadjusters' responses on the modified Geschwind-Galaburda questionnaire were compared. The reported information is summarized in Table 4. Examination of group data on each of the questionnaire items showed that the two groups did not differ in number and type of symptoms reported.

Exposure to and Attitude Toward Foreign Languages, Foreign Accents, and Foreign Speakers

The third set of analyses was carried out to compare good adjusters and all nonadjusters on the exposure and attitude measures. Recall that for the purpose of analyzing the cognitive and linguistic measures, the adjusters and nonadjusters groups had been matched for exposure and attitude scores. For the analyses discussed here, however, we compared the seven good adjusters to the rest of the

Table 3. Individual Scores on Cognitive- and Linguistic-Flexibility Tasks: Seven Adjusters and Seven Nonadjusters

Ss/task	Trails-B #errors/26	Rigidity #rigid/15	Phonology #correct/36	Coreference #correct/10	Morphology #errors/20	Ambiguity #correct/24	Stress Pattern #correct/24	WCST* #errors
Adjusters								
1	0	14	27	8	5	18	22	22
2	0	14	17	10	6	17	0	24
3	0	7	29	9	6	16	10	18
4	1	7	29	10	3	11	21	27
5	0	7	19	6	9	14	5	14
6	0	8	36	11	3	15	20	14
7	0	11	14	9	7	14	1	27
mean	0.1	9.7	24.4	9	5.6	15	11.1	20.9
Nonadjusters								
1	0	13	26	11	4	12	20	11
2	0	5	26	8	5	12	9	19
3	0	7	27	10	3	19	4	11
4	1	2	21	9	3	16	5	19
5	1	8	33	11	4	17	8	26
6	1	12	32	10	4	21	13	27
7	13	7	30	10	4	18	3	52
mean	1.9	7.7	27.9	9.9	3.9	16.4	8.9	23.6

* WCST = Wisconsin Card Sorting Test

Table 4. Performance of Good Adjusters and Matched Nonadjusters on the Geschwind-Galaburda Questionnaire

Item/Number of Students		Adjusters (n = 7)	Nonadjusters (n = 7)
Handedness	Right-handed	5	7
	Left-handed	1	0
	Ambidextrous	1	0
	Switched to right	1	1
Familial Handedness	Right-handed (%)	22/30 (73)	16/21 (76)
	Left-handed (%)	6/30 (20)	4/21 (19)
	Ambidextrous (%)	2/30 (7)	1/21 (5)
Birth	Single	7	7
	Twins	0	0
Early Graying		0	0
Allergies	Asthma	1, 4 fam.*	1, 1 fam.*
	Hay fever	2, 4 fam.*	2, 6 fam.*
	Eczema	0	1 fam.
	Other	0	0
Hx of Immune Diseases	(Total Reports)	0	2
Fam. Hx. Immune Diseases	(Total Reports)	2	9
Special Talents	(Total Reports)	2	5
Familial Special Talents	(Total Reports)	3	4
Hx. of Language Developmental Difficulties		0	0
Fam. Hx. of Language Developmental Difficulties		1	6
Hx. of Developmental Behavior Disorders		0	0
Fam. Hx. of Developmental Behavior Disorders		0	0

* #, # fam. = Number of individuals reported, number of family members reported.

students ($n = 97$) on the exposure and attitude scores. We conducted sign tests to determine the overall pattern of responses and t-tests on the individual items, using $\alpha = 0.01$ to correct for multiple comparisons.

Exposure to Foreign Languages and Foreign Accents

The comparison using a sign test between the exposure scores of the seven good adjusters and the rest of the students revealed no overall differences between the groups ($p = 1$). We then separated those items that clearly concerned exposure to foreign languages ($n = 10$) from those concerning exposure to English spoken with foreign accents ($n = 9$). As was found for the overall exposure scores, when the two groups were compared on each of the clusters separately, there was no significant difference between the two groups on either cluster ($p = 0.34$; $p = 0.5$). Previous exposure to NNSTAs, as measured by two items on the questionnaire, also did not differ between the two groups. Item analysis using post-hoc multiple t-tests was performed to explore potential differences in specific types of exposure to foreign languages and foreign accents. Power was low due to the small size of the adjusters sample; none of the individual exposure items showed significant differences between the groups (with the lowest $p > 0.09$).

Because the participating students varied considerably in terms of their exposure to languages besides English, we used the language-exposure items on the questionnaire to assess whether students' monolingual versus bilingual status[2] predicted their adjustment to accented speech. The average score of the four relevant items on the questionnaire was calculated for each student. Possible average scores ranged from 0 to 4. Based on these scores, 49 students were identified as monolingual English speakers with no or minimal knowledge of any other language beside English (average score of 0 to 1), 30 students comprised an intermediate group with some knowledge of another language or languages in addition to English (average score of 1.25 to 2.75), and 19 students were identified as bilinguals, that is, students who can speak and understand another language in addition to English (with an average score of 3 to 4). An additional 6 students who did not answer the relevant questionnaire items consistently were excluded from the following analysis. To assess whether exposure factors as reflected by bilingual status further explain superior ability to adjust to accented English we considered the data from the three separate subgroups: monolinguals, intermediate, and bilinguals.

Two (out of the 49, 4%) monolingual students, 2 (out of the 30, 7%) intermediate students, and 3 (out of the 19, 16%) bilinguals were identified as good adjusters based on their performance on the discrimination task. In other words, of the seven good adjusters, two were monolingual students, two were intermediate, and three were bilingual speakers.

The overall adjusters and nonadjusters groups were thus divided into (1) two monolingual adjusters to accented English and two monolingual nonadjusters, (2) two intermediate adjusters and one intermediate nonadjuster, and (3) three bilingual adjusters and four bilingual nonadjusters subgroups. The distribution of the students and their mean adjustment scores in the three subgroups are shown in Table 5.

Considering these data it can be seen that the proportion of bilingual adjusters (16%) was greater than that of the intermediate and monolingual students (4% and 7%, respectively). However, one bilingual subject reported previous exposure to the particular accent used in the study. If this subject is excluded, there would be two bilingual adjusters (out of 19, 11%), which would be closer to, yet still higher than, the other proportions.

Average attitude scores among the monolingual, intermediate, and bilingual adjusters subgroups did not differ (see Table 6). Mean attitude scores for the monolingual students were 56.5, 72.5 for the intermediate group, and 61.0 for the

---

[2] The term *bilinguals* is used here in its broader meaning, i.e., including speakers of more than two languages. Because our target population was monolingual speakers, our questionnaire did not allow for more detailed information regarding variables such as the number of languages spoken and degree of proficiency in each of these languages.

bilingual students. Statistical analysis using a one-way ANOVA indicated that there were no significant differences among these scores of the three groups ($F = 0.9$, $p = 0.47$).

Attitude Toward Foreigners and Speakers of Accented English

The comparison using a sign test between attitude scores of the adjusters and the rest of the students revealed significant differences between the groups, whereby the adjusters showed a more positive attitude toward learning foreign languages and toward foreigners in general ($p = 0.029$). Post-hoc multiple t-test analysis did not reveal significant differences between the adjusters and the rest of the students on any of the individual attitude items.

<u>Table 5</u>. Distribution and Mean Discrimination Improvement of Three Subgroups: Monolingual, Intermediate, and Bilingual

Group	Number of Nonadjusters (%)	Mean Adjustment Score	Number of Adjusters (%)	Mean Adjustment Score*
Monolinguals ($n = 49$)	47 (96)	0	2 (4)	5
Intermediate ($n = 30$)	28 (93)	0	2 (7)	6
Bilinguals ($n = 19$)	16 (84)	–1	3 (16)	7

*Mean adjustment score = mean of score differences from list 1 to list 3

<u>Table 6</u>. Mean Exposure and Attitude Scores for Monolingual, Intermediate, and Bilingual Adjusters and Nonadjusters

Group	Exposure			Attitude		
	Mean	Range	SD	Mean	Range	SD
Monolingual						
Adjusters ($n = 2$)	10	8-12	2.83	56.5	41-72	21.9
Nonadjusters ($n = 2$)	18.5	11-26	10.6	61	52-70	12.7
Intermediate						
Adjusters ($n = 2$)	26.5	26-27	0.7	72.5	66-79	9.2
Nonadjusters ($n = 1$)	29	29		64	64	
Bilingual						
Adjusters ($n = 3$)	50.7	44-53	5.86	61	56-65	4.6
Nonadjusters ($n = 4$)	44.5	39-49	4.12	60	44-73	12.1
Total						
Adjusters ($n = 7$)	32.14	8-53	18.9	63	41-79	12.1
Nonadjusters ($n = 7$)	34.86	11-49	13.6	60.9	44-73	10.1

DISCUSSION

Varying ability to comprehend English spoken by nonnative speakers was previously found to play a role in undergraduate students' evaluation of nonnative speakers of English teaching assistants. In the present study, various factors that may account for this variability in ability to adjust to a new accent were explored. One hundred and twelve undergraduate students were tested for their ability to adjust to accented English. Variability in adjusting performance was analyzed in relation to measures of cognitive and linguistic flexibility, special talent in adjusting to accents based on neuroimmunoendocrinological characteristics, and students' exposure to and attitude toward foreign languages, accents, and foreign speakers.

In the first stage of the study, we tested undergraduate students for their ability to adjust to accented English. Out of the 112 undergraduate students tested, 104 students who were identified as native speakers of English were considered. Students' adjustment to the accented speech, as measured by their improvement in comprehending a nonnative speaker following a 12-minute period of exposure to the speaker's accented speech, was evaluated.

Ability to adjust to a new accent was measured based on students' performance on a word-discrimination task, administered in three time intervals with increasing amount of exposure to the accented speech. The results of the discrimination tasks revealed a range of ability to discriminate single words when spoken with accented speech. Moreover, a varying degree of improvement in performance with increased exposure to the accent was evident. Students who demonstrated a sizable improvement in their performance from the first administration of the task to the last administration were considered good adjusters. By our criteria, seven students (7%) were deemed to be particularly good adjusters.

In the second stage, we considered four factors that may account for differences found in the adjusting ability. The first factor was cognitive and linguistic flexibility. The seven good adjusters were compared to seven matched nonadjusters on a battery of cognitive and linguistic tests. No significant differences were found between the two groups. Moreover, on several tasks, great variability in performance among members of the two groups was observed.

The linguistic-related tests included tasks that measured metalinguistic skills (e.g., the phonological subtest of the Gjerlow-Johnson Metalinguistic Battery), as well as tasks that measured flexibility in language processing (e.g., the ambiguity detection subtest in the Gjerlow-Johnson battery). Metalinguistic ability has been suggested as a contributing factor in the process of learning a second language (Paradis, 1996), although Obler (1996) has pointed out that metalinguistics may be defined as conscious rule acquisition by some researchers. But for others (e.g., Gjerlow-Johnson) it is less conscious rule-inferring that constitutes metalinguistic ability and that allows speakers to use their linguistic knowledge in new contexts. The metalinguistic measures in the present study did not reveal differences between the two groups.

As for linguistic flexibility, in accordance with special talent theories concerning linguistic ability (such as that of Fein & Obler, 1988; Schneiderman & Desmarais, 1988), it would be hypothesized that the ability to process linguistic material independently of previous language processing procedures may contribute to the ability to learn a new language or, by way of analogy, to adjust to a new variety of a known language. Alternatively, more general neurocognitive flexibility would be expected to underlie superior ability to adjust to a new or modified linguistic system (Schneiderman & Desmarais, 1988b). Thus, based on theories of talent and neurocognitive flexibility as described above, good adjusters were expected to show superior performance on cognitive and/or linguistic flexibility measures. However, no consistent differences between the two groups were found in this study for any of the flexibility measures. Overall, adjusters could not be distinguished from nonadjusters based on their performance on cognitive or linguistic flexibility tasks, nor did data inspection suggest that individual tests might differentiate the groups.

The second factor considered concerned Geschwind and Galaburda's neuroanatomical theory of talent (Geschwind & Galaburda, 1985). In their theory, Geschwind and Galaburda linked familial immune disorders, handedness, neuropsychological deficit, and special talents. We used a modified version of the Geschwind-Galaburda questionnaire to evaluate whether the theory can account for good adjustment to accented speech.

A comparison of the good adjusters and the nonadjusters on the modified Geschwind-Galaburda questionnaire did not provide any support for such a hypothesis. However, self-reporting of talents may not be sufficient to evaluate the interrelationship among the relevant factors. While no differences on the modified Geschwind-Galaburda questionnaire were observed, a more detailed investigation may be needed before dismissing talent theories as an account for differences among comprehenders of accented speech.

In addition, measures of exposure to and attitude toward foreign languages, accents, and foreigners in general were considered. For the purpose of the first two comparisons, it was crucial to control for various independent variables including exposure and attitude factors, and thus the adjusters and the nonadjusters were matched on their overall exposure and attitude scores. However, in order to investigate the role that exposure and attitude variations may play in the ability to adjust to accented speech, further detailed analysis of these measures was conducted on the entire population studied.

As to exposure variables, previous experience with more than one language has been reported to facilitate the learning of additional languages (Eisenstein, 1980; Klein, 1995). Theories that account for second language acquisition processes in terms of parameter setting (within the Chomskian framework of UG) may predict that practice with adjusting the new settings for a second language would increase speakers' flexibility and hence facilitate further second language learning (Schneiderman & Desmarais, 1988a; 1988b). Alternatively, the model may predict that experience with parameter setting may result in enhanced awareness of required triggering data and in faster application of the new setting (Klein, 1995). Based on such theories, it could be expected that greater experience with foreign languages may account for flexibility in processing language variations including comprehending language spoken with foreign accents. In the present study, past experience and exposure to languages other than English did not differ between the adjusters and the nonadjusters. However, when measuring the proportion of good adjusters with respect to their bilingual status, a somewhat greater proportion of bilingual adjusters (16%, or 11% – if excluding the one student who reported exposure to the accent in question) was found than that of the intermediate group (7%) and the monolinguals (4%) (Galletta, Goral, & Obler, 1995).

Interestingly, exposure to foreign accents per se also did not differ between the two groups. Furthermore, previous experience with foreign teaching assistants or instructors, while found to correlate with listening comprehension performance in previous studies (e.g., Rubin & Smith, 1990), did not significantly distinguish between the two groups in the present study.

With regard to attitude variables, a number of studies focusing on the NNSTAs problem found that attitude toward foreign people and cultures influenced students' evaluation of NNSTAs (e.g., Brown, 1992). When the adjusters in the present study were compared to the rest of the students on their attitude scores, as measured on a self-report five-point-scale questionnaire, an overall more positive attitude toward foreign languages and foreign speakers was found among the good adjusters than the nonadjusting students. This finding is consistent with previous findings concerning the role of attitude in ability to comprehend accented speech (e.g., Rubin, 1992). Positive attitude toward foreign speakers may contribute to decreased resistance and increased motivation in the process of listening to the accented speech as English and to the ability to successfully match the heard input with meaningful information.

In summary, differences in ability to adjust to a new accent were found to be related to students' overall attitude toward foreign languages and foreign speakers. Adjusters and nonadjusters, however, did not differ on talent measures including cognitive and linguistic flexibility measures and neuroimmunoendocrinological characteristics, nor, surprisingly, on their overall previous exposure to foreign languages and foreign accents. While general exposure to foreign languages was not found here to play a role in ability to adjust to accented speech, the relation between ability to learn a new language and ability to comprehend accented English was not directly investigated. Further research is needed to evaluate the relation between talent in acquiring foreign languages and talent in comprehending foreign accents. Furthermore, for the purpose of the present study, varying comprehension skills were obtained based on discrimination scores at the single-word level. Further study is needed to address issues of comprehending accented speech as evident in ability to understand words in context. Further research can address additional aspects of adjustment to accented speech as well as the effects of longer periods of exposure to accented speech.

ACKNOWLEDGMENTS

Thanks to Dr. Ron Bloom, his colleagues, and their students at the department of Speech, Language and Hearing Sciences at Hofstra University and to Dr. Nancy Eng and the department of Speech and Communication Sciences at St. John's University for help in facilitating our testing of students in their departments. We also thank Dr. Eng for her careful reading of an earlier version of this paper. We thank Elmera Goldberg for helping us generate the minimal pair stimuli. Thanks to Dr. Mark Weiss for help in digitizing the words for the minimal pair discrimination lists. We appreciated Dr. Kris Gjerlow's consulting concerning our using her metalinguistic battery. Thanks to Dr. Don Rubin for sending us the background questionnaire used in Rubin and Smith (1990), which inspired our questionnaire. We thank John Shin and Dr. Lisa Connor of the Language and the Aging Brain Lab in the Boston VA Medical Center for advising us on data and statistical analyses. Thanks to Valeriy Shafiro and Melissa Bortz for help in data analysis. Thanks to Rick de Graaff for his suggestion with respect to the MLAT subtest. This study was supported by PSC-CUNY grants #665488 and #666536.

REFERENCES

Benbow, C. P. (1988). Neuropsychological perspectives on mathematical talent. In L. K Obler and D. Fein (Eds.), *The exceptional brain: Neuropsychology of talent and special abilities*. New York: Guilford Press.

Breskin, S. (1968). Measurements of rigidity, a non-verbal test. *Perception and Motor Skills, 27*, 1203-1206.

Brooks, A. (1980). *Cognitive rigidity and the ability to detect linguistic ambiguity*. Unpublished manuscript.

Brown, K. (1992). American college student attitudes toward nonnative instructors. *Multilingua, 11* (3), 249-265.

Eisenstein, M. (1980). Childhood bilingualism and adult language aptitude. *International Review of Applied Psychology, 29*, 159-174.

Fein, D. & Obler, L. K. (1988). Neuropsychological study of talent: A developing field. In L. K. Obler and D. Fein (Eds.), *The exceptional brain: Neuropsychology of talent and special abilities*. New York: Guilford Press.

Francis, W. N. & Kucera, H. (1982). *Frequency analysis of English usage: Lexicon and grammar*. Boston: Houghton Mifflin Company.

Galletta, E., Goral, M., & Obler, L. K. (1995). *Factors underlying comprehension of accented English*. SLRF (Second Language Research Forum), Ithaca, NY.

Geschwind, N. & Galaburda, A. (1985). Cerebral lateralization: Biological mechanisms, associations and pathology. *Archives of Neurology, 42*, 428-459, 521-552, 634-654.

Gjerlow-Johnson, K. (1991). *Metalinguistic abilities in literate adults*. Unpublished doctoral dissertation, CUNY Graduate School, New York City.

Gleitman, H. & Gleitman, L. (1971). *Phrases and paraphrases*. New York: W. W. Norton & Co.

Heaton, R. K. (1993). *Wisconsin card sorting test*. Psychological Assessment Resources Inc.

Hofstede, G. (1986). Cultural differences in teaching and learning. *International Journal of Intercultural Relations, 10* (3), 301-320.

Klein, E. (1995). Second versus third language acquisition: Is there a difference? *Language Learning, 45* (3), 419-465.

Mettler, S. (1991). The discredited speaker: Listener reactions to ESL discourse. *College ESL, 1*, 9-20.

Nayak, N., Hansen, N., Krueger, N., & McLaughlin, B. (1990). Language-learning strategies in monolingual and multilingual adults. *Language Learning, 40*, 221-244.

Norris, T. (1991). Nonnative English-speaking teaching assistants and student performance. *Research in Higher Education, 32*, 433-488.

Novoa, L., Fein, D., & Obler, L. K. (1988). Talent in foreign languages: A case study. In L. K. Obler and D. Fein (Eds.), *The exceptional brain: Neuropsychology of talent and special abilities*. New York: Guilford Press.

Obler, L. K. (1996, November). *Comments on Paradis's "What bilingual aphasia tells us about the brain."* Paper presented at the International Workshop on Language, Brain, and Verbal Behavior, Barcelona, Spain.

Obler, L. K. & Fein, D. (Eds.). (1988). *The exceptional brain: Neuropsychology of talent and special abilities*. New York: Guilford Press.

Paradis, M. (1996, November). *What bilingual aphasia tells us about the brain*. Paper presented at the International Workshop on Language, Brain, and Verbal Behavior, Barcelona, Spain.

Rubin, D. L. (1992). Nonlanguage factors affecting undergraduates' judgments of nonnative English-speaking teaching assistants. *Research In Higher Education, 33*, 511-531.

Rubin, D. L. & Smith, K. A. (1990). Effects of accent, ethnicity, and lecture topic on undergraduates' evaluation of nonnative English-speaking teaching assistants. *International Journal of Intercultural Relations, 14,* 337-353.

Schneiderman, E. I. & Desmarais, C. (1988). A neuropsychological substrate for talent in second-language acquisition. In L. K. Obler and D. Fein (Eds.), *The exceptional brain: Neuropsychology of talent and special abilities.* New York: Guilford Press.

Schneiderman, E. I. & Desmarais, C. (1988). The talented language learner: Some preliminary findings. *Second Language Research, 4,* 91-105.

Scholes, R. J. & Willis, B. (1988). The illiterate native speaker of English: Oral language and intensionality. *Proceedings of the Florida Reading Association,* 33-42.

LANGUAGE IN BRAIN DAMAGE: DEMENTIA

WORD AND PSEUDOWORD REPETITION IN ALZHEIMER'S DISEASE

Marie-Claire Goldblum, Catherine Tzortzis,
Thérèse Jahchan, and François Boller

INTRODUCTION

In its beginning stage, AD is, from a neuropsychological point of view, a heterogeneous condition (Martin et al., 1986; Celsis et al., 1987; Boller et al., 1992) with symptoms associated with either language or visuospatial impairment being more prominent in some cases. However, the general profile of the majority of patients includes memory disorders in addition to visuospatial disorientation and language disorders. In regard to language function, while AD is characterized by widespread neuronal impairment, the observed deficits are not an across-the-board phenomenon. The consensus is that some linguistic levels of knowledge are less impaired than others. Syntax, morphology, phonology, and articulatory levels are considered to be almost preserved (Bayles, Tomoeda, & Trosset, 1992; Cummings et al., 1985; Nebes, 1992), while lexical and semantic knowledge are severely disturbed (Schwartz, Marin, & Saffran, 1979; Bayles & Tomoeda, 1983; Diesfeld, 1989; Murdoch & Chenery, 1987; Nebes, 1992). As a consequence, in addition to the fact that abilities outside the language domain are usually required to correctly execute a task, patients may show dissociations in language activities relative to the degree of involvement of these linguistic levels. For instance, as underlined by Obler and Albert (1984) in their description of language disturbances in aging, repetition disorders may appear in mild AD patients as soon as "one gives them very long sentences" (Albert, 1984). This suggests that, besides linguistic factors such as lexical frequency, short-term memory limitations contribute to the repetition disorder of AD patients. Even restricting our scope to activities that only require single word production (e.g., naming tasks) there is indeed a large variability in performance.

Naming from visual confrontation is moderately to severely disturbed, though less impaired than word production in a categorical verbal fluency task (Rosen, 1980; Martin & Fedio, 1983; Ober et al., 1986). In contrast, oral naming of written words (reading) is relatively spared. Naming from auditory (word) confrontation with graphic production (writing or dictation) is more impaired than reading (Horner et al., 1988), though this situation is mostly observed in language with complex writing systems such as French or English. Naming from auditory (word) confrontation with oral production (repetition) is reported to be nearly flawless. Although some studies have dealt with single word repetition and have taken into account meaningfulness of stimuli (Appel, Kertesz, & Fisman, 1982; Cummings et al., 1985; Glosser et al., 1997), available data come mostly from sentence (Holland et al., 1986; Obler & Albert, 1984) or word-list stimuli (Hulme et al., 1993).

Psychological models, such as Morton's logogen (Morton & Patterson, 1980; Patterson & Morton, 1985) and related models, provide ways to interpret this variability in AD patients. All of these models have been based on reading and writing abilities and include two ways of processing a verbal input stimulus, hence they are called *dual route* models (auditory or visual). The first processing mode, or route, includes a stage of sensory analysis before contact is made with a device (input logogen in Morton's terminology); this makes available the recognition of a corresponding lexical entry (word or morpheme) which eventually makes contact with a general knowledge store (cognitive system) containing semantic information associated to that stimulus. The output from this store is sent to a device (the output logogen) that activates the abstract phonological output corresponding to the input stimulus. This information is sent to a *response buffer* before achieving a stage where other articulatory specifications take place for correct oral production. This routine is assumed to be the only one available for picture naming, except that the first stage is a separate visual perceptive analysis that contacts an *input pictogen* sending information to the semantic store.

A second processing mode, or route, has been proposed where reading is concerned. This processing mode was hypothesized to account for the obvious ability of every normal reader to read pseudowords without any lexical and corresponding semantic representation. It also received support from the neuropsychological description of either *deep* (Coltheart, Patterson, & Marshall, 1980) or *phonological* dyslexics (Beauvois & Derouesné, 1979; Miceli, Capasso, & Caramazza, 1994) with selective difficulty in reading meaningless stimuli.

The second routine for reading is hypothesized to work independently of the lexico-semantic processing mode and to include *en route* a set of abstract rules of conversion between graphemes and phonemes. Moreover, the observation that in languages with non-transparent orthographic systems (e.g., French or English), irregular or inconsistent words (such as *yacht* and *bear*) cause particular difficulties to patients (identified under a general label as *surface* dyslexics (Patterson, Marshall, & Coltheart, 1985)), entailed a further fractionation of the phonological non-semantic reading procedure: a lexical routine directly linking abstract lexical entry to lexical output for reading of both regular and irregular words was added to the aforementioned non-lexical procedure available for reading of both regular words and pseudowords.[1]

Authors such as Wernicke, Lichtheim, Freud, Goldstein, and Luria, and, more recently, Warrington and Shallice (1969), Tzortzis and Albert (1974), and Strub and

---

[1] Actually, the existence of these two independent routes has been criticized by authors such as Glushko (1979), who proposed a single mechanism in which pseudowords are processed by analogy to real words, and Henderson (1985), who also proposed a single multi-level procedure for processing of both words and pseudowords (see Humphreys and Evett, 1985, for a discussion of this topic).

Gardner (1974), have given considerable attention to repetition disorders in conduction and transcortical sensory aphasia. However, this activity has not received a comparably refined analysis and debate about how to model it. Indeed, repetition is indifferent to pedagogical theories, and, contrary to reading and writing, it enjoys *a priori* unambiguous, simple phonological rules of correspondence between segments at input and output, be they phonemes or larger components. Yet pseudowords may exist in the auditory modality as well as in the visual modality (reading), and neuropsychological cases of *deep dysphasia* (for a review see Katz & Goodglass, 1990, and Howard & Franklin, 1988) as well as *phonological dysphasia* have been reported (Pate, Saffran, & Martin, 1987; Kohn & Smith, 1991; Wilshire & McCarthy, 1996; Sartori, Barry, & Job, 1984; Hanley & Kay, 1997). Thus, dual routes (McCarthy & Warrington, 1984) or even *triple routes* with two phonological processes (Coslett et al., 1987) have been suggested for auditory processing of words.

Within the framework of the models outlined above, and given that AD patients suffer a decline of lexico-semantic knowledge while retaining good phonological abilities, it may be possible to explain the differential difficulties encountered in naming tasks. Both tasks of verbal fluency and naming from visual confrontation require processing through semantic memory and search of the output lexicon. Thus, both tasks would be severely impaired. However, naming from visual confrontation, which provides perceptual information, could make this task easier than verbal fluency. The other naming tasks that do not require semantic mediation would show relative preservation. Yet, reading and writing, which present irregularities or inconsistencies and require lexical mediation in some languages, would be more disturbed than repetition which is totally regular.

Even though repetition is considered to be a well-preserved activity, the fact that AD patients suffer a degradation in lexico-semantic knowledge offers the possibility of studying the functioning of hypothesized lexical and non-lexical processing of linguistic material in the auditory modality. This may contribute to a better understanding of lexico-phonological disorders in these patients and to the assessment of proposed models of normal repetition ability.

Recently, Glosser et al. (1997) studied repetition of single words and pseudowords in a group of AD patients. Their results showed that AD patients had a significant impairment relative to controls for the two types of stimuli, although both groups performed worse on pseudowords than word repetition. In a second experiment using low frequency words and matched pseudowords, no correlation emerged between repetition accuracy and severity of dementia in the AD group. The analysis of lexicalization and nonword errors showed a similar pattern in the two groups, with an equivalent proportion of the two types of errors in word repetition and a prevalence of nonword errors in pseudoword repetition. Finally, the performance on word and pseudoword repetition showed a significant correlation in both AD patients and control subjects. The authors conclude that models with two independent phonological routes cannot explain this correlation and that their data are most compatible with the notion that a single lexical phonological system is responsible for processing of the two classes of stimuli.

The aim of our study was manifold. We first wanted to confirm that repetition is remarkably preserved compared to other language functions and to seek for possible relationships between repetition disorders and severity of the disease or verbal comprehension disorders. Second, although Auditory Verbal Short-Term Memory seems minimally involved in single-item repetition, we sought to investigate its influence on repetition of long stimuli. Finally, we sought to replicate the results of Glosser et al. and, in particular, to examine whether a correlation exists between word and pseudoword repetition, which the authors take as an indicator of non-independence between lexical and non-lexical phonological processing and as a piece of evidence in support for a multilevel single phonological processing.

SUBJECTS

Twenty-five patients with AD (17 women and 8 men: *mean* age of 76; *SD*, 5.8; *range*, 66 to 85), with a *mean* Mini-Mental Status Examination (MMSE) score of 19 (*SD*, 2.9; *range*, 11 to 23), entered the study. The diagnosis of probable AD was made according to the NINCDS-ADRDA criteria (McKhann et al., 1984). MRI or CT scanning, together with blood analysis, showed no evidence for another etiology. Patients with a history of head injury, alcoholism, or serious psychiatric illness were excluded from this group. Patients with a score of four or higher on the Hachinski scale (Hachinski et al., 1975) were excluded to reduce the possibility of including multi-infarct dementia. Patients who scored under ten on the MMSE (Folstein et al., 1975) were also excluded from the study.

Twenty-five normal subjects (21 women and 4 men: *mean* age of 75; *SD*, 6; *range*, 67 to 90), with a *mean* MMSE score of 29.6 (*SD*, 0.6; *range*, 28 to 30), constituted a control group (NC). They were either spouses of patients or other individuals who volunteered to participate in the research projects of our laboratory. Informed consent was obtained from all subjects participating in the study.

Group comparisons indicated that, as expected, AD patients had MMSE scores significantly lower than NC ($t = 18.03$; $p < 0.0001$). No significant difference emerged in gender distribution between the groups ($X^2 = 0.845$, ns). Statistical analysis of the distribution of patients and NC subjects according to three levels of education (*level 1*: five years of schooling; *level 2*: between five and 12 years of schooling, and *level 3*: over 12 years of schooling) showed that there were more AD patients than NC subjects with a low or average level of education ($X^2 = 8.02$, $p < 0.02$). Because of the known auditory acuity loss associated with advancing age, it is important to underscore that the two groups were quite comparable according to age (NC: *mean* of 75, *SD*, 6.08, *range*, 67 to 90; AD: *mean* of 76, *SD*, 5.83, *range*, 66 to 85; $t = 0.784$, $p > 0.45$).

Neuropsychological Evaluation

The AD patients and NCs performed a comprehensive set of neuropsychological tasks (Boller & Hécaen, 1979). The repetition task from this battery included nine words: three one-syllable words (i.e., *chat*, cat; *oeuf*, egg; *tronc*, trunk), three two-syllable words (i.e., *brouillard*, fog; *époux*, spouse; *acteur*, actor), and three four-syllable words (i.e., *mécanicien*, mechanic; *hélicoptère*,

Table 1.

Groups	Sentence Repetition	Digit Span	Comprehension of Oral Commands
NC subjects			
mean score	100	6.2	100
SD		0.5	
AD patients			
mean score	98.6	5.2	95
SD	4.09	1.3	8.2
t test	1.78	3.16	3.06
	$p > 0.08$	$p < 0.003$	$p < 0.004$

helicopter; *aérodrome*, airport). Nine pseudowords were obtained by changing some vowels and consonants from the word stimuli and comprised three one-syllable stimuli (i.e., *chon*, *anfe*, and *tra*), three two-syllable stimuli, (i.e., *traillar*, *ékou*, and *aptice*), and three four-syllable stimuli (i.e., *nérovicien*, *manisbolère*, and *aémodrope*).

The words and pseudowords were presented to subjects in separate tasks with word repetition being performed first. Prior to presentation of each task, subjects were told whether they were going to hear real words or pseudowords.

In addition to word and pseudoword repetition, the performance of subjects on various tasks from the language evaluation was analyzed. These were selected on the basis of their potential relationship to or influence on the repetition test, and included sentence repetition, auditory verbal short-term memory (digit span), and oral comprehension of commands.

RESULTS

Scores obtained by the two groups of subjects on these tasks are shown in Table 1. Group comparisons (see last row) showed that AD patients obtained lower scores than NC subjects on the digit span and oral comprehension tasks. Although they also obtained lower scores than NCs on the sentence repetition tests, that difference is only marginally significant.

Table 2 shows the mean scores obtained by the two groups in the repetition task according to meaningfulness and length of the stimuli.

Individual scores were submitted to repeated measures of analyses of variance (ANOVAs) with group (AD and NC) as the inter-subject factor and meaningfulness (words or pseudowords) and length of stimuli (one, two, or four syllables) as intra-subject factors.

AD patients obtained overall lower scores than NC subjects ($F[1, 48] = 10.26$; $p < 0.003$). Meaningfulness affected repetition of the stimuli, with higher scores on words than pseudowords ($F[1, 48] = 26.86$; $p < 0.0001$). No significant main effect of length emerged. However, meaningfulness entered into a significant interaction

Table 2. Repetition scores in AD and NC subjects (mean % correct)

Groups	Words			Pseudowords		
	1 Syllable	2 Syllable	4 Syllable	1 Syllable	2 Syllable	4 Syllable
NC subjects						
mean score	100	97.3	100	97.3	93.3	97.3
SD		1.85		1.85	2.7	1.85
AD patients						
mean score	96	100	97.3	85.3	85.3	76
SD	11.06		9.3	25.6	21.7	32.7

Table 3. Distribution of different types of repetition errors for pseudoword stimuli

	AD patients		NC subjects	
	Lexicalizations	Nonword substitutions	Lexicalizations	Nonword substitutions
1 syllable	10	1	2	0
2 syllables	5	6	2	3
4 syllables	0	18	0	2

Figure 1. Repetition scores (% correct) according to severity of dementia (MMSE)

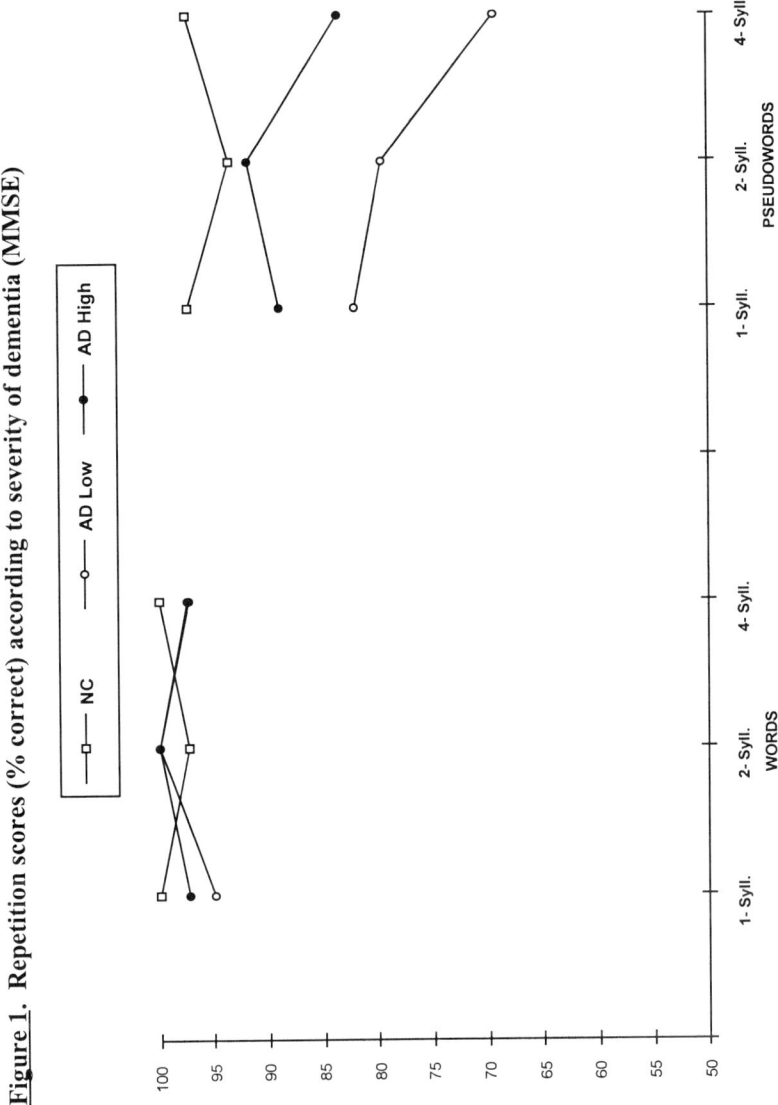

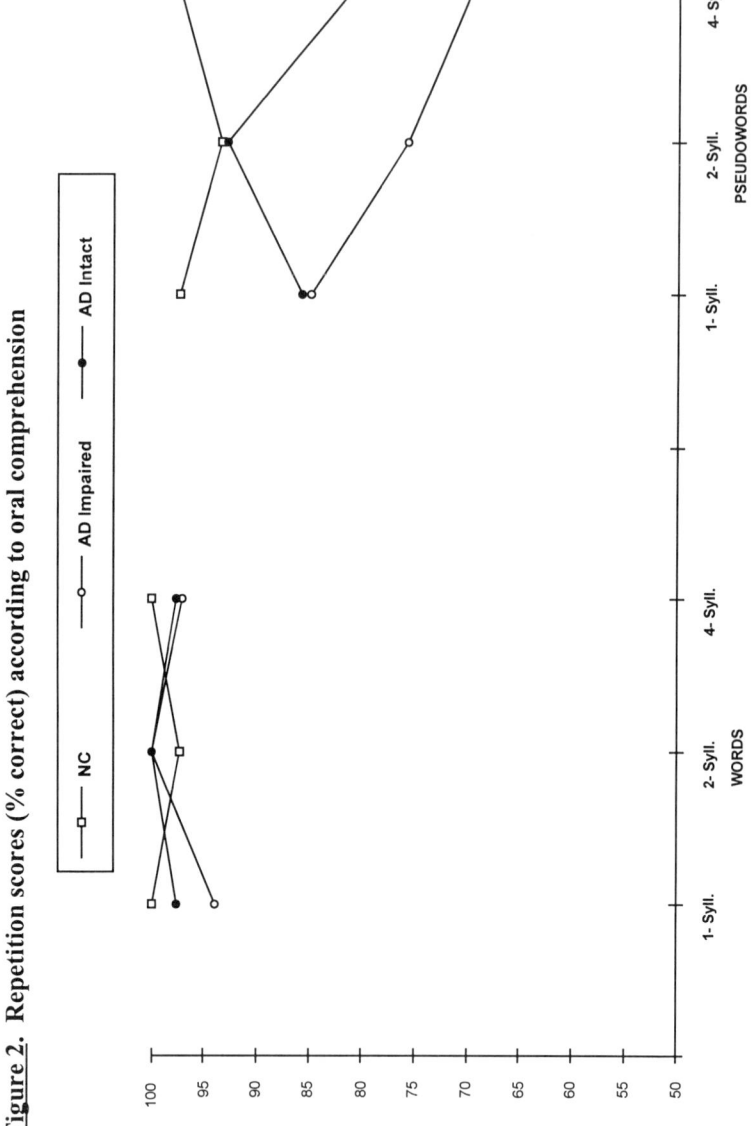

Figure 2. Repetition scores (% correct) according to oral comprehension

Figure 3. Repetition scores (% correct) according to Auditory Verbal STM (Digit Span)

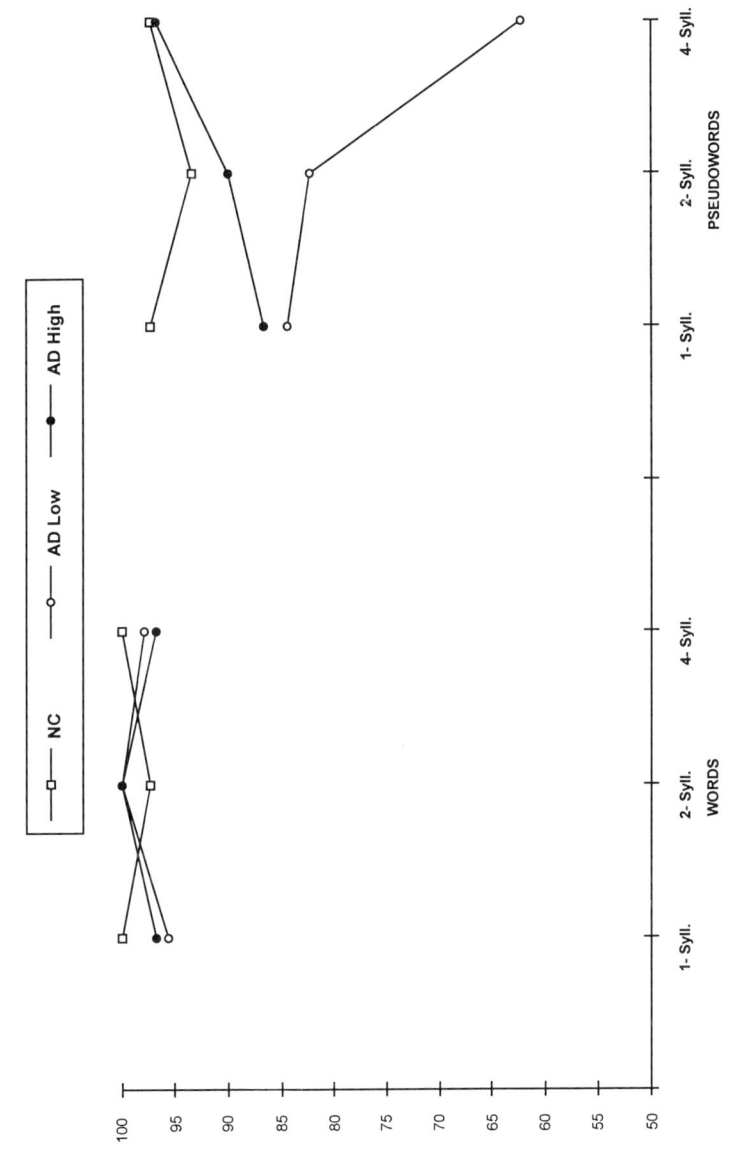

with the group factor (F [1, 48] = 11.94; $p < 0.002$), and a similar trend emerged for length (F [1, 48] = 3.06; $p < 0.06$).

Because of the observed interactions, separate analyses of variance were conducted within each group. Within the NC group, words yielded higher scores than pseudowords, but this advantage was only marginally significant (F [1, 24] = 4.26; $p < 0.06$). Two-syllable words and pseudowords were less well-repeated than one- and four-syllable words and pseudowords, which resulted in a marginally significant effect of length (F [1, 24] = 3; $p < 0.06$). Within the AD patients group, words yielded significantly higher scores than pseudowords (F [1, 24] = 22.61; $p < 0.0001$), but length of the stimuli had no main effect, and no interaction with meaningfulness of the stimuli was observed (words versus pseudowords: one-syllable: t = 1.99, $p < 0.06$; two-syllable: t = 3.38, $p < 0.003$; four-syllable: t = 3.36, $p < 0.003$). Between-group comparisons confirmed that AD patients performed similarly to NC for word repetition (t = 1.5) and that their repetition deficit was limited to pseudowords (t = 3.44, $p < 0.002$).

In order to evaluate the influence of severity of the disease, the AD patients were further separated into two groups with high scores versus low scores on the MMS. Thirteen patients with MMS under 20 constituted the *low MMS* group (*mean* score, 16.69; *SD*, 2.02; *range*, 11 to 19) and 12 patients with MMS of 20 or above constituted the *high MMS* group (*mean* score, 21.42; *SD*, 0.99; *range*, 20 to 23). Results (see Figure 1) showed that although repetition was less well-executed in the low MMS group than in the high MMS group, the difference did not reach statistical significance (F [1, 23] = 1.88, $p > 0.1$). Words entailed higher scores than pseudowords (F [1, 23] = 23.5, $p < 0.0001$). Length of the stimuli did not affect the performance of subjects (F [1, 23] = 1.5, ns). No significant interaction was observed with the group factor.

Because oral comprehension might differently affect word- as opposed to pseudoword-repetition, a similar analysis was conducted taking into account the performance of the patients on the comprehension of oral commands. Eleven patients with a maximum score of 95% correct constituted the *impaired comprehension* group (*mean* score, 89.1; *SD*, 9.44; *range*, 65% to 95%), and 14 patients constituted the *intact comprehension* group (*mean* score, 100%). Results are shown in Figure 2. Although repetition was less well-executed in the impaired comprehension group than in the intact comprehension group, the difference did not reach statistical significance (F [1, 23] = 1.67, $p > 0.2$). Once again, words entailed higher scores than pseudowords (F [1, 23] = 24.36, $p < 0.0001$). Length of the stimuli did not affect the performance of subjects (F [1, 23] = 1.47, ns). No significant interaction was observed with the group factor.

A third analysis was performed considering the possible effect of Auditory Verbal Short-Term Memory (STM) impairment of patients as measured by their digit span scores. Fifteen patients with a maximum digit span of five entered the *low STM* group (*mean* score, 4.33; *SD*, 0.62; *range*: 3 to 5), and ten patients with a digit span above five entered the high STM group (*mean* score, 6.5; *SD*, 0.71; *range*, 6 to 8). Results showed that, although the low STM group achieved lower scores than the high STM group, this difference resulted in only a trend to significance (F [1, 23] = 3.02, $p < 0.1$). As in previous analyses, words yielded higher scores than pseudowords (F [1, 23] = 21.43, $p < 0.0001$). Unlike previous analyses, a significant interaction between the group factor and meaningfulness of stimuli emerged ($F\,[1, 23] = 5.93, p < 0.03$). Group comparisons showed that while the two groups performed equally on word repetition, the low STM group obtained significantly lower scores than the high STM group on pseudoword repetition ($t = 2.11, p < 0.05$). The length of stimuli showed a trend to a significant interaction with the group factor ($F\,[2, 46] = 2.85, p < 0.07$) and with both the group of patients and meaningfulness of the stimuli ($F\,[2, 46] = 3.13, p < 0.06$). As illustrated in Figure 3 below, whereas both groups achieved lower scores on pseudoword- than word- repetition (low STM group: ($F\,[1, 14] = 21.25, p < 0.0005$); high STM group: ($F\,[1, 9] = 7.36, p < 0.03$), the length of the stimuli affected only the low STM group ($F\,[2, 28] = 3.27, p < 0.06$), and this effect was limited to pseudoword repetition ($F\,[2, 28] = 3.84, p < 0.04$)). Group comparisons revealed that the low STM group had significantly lower scores than the high STM group for four-syllable pseudowords ($F\,[1, 23] = 8.85, p < 0.007$).

Finally, with the two groups combined, word- and pseudoword-repetition were significantly correlated ($r = 0.47, p < 0.01$). But when examined separately, no significant correlation emerged in the NC group ($r = 0.27$, ns), while the correlation remained significant in the patient group ($r = 0.50, p < 0.02$).

Analysis of Errors in Pseudoword Repetition

Since word repetition was well preserved (for AD patients, five errors: three real words and two nonwords; for NC subjects, two errors: one real word and one nonword), no qualitative analysis was attempted for these stimuli. Errors in pseudoword repetition were classified as either lexicalizations (*époux* for *ékou*) or erroneous nonwords (*aktice* for *aptice*). AD patients produced 15 lexicalizations and 25 erroneous nonword substitutions, whereas NC subjects produced four lexicalizations and five erroneous nonword substitutions. Chi-square analysis revealed that the distribution of the two kinds of errors was similar in the two groups ($X^2, 0.0003; p > 0.9$). The type of error was further analyzed in the AD and NC groups according to the length of stimuli (see Table 3).

Chi-square analyses revealed that the distribution of the two kinds of errors was significantly different with regard to length of the pseudowords in the AD group ($X^2, 24.4; p < 0.0001$). Lexicalizations were predominant for one-syllable stimuli whereas nonword substitutions characterized four-syllable stimuli. No significant difference in the distribution of errors was observed in the NC group, possibly because of the small number of errors. However, inasmuch as the NC subjects produced only lexicalizations for one-syllable pseudowords and only nonword substitutions for four-syllable pseudowords, whereas for two-syllable stimuli they produced an equal number of the two types of errors, their error distribution pattern is relatively comparable to that of AD patients.

DISCUSSION

Our data show that AD patients were globally impaired relative to NC subjects on a repetition task. However, their deficit appeared to be limited to pseudowords.

AD patients obtained scores comparable to NCs for single word and sentence stimuli, which is in agreement with former reports that repetition is a largely preserved function in AD (Appel et al., 1982; Cummings et al., 1985). Both groups showed a lower performance for pseudoword stimuli. The word advantage is small in NC subjects, while it is highly significant in AD patients. This discrepancy may be surprising in the light of the semantic deficits associated with AD, which should reduce any advantage for words due to their having a long-term lexical and semantic representation. Results from Glosser et al. (1997) also showed this paradoxical effect in that the lexical advantage was present even for low frequency, unfamiliar words.

No significant difference was found between groups of patients with or without comprehension disorders, or between patients classified according to severity of the disease as measured by their scores on the MMSE. Results obtained by Glosser et al. also showed that the severity of dementia was unrelated to repetition disorders. Altogether, these results suggest that, in agreement with models such as those described in the introduction section, semantic interpretation is not mandatory for word repetition and that, for this reason, repetition of meaningful stimuli is not affected by AD patients' semantic memory disorders. Moreover, our results also indicate that the cognitive decline associated with progression of the illness has no direct influence on repetition ability, even for meaningless stimuli.

By contrast, patients with a reduced digit span, when compared with patients with a normal span, showed a significant deficit on pseudoword repetition, which was related to the length of the stimuli. This result confirms earlier observations by Obler and Albert (1984) that, in mild or mid-stage, AD repetition is impaired for material containing either low-frequency words or long stimuli. It also suggests that integrity of Auditory Verbal Short-Term Memory plays a major role in repetition of pseudowords, and, because pseudoword repetition is independent of severity of the disease, it may be specifically impaired even in the beginning stage of AD. Such a view is in agreement with the notion of heterogeneity of symptoms in AD and gives support to already reported results that variability may be present within the language domain. For instance, Becker et al.'s (1988) results suggest that the language impairment in AD may be associated with two distinct neuropsychological abnormalities because they found that a lexico-semantic impairment is unrelated to age at onset or progression of symptoms, while a syntactic impairment may be associated with earlier onset and more rapid progression of dementia.

Like Glosser et al. (1997), we found that errors in pseudoword repetition evidenced a similar pattern in AD and NC subjects. Both groups produced more nonword substitution than lexicalization errors, although this distribution was less clear-cut in NC subjects than in AD patients. However, when these two types of errors were analyzed separately, according to the length of the pseudoword stimuli, lexicalizations were mostly confined to short pseudowords. This suggests that there may be a bias associated with language structure rather than a genuine difference in error type. Indeed, in French, as in most languages, substitution of a single phoneme in a short pseudoword (or word as well) has very high probability to result in a real word and to be mistakenly interpreted as a lexicalization. This possibility becomes very low with longer phoneme strings. For this reason, we propose, rather, that patients produce mainly phonological errors and that these become more frequent with increasing length of meaningless stimuli. As emphasized by studies that focused on error type in naming from visual confrontation in AD patients (Nicholas et al., 1996) and in normal elderly subjects (Hodgson & Ellis, 1998), a given category of errors defined *a priori* may have various origins, and one should be cautious with regard to their interpretation.

Unlike Glosser et al. (1997), on our stimulus set we found that AD patients were not impaired on word repetition and that, in this case, length of the stimuli had no significant effect on the performance of subjects, even in the subgroup with a low digit span^2. Nonetheless, like Glosser et al., we found a significant positive correlation between word and pseudoword repetition, at least in the patient group. This type of result is taken by Glosser et al. as a point in support for non-independence between lexical and non-lexical phonological processes in repetition and in favor of single lexical multilevel models.

However, the original dual route models have been considerably modified. As amply discussed in Humphreys and Evett (1985), independence between the two processes is no longer considered to be a strong component of the model. The debate about the size of the graphemic-phonological elements entering the correspondence rules (be they phonemes, morphemes, or words) has also been considerably revised by supporters of dual route models. Indeed lexical influences on sublexical processing are admitted to the point that some authors propose an interactive *Summation Hypothesis* (Hillis & Caramazza, 1991; Miceli et al., 1994). These modifications blur the original differences between dual route, lexical analogy (Glushko, 1979; Kay & Marcel, 1981) or multi-level (Henderson, 1985) models.

Moreover, a raw correlation between word- and pseudoword- repetition may emerge as a consequence of a common impairment at various levels (e.g., input level, output level, or response buffer problems), even within the frame of models encompassing relatively separate processes. The preservation of word repetition, opposed to the compromised long pseudoword repetition, does not refute alternative single models, but, in our view, it is also compatible with *revised* dual route models. Our results with AD patients with limited digit span, who show impairment with long meaningless stimuli, may reflect different, though interactive, processing for words and pseudowords. Indeed, even though STM is compromised for word repetition, the phonological route (or processing mode) can take advantage of the phonological lexical route that involves long-term representations, whereas for pseudoword repetition, the phonological route has to rely almost exclusively on the use of correspondence rules and on an intact short-term memory process.

ACKNOWLEDGMENTS

This research was supported by the Villa d'Epidaure and the AGIRC retirement agency. The authors are grateful to Anne Petrov for the revision of the English manuscript.

---

^{2} Although these discrepant results should be taken with caution because our stimulus set was markedly smaller than that of Glosser et al.

REFERENCES

Albert, M. L. (1984). *Clinical neurology of aging*. New York: Oxford University Press.
Appell, J., Kertesz, A., & Fisman, M. (1982). A study of language functioning in Alzheimer patients. *Brain and Language, 17*, 73-91.
Bayles, K. A. & Tomoeda, C. K. (1983). Confrontation naming impairment in dementia. *Brain and Language, 19*, 98-114.
Bayles, K. A., Tomoeda, C. K., & Trosset, M. W. (1992). Relation of linguistic communication abilities of Alzheimer's patients to stage of disease. *Brain and Language, 42*, 454-472.
Beauvois, M. F. & Derouesné, J. (1979). Phonological alexia: Three dissociations. *Journal of Neurology, Neurosurgery and Psychiatry, 42*, 1115-1124.
Becker, J. T., Huff, F. J., Nebes, R. D., Holland, A., & Boller, F. (1988). Neuropsychological function in Alzheimer's disease: Pattern of impairment and rates of progression. *Archives of Neurology, 45*, 263-268.
Boller, F. & Hécaen, H. (1979). L'évaluation des fonctions neuropsychologiques: Examen standard de l'Unité de Recherches Neuropsychologiques et Neurolinguistiques (U.111) I.N.S.E.R.M. *Revue de Psychologie Appliquée, 29* (3), 247-266.
Boller, F., Forette, F., Khachaturian, Z., Poncet, M., & Christen, Y. (1992). *Heterogeneity of Alzheimer's disease*. Paris: Springer-Verlag.
Celsis, P., Agniel, A., Puel, M., Rascol, A., & Marc-Vergnes, J. P. (1987). Focal cerebral hypoperfusion and selective deficit in dementia of the Alzheimer type. *Journal of Neurology, Neurosurgery and Psychiatry, 50*, 1602-1612.
Coltheart, M., Patterson K. A., & Marshall, J.C. (1980). *Deep dyslexia*. London: Routledge and Kegan Paul.
Coslett, H. B., Roeltgen, D. R., Gonzalez-Rothi, L. J., & Heilman, K. M. (1987). Transcortical sensory aphasia : Evidence for subtypes. *Brain and Language, 32*, 362-378.
Cummings, J. L., Benson, F. D., Hill, M. A., & Read, S. (1985). Aphasia in dementia of the Alzheimer type. *Neurology, 35*, 394-397.
Diesfeldt, H. F. A. (1989). Semantic impairment in senile dementia of the Alzheimer type. *Aphasiology, 3*, 41-54.
Folstein, M. F., Folstein, S. E., & McHugh, P. R. (1975). "Mini-Mental State": A practical method for grading the mental state of patients for the clinician. *Journal of Psychiatric Research, 12*, 189-198.
Glosser, G., Kohn, S. E., Friedman, R. B., Sands, L., & Grugan, P. (1997). Repetition of single words and nonwords in Alzheimer's disease. *Cortex, 33*, 653-666.
Glushko, R. J. (1979). The organisation and activation of orthographic knowledge in reading aloud. *Journal of Experimental Psychology: Human Perception and Performance, 5*, 674-691.
Hachinski, V. C., Iliff, L. D., Zilhka, E., Du Boulay, G. H., McAllister, V. L., Marshall, J., Russell, R. W. R., & Symon, L. (1975). Cerebral blood flow in dementia. *Archives of Neurology, 32*, 632-637.
Hanley, J. R. & Kay, J. (1997). An effect of imageability on the production of phonological errors in auditory repetition. *Cognitive Neuropsychology, 14*, 1065-1084.
Henderson, L. (1985). Issues in the modeling of pronunciation assembly in normal reading. In K. E. Patterson, J. C. Marshall, & M. Coltheart (Eds.), *Surface dyslexia: Neuropsychological and cognitive studies of phonological reading* (pp. 459-508). London: Lawrence Erlbaum.
Hillis, A. & Caramazza, A. (1991). Mechanisms for accessing lexical representations for output: Evidence from a category-specific semantic deficit. *Brain and Language, 40*, 106-144.
Hodgson, C. & Ellis, A. W. (1998). Last in, first to go: Age of acquisition and naming in the elderly. *Brain and Language, 64, 146-163.*
Holland, A. L., Boller, F., & Bourgeois, M. (1986). Repetition in Alzheimer's disease: A longitudinal study. *Journal of Neurolinguistics, 2*, 163-176.
Horner, J., Heyman, A., Dawson, D., & Rogers, H. (1988). The relationship of agraphia to the severity of dementia in Alzheimer's disease. *Archives of Neurology, 45*, 760-763.
Howard D. & Franklin, S. (1988). *Missing the meaning?* Cambridge, MA: MIT Press.
Hulme, C., Lee, G., & Brown, G. D. A. (1993). Short-term memory impairment in Alzheimer-type dementia: Evidence for separable impairment of articulatory rehearsal and long-term memory. *Neuropsychologia, 31*, 161-172.

Humphreys, G. W. & Evett, L. J. (1985). Are there independent lexical and nonlexical routes in word processing? An evaluation of the dual-route theory of reading. *The Behavioral and Brain Sciences*, *8*, 689-740.
Katz, R. B. & Goodglass, H. (1990). Deep dysphasia: Analysis of a rare form of repetition disorder. *Brain and Language*, *39*, 153-185.
Kay, J. & Marcel, A. J. (1981). One process, not two, in reading aloud: Lexical analogies do the work of nonlexical rules. *Quarterly Journal of Experimental Psychology, 33A*, 397-414.
Kohn, S. E. & Smith, K. L. (1991). The relationship between oral spelling and phonological breakdown in conduction aphasia. *Cortex*, *27*, 631-639.
Martin, A. & Fedio, P. (1983). Word production and comprehension in Alzheimer's disease: The breakdown of semantic knowledge. *Brain and Language*, *19*, 124-141.
Martin, A., Brouwers, P., Lalonde, F., Cox, C., Teleska, P., & Fedio, P. (1986). Towards a behavioral typology of Alzheimer's patients. *Journal of Clinical and Experimental Neuropsychology*, *8*, 594-610.
McCarthy, R. & Warrington, E. K. (1984). A two-route model of speech production. *Brain*, *107*, 463-485.
McKhann, G., Drachman, D., Folstein, M., Katzman, R., Price, D., & Stadlan, E. M. (1984). Clinical diagnosis of Alzheimer's disease: Report of the NINCDS-ADRDA Work Group under the auspices of the Department of Health and Human Services Task Force on Alzheimer's Disease. *Neurology*, *34*, 939-944.
Miceli, G., Capasso, R., & Caramazza, A. (1994). The interaction of lexical and sublexical processes in reading, writing and repetition. *Neuropsychologia*, *32*, 317-333.
Morton, J. & Patterson, K. E. (1980). A new attempt at an interpretation or an attempt at a new interpretation. In M. Coltheart, K. E. Patterson, & J. C. Marshall (Eds.), *Deep dyslexia* (pp. 91-118). London: Routledge and Kegan Paul.
Murdoch, B. E. & Chenery, H. J. (1987). Language disorders in dementia of the Alzheimer type. *Brain and Language*, *31*, 122-137.
Nebes, R. (1992). Cognitive Dysfunction in Alzheimer's disease. In C. Craik & T. Salthouse (Eds.), *The Handbook of aging and cognition* (pp. 373-445). New Jersey: Lawrence Erlbaum.
Nicholas, M., Obler, L. K., Au, R., & Albert, M. L. (1996). On the nature of naming errors in aging and dementia: A study of semantic relatedness. *Brain and Language*, *54*, 184-195.
Ober, B. A., Dronkers, N. S., Kos, E., Delis, D. C., & Friedland, R. P. (1986). Retrieval from semantic memory in Alzheimer-type dementia. *Journal of Clinical and Experimental Neuropsychology*, *8*, 75-92.
Obler, L. K. & Albert, M. L. (1984). Language in aging. In M. L. Albert (Ed.), *Clinical neurology of aging* (pp. 245-253). New York: Oxford University Press
Pate, D. S., Saffran, E. M., & Martin, N. (1987). Specifying the nature of the production impairment in a conduction aphasic: a case study. *Language and Cognitive Processes*, *2*, 43-84.
Patterson, K. E., Marshall, J. C., & Coltheart, M. (1985). *Surface dyslexia: Neuropsychological and cognitive analyses of phonological reading*. London: Lawrence Erlbaum.
Patterson, K. E. & Morton, J. (1985). From orthography to phonology: An attempt at an old interpretation. In K. E. Patterson, J. C. Marshall, & M. Coltheart (Eds.), *Surface dyslexia: Neuropsychological and cognitive studies of phonological reading* (pp. 335-359). London: Lawrence Erlbaum.
Rosen, W. G. (1980). Verbal fluency in aging and dementia. *Journal of Clinical Neuropsychology*, *2*, 135-146.
Sartori, G., Barry, C., & Job, R. (1984). Phonological dyslexia: A review. In R. N. Malatesha & H. A. Whitaker (Eds.), *Dyslexia: A global issue* (pp. 339-356). Nijhoff: The Hague.
Schwartz, M. F., Marin, O. S. M., & Saffran, E. M. (1979). Dissociations of language function in dementia: A case study. *Brain and Language*, *7*, 277-306.
Strub, R. L. & Gardner, H. (1974). The repetition defect in conduction aphasia: Mnestic or linguistic? *Brain and Language*, *1*, 241-255.
Tzortzis, C. & Albert, M. L. (1974). Impairment of memory for sequences in conduction aphasia. *Neuropsychologia*, *12*, 355-366.
Warrington, E. K. & Shallice, T. (1969). The selective impairment of auditory verbal short-term memory. *Brain*, *92*, 885-896.
Wilshire, C. E. & McCarthy, R. A. (1996). Experimental investigation of an impairment in phonological encoding. *Cognitive Neuropsychology*, *13*, 1059-1098.

SENTENCE COMPREHENSION IN ALZHEIMER'S DISEASE

David Caplan and Gloria Waters

INTRODUCTION

Patients with early Alzheimer's disease are known to have semantic problems at the lexical level that are out of proportion to their problems producing and recognizing the forms of language. We describe a comparable disorder at the sentence level with good ability to structure sentences syntactically. We use that structure to determine literal propositional meaning and difficulties using the propositional content so derived to accomplish tasks.

SENTENCE COMPREHENSION IN ALZHEIMER'S DISEASE

Sentences are the level of the language code at which the meanings of individual words are related to each other to express the intended idea or propositional content. This includes information about events and states in the world, such as the actors and recipients of an action, the features that are associated with an item, etc. This propositional information can be stored in long-term semantic memory to increase a person's knowledge of the world and is used for reasoning and planning action. The ability to represent propositional information thus contributes in an important way to the power that human language has as a vehicle for thought and communication.

The propositional content of a sentence is determined by the syntactic structure of that sentence in conjunction with its lexical content (Chomsky, 1981; 1986; 1994). For instance, the sentence "The dog that scratched the cat chased the bird" means that *the dog*, and not *the cat*, is doing the chasing, even though the sequence of words "the cat chased the bird" occurs in the sentence. The sentence is understood this way because of the position of the words *dog* and *cat* in the syntactic structure of the sentence. *The dog* is the subject of *chased* and *the cat* is the object of *scratched*; *the cat* has no syntactic relationship to *chased*.

Psychologists and computational scientists have developed a variety of models of sentence comprehension that include syntactic analysis (parsing) as part of the process of determining the propositional content of a sentence (Berwick & Weinberg, 1984; Frazier & Clifton, 1996; MacDonald, Perlmutter, & Seidenberg, 1994). We may contrast the process of extracting the propositional content of a sentence from the signal, which we will call *sentence interpretation*, with the process of using the meaning that has been extracted to perform other tasks. The contrast can be appreciated intuitively by considering the difference between understanding a sentence like (1) and accomplishing the requested action: (1) "Please pick up four tomatoes, a pound of apricots, prune juice, shallots, six apples, and a bag of carrots on the way home." The memory requirements associated with carrying out the request are such that the sentence may not be the basis for effective action, even though it is easily understood. We therefore draw a distinction between using the meaning of a sentence to plan action, to reason, and to do other tasks in what we call *post-interpretive processing* and sentence interpretation.

This distinction may be relevant to the nature of the problems that Alzheimer's patients have in sentence processing. Many studies suggest that Alzheimer's patients retain the ability to structure a sentence syntactically but have impaired abilities to process words and sentences semantically (Bayles, 1982; Hier, Hagenlocker, & Shindler, 1985; Irigaray, 1973; Kempler, Curtiss, & Jackson, 1987; Schwartz, Marin, & Saffran, 1979; Whitaker, 1976). The verbal output of Alzheimer's patients is characteristically fluent, suggesting that syntactic abilities are preserved in these patients, at least in the early stages of the illness (Blanken, Dittmann, Haas, & Wallesch, 1987; Illes, 1989; Kirschner, 1982). Fluent, syntactically well-formed speech has also been found in Alzheimer's patients in picture description (Hier, Hagenlocker, & Shindler, 1985; Kemper, Anagnopoulos, Lyons, & Heberlein, 1994) and sentence construction tasks (Schwartz et al., 1979). Alzheimer's patients have also been found to correct errors of syntax and phonology but not semantic errors in anomalous sentences (Bayles, 1982). They make better use of syntactic than semantic cues in disambiguating spoken homophones and while writing them to dictation (Kempler et al., 1987; Schwartz et al., 1979). The responses of Alzheimer's patients on a picture description task have been described as "syntactically well-structured but semantically disorganized and vague" (Kemper et al., 1994). These studies suggest good syntactic processing in Alzheimer's disease, at least in speech production.

While Alzheimer's patients have been shown to produce both oral and written language that is syntactically well-structured, the sentence production of these patients does differ from that of age-matched controls in other important respects. In one study, over 350 Alzheimer's patients were asked to write a single sentence, and these productions were scored for their length in words and clauses, the number of propositions produced, and six categories of grammatical constituents including pronouns, main verbs, secondary verbs, negatives, conjunctions, and questions (Kemper et al., 1993). Results showed that 89% of the variance in the clinical rating of dementia severity could be accounted for by sentence length in clauses and propositional content. This suggests that the ability to produce propositions in written form is reduced as the severity of dementia increases. Furthermore, estimates of these linguistic abilities early in life appear to be powerful predictors of cognitive function and Alzheimer's disease later in life. In a longitudinal study, Snowdon et al. (1996) analyzed autobiographies written by 93 nuns when they entered a convent and evaluated the cognitive performances of these women when they were between 75 and 95 years of age (a span of some 58 years). Alzheimer's disease was assessed neuropathologically in a sample of 25 participants who died. A stronger and more consistent association was found between cognitive function later in life and the density of propositions in these early narratives than between cognitive functions and the grammatical complexity of the narratives. Strikingly, low idea density was present in the autobiographies of 90% of women with neuropathologically proven Alzheimer's disease but only in 13% of those without Alzheimer's disease. Further studies have shown that measures of idea density and grammatical complexity are highly stable over the life span ($r = 0.62$ to 0.74) (Kemper, Snowdon, & Greiner, 1996). The authors hypothesize that low linguistic ability early in life may be an early expression of Alzheimer's disease neuropathology.

We believe that these results suggest a finer distinction. The greater relationship between measures of propositional density and the severity of Alzheimer's disease than between measures of grammatical well-formedness and the severity of Alzheimer's disease is consistent with the view that these patients are impaired in formulating concepts but are able to use the forms of language to convey the concepts that they do activate. This is a division of function related to language production that corresponds to what we have suggested between post-interpretive and interpretive aspects of the comprehension process.

Compared to sentence production, the sentence comprehension abilities of Alzheimer's patients have been the subject of fewer studies, and findings have been more contradictory. Some authors have asserted that sentence comprehension is impaired (Emery, 1985; Kontiola, Laaksonen, Sulkava, & Erkinjuntti, 1990; Tomoeda, Bayles, Boone, Kaszniak, & Slauson, 1990) and others have asserted that it is preserved (Schwartz, Marin, & Saffran, 1979; Sherman et al., 1988; Smith, 1989). We have argued that the differences between the studies reflect the degree to which the tasks on which patients were tested required complex post-interpretive processing (Rochon et al., 1994; Waters et al., 1995; Waters, Rochon, & Caplan, 1998). Careful examination of the results of these studies suggests that Alzheimer's patients may have performed poorly because of deficiencies in their ability to access semantic knowledge, to enact responses, and to accomplish other post-interpretive requirements of many of these tasks (see Rochon, Waters, and Caplan, 1994, for discussion). The studies that show few or no sentence comprehension impairments in Alzheimer's disease have tended to use tasks with simpler demands, such as sentence-picture matching (Schwartz, Marin, & Saffran 1979; Sherman et al., 1988; Smith, 1989) (although see Grober and Bang, 1995). Evidence for the view that Alzheimer's patients can also accomplish sentence interpretation normally comes from recent work by MacDonald and her colleagues. Using an on-line cross-modal naming task, these researchers have shown that Alzheimer's patients have preserved sensitivity to grammatical violations and that they are as able as age-matched controls to use frequency information and semantic and syntactic contexts to resolve syntactic ambiguities (Lalami et al., 1996; Stevens et al., 1996). The entire pattern of performances suggests that Alzheimer's patients have relatively preserved abilities to structure sentences syntactically in sentence interpretation and an impairment in aspects of post-interpretive sentence comprehension.

Our own work provides evidence for the integrity of syntactic comprehension and some degree of impairment of post-interpretive processing in Alzheimer's disease. In our first study with Alzheimer's patients, we tested 22 patients and age- and education-matched controls for their ability to comprehend nine different syntactic structures using a sentence-picture matching test (Rochon, Waters, &

Caplan, 1994). The stimulus materials (Table 1) were designed to contrast sentences that were matched for length and other relevant variables but differed in syntactic complexity, and sentences that were matched for syntactic complexity but differed in terms of number of propositions. Sentences were considered syntactically complex if they contained a *trace* in object position according to Chomsky's (1981; 1986; 1994) theory and if there was a parsing model in which the memory storage and computational requirements were greater in these sentences than in their matched pair. Overall, the Alzheimer's patients performed more poorly than the controls. However, examination of their performance on the various sentence types showed that they did not perform more poorly on the syntactically more complex sentences but rather, that their performance was poorer than controls on sentences with two propositions (Figure 1).

This basic pattern of an absence of an effect of syntactic complexity but the presence of an effect of the number of propositions for Alzheimer's patients on sentence picture matching has been replicated in several studies (Rochon & Saffran, 1995; Waters et al., 1995; 1998). In some studies, an effect of the number of propositions has also been found for the elderly control subjects, although the magnitude of this effect is smaller than that seen in the patients (Rochon & Saffran, 1995; Waters, Rochon, & Caplan, 1998). The patients and controls in these studies have tended to be older than those in studies where the effect was not seen in the control group. This basic pattern suggests that the difficulty these subjects have is not with syntactic analysis and sentence interpretation but rather with matching propositions to pictures, a post-interpretive aspect of the comprehension process. It should be noted that in all of our studies with patients, the pattern of performance seen for the group as a whole is also seen in the vast majority of individual patients.

One possible reason for the failure to find an effect of syntactic complexity using the sentence-picture matching test is that the task is simply too easy for such effects to emerge, particularly in the control subjects. Therefore, it is important to note that the performance of patients and controls is below ceiling on the sentences with two propositions and that the comparison of syntactically simple and complex sentences with two propositions did not result in a significant effect of syntactic complexity for either patients or controls. However, it may be that differences between the groups would emerge if processing time and not only accuracy were measured.

We addressed this possibility in three additional experiments using timed sentence-acceptability judgments, all of which failed to find a difference between patients and controls in processing syntactically complex compared to syntactically simple sentences. In two separate studies, Alzheimer's patients and controls were tested on a subset of the syntactically simple and complex sentence types used in our sentence-picture matching experiments in a timed acceptability-judgment task. In both studies, reaction times for syntactically complex sentences were longer than for syntactically simple sentences, but the differences between simple and complex sentences were not any greater for the patients than for the controls (Figure 2). This same result was found in a third study in which the stimuli tested subjects' abilities to perform the syntactic operation of finding the antecedent for a pronoun or a reflexive, rather than their abilities to assign thematic roles (e.g., determine whether "The man with the woman cut himself" versus "The man with the woman cut

Table 1. Sentence Types Used in Sentence-Picture Matching Task

Sentence Structure	Number of Words	Number of Propositions and Verbs	Number of Thematic Roles	Canonicity of Thematic Roles
Active (A) *The lion kicked the elephant*	5	1	2	Canonical
Active Conjoined Theme (Acth) *The pig chased the lion and the cow*	8	1	2	Canonical
Dative (D) *The elephant pulled the dog to the horse*	8	1	3	Canonical
Passive (P) *The elephant was pushed by the cow*	7	1	2	Non-canonical
Truncated Passive (TP) *The pig was touched*	4	1	2	Non-canonical
Cleft Object (CO) *It was the dog that the horse passed*	8	1	2	Non-canonical
Object Subject (OS) *The horse kicked the elephant that touched the dog*	9	2	4	Canonical
Conjoined (C) *The elephant followed the lion and pulled the dog*	9	2	4	Canonical
Subject Object (SO) *The dog that the pig followed touched the horse*	9	2	4	Non-canonical

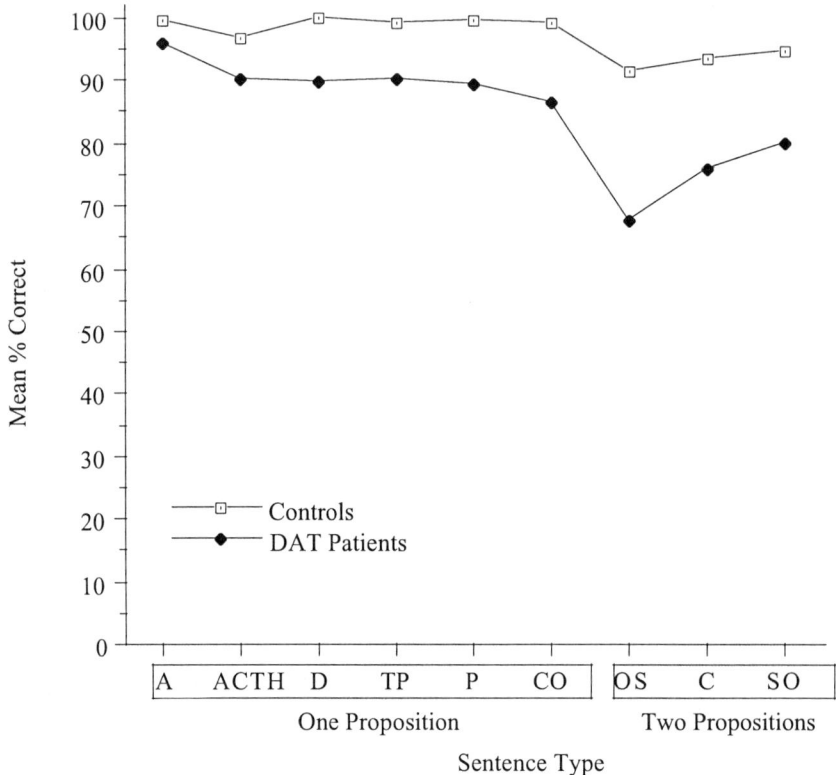

Figure 1. Sentence-Picture Matching Task. Sentence-picture matching performances of Alzheimer's patients and controls on sentences shown in Table 1 showing the effect of the number of propositions but not of syntactic complexity.

herself" is acceptable) (Waters & Caplan, 1997) (Figure 3). These studies using RT measures are not subject to the concern that ceiling effects affected results, since there were effects of syntactic structure in the RT data that were not greater in the Alzheimer's patients than the controls.

Finally, we have recently carried out a study in which Alzheimer's patients in the mild to moderate stages of the disease were tested in an auditory self-paced listening task. In this task, subjects pushed a key to hear successive auditory segments of sentences. The sentence types presented were either syntactically complex (containing object relative clauses) or syntactically simple (containing subject relative clauses). Participants paced their way through the sentences and made plausibility judgments at the end of each sentence. All participants showed longer listening times on the more demanding portions of the complex sentences than on the corresponding segments of the simple sentences, and the increase in listening times was not greater in the Alzheimer's patients than in the controls. Preliminary results for 10 Alzheimer's patients and 50 control subjects are shown in Figure 4.

In three additional experiments, we have examined the effect of manipulating the non-linguistic visual and memory demands of the sentence-picture matching task on the performance of Alzheimer's patients and controls (Waters et al., 1998). In one experiment, subjects matched the spoken sentence to one of two pictures that either appeared before or immediately following the presentation of the sentence. The second experiment employed a video-verification task in which subjects were required to determine whether the spoken sentence matched a videotaped depiction of the action in the sentence or a syntactic foil. In this task, the spoken sentence sometimes ended before the action was completed, thereby requiring the propositional content of the sentence to be maintained in memory while the action in the video unfolded. In the third experiment, in different conditions, subjects were required to determine whether the spoken sentence matched a single picture or to choose the picture that matched the sentence from an array of two or three pictures. In all tasks, Alzheimer's patients were affected by the number of propositions in the presented sentence but not by the syntactic complexity of the sentence (Figure 5).

Comparison across the one-, two-, and three-picture versions of the task showed that the magnitude of the effect of number of propositions increased as the number of pictures in the array increased (Figure 6). In addition, analysis of the data from each of the tasks separately showed that the effect of the number of propositions did not occur when the foil depicted an incorrect lexical item but only when subjects were attempting to match the target to a foil that required a syntactic analysis by depicting reversed thematic roles. These results once again support the view that Alzheimer's patients do not have disturbances in syntactic processing. In addition, they suggest that the effect of the number of propositions arises at a later stage of the broader comprehension process, such as in holding a representation of the sentence in memory until the pictures can be analyzed and/or in comparing the results of the picture analysis with the stored representation of the sentence meaning.

In another study (Rochon et al., under review), we examined the relationship between the magnitude of the proposition effect and Alzheimer's patients' performance on tasks that assessed primary memory (digits forward, Corsi block,

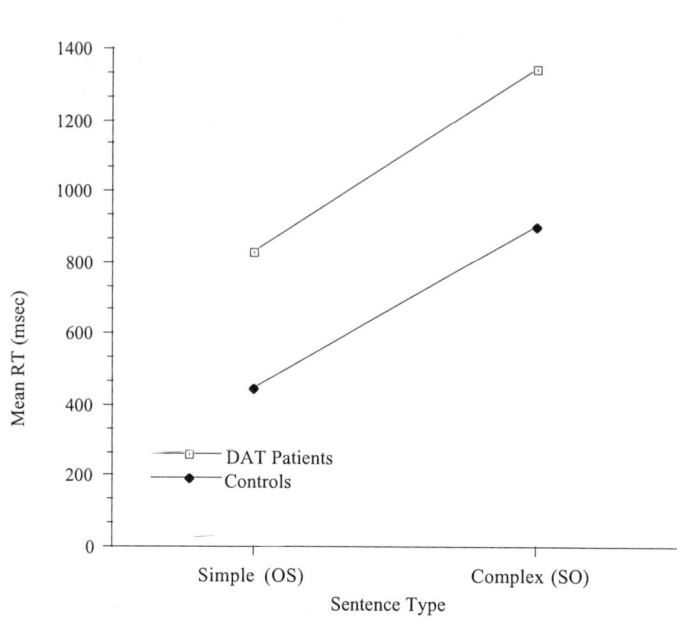

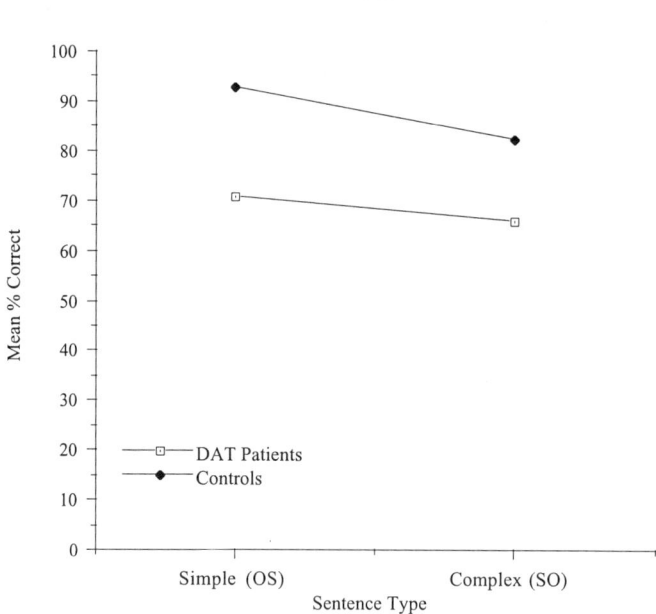

Figure 2. Sentence-Acceptability Task. Sentence-acceptability (plausibility) judgment performances of Alzheimer's patients and controls on sentences containing relative clauses, showing equivalent effects of syntactic complexity in the two groups.

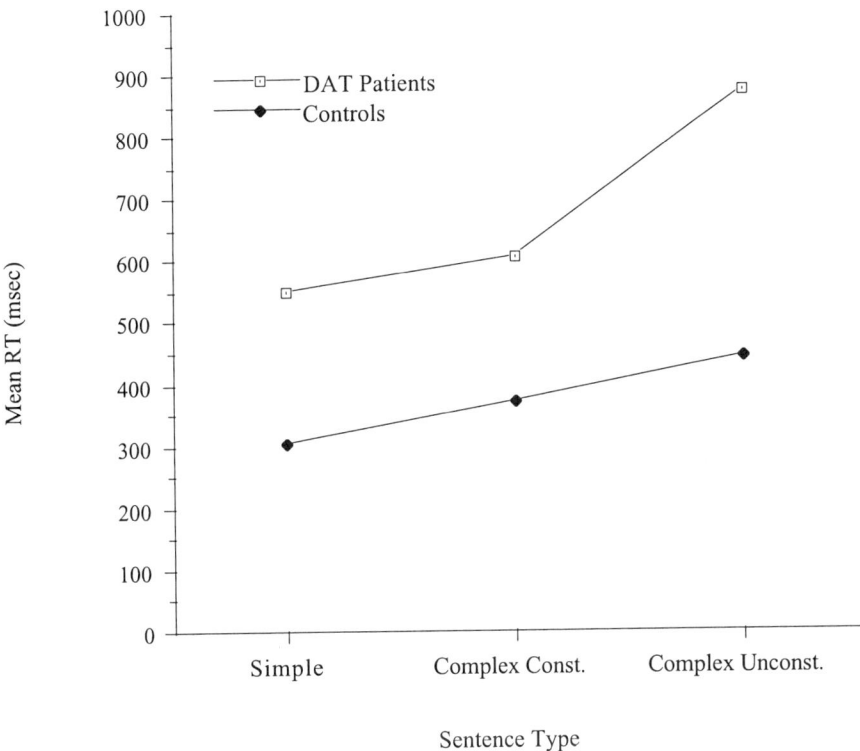

Figure 3. **Coindexation of Reflexives.** Sentence-acceptability judgment performances of Alzheimer's patients and controls on sentences containing reflexives, showing equivalent effects of syntactic complexity in the two groups.

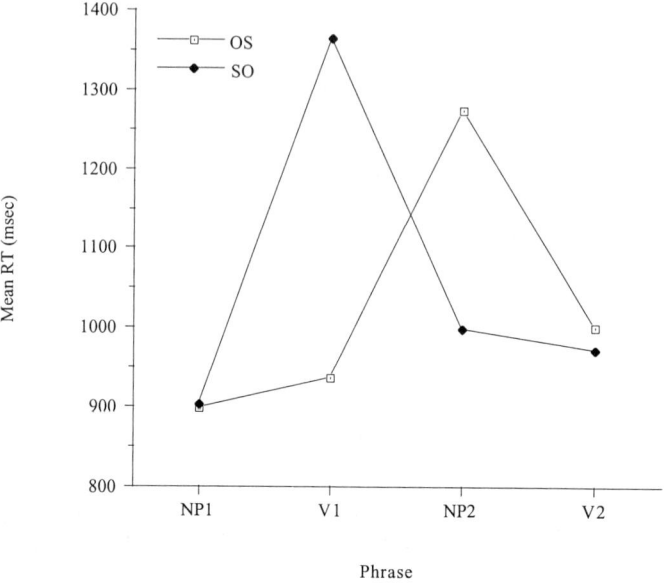

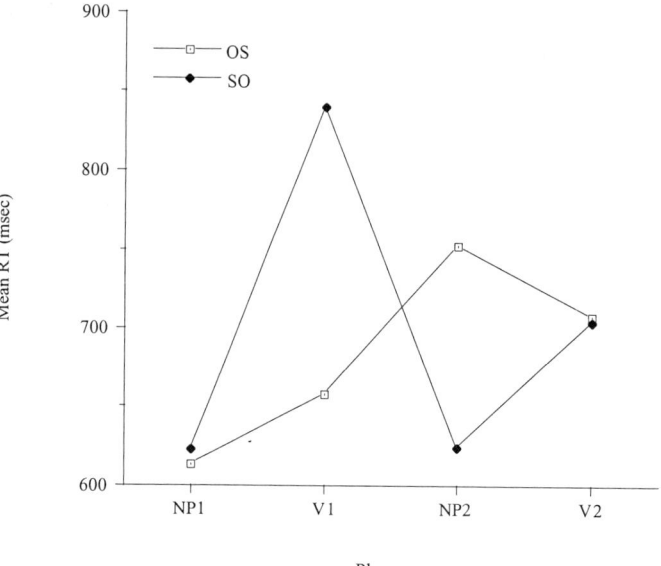

Figure 4. Performances of Alzheimer's patients and controls on self-paced listening (auditory moving windows) for sentences containing relative clauses, showing equivalent effects of syntactic complexity in the two groups.

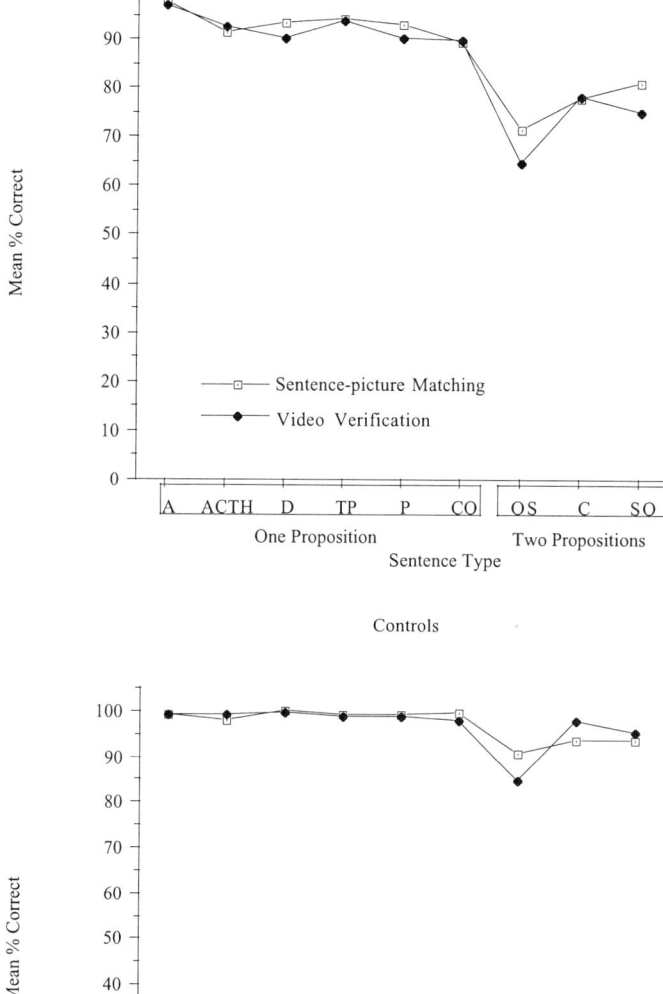

Figure 5. Video-verification performances of Alzheimer's patients and controls on sentences shown in Table 1, showing the effect of the number of propositions but not of syntactic complexity.

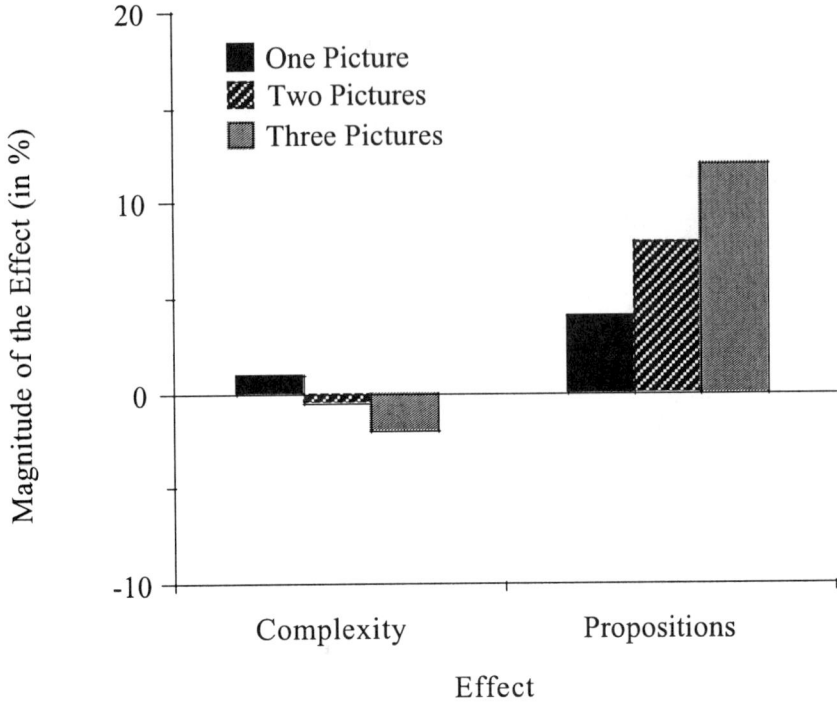

Figure 6. **Effect of Number of Pictures on Complexity and Proposition Effects.** Sentence-picture matching performances of Alzheimer's patients and controls on sentences shown in Table 1, showing an effect of the number of pictures on the effect of number of propositions but not that of syntactic complexity.

and auditory and visual word span), articulatory rehearsal/phonological storage processes in STM (auditory and visual phonological similarity and word length), and measures of working memory function (digits backward) (Case et al., 1982) (working memory span, and dual-task performance). The magnitude of the effect of number of propositions was unrelated to all of the measures of primary memory and phonological storage/articulatory rehearsal (except visual word span) but was significantly correlated ($r = -0.62$ to 70) to all three working memory measures.

Finally, we have examined the pattern of interference of a concurrent verbal memory load, which imposes an additional load on a working memory system, on sentence comprehension in Alzheimer's disease. In one study, Alzheimer's patients performed the sentence-picture matching task while retaining a concurrent memory load that was equivalent to their span or one less (Waters et al., 1995). Overall, performance was poorer with the digit load, but comparisons of matched sentences showed that the concurrent memory load exacerbated the effect of the number of propositions but not the effect of syntactic complexity (Figure 7). In a second study, we examined the ability of patients with Alzheimer's disease and normal controls to perform a timed sentence acceptability judgment task that required the

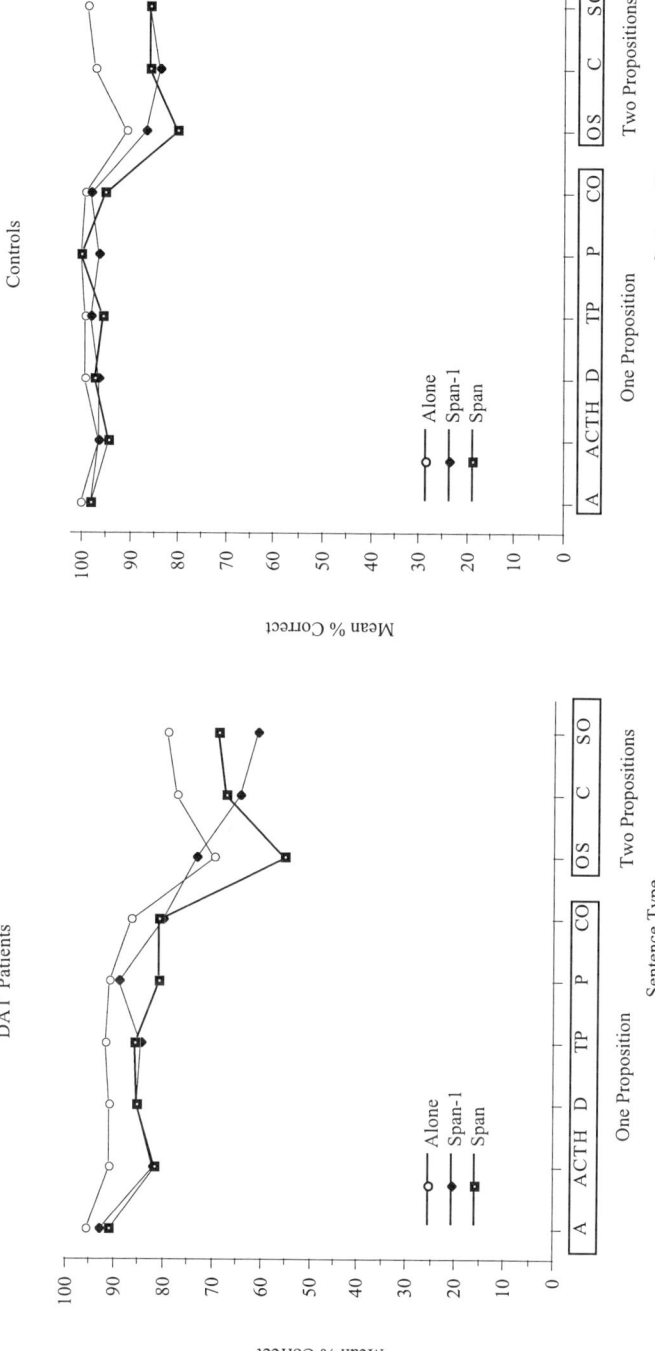

Figure 7. Digit Load Experiment Performance on the Sentence Task. Sentence-picture matching performances of Alzheimer's patients and controls on sentences shown in Table 1 under concurrent digit load equal to each subject's span, showing an increase in the effect of the number of propositions but not of syntactic complexity in the patients.

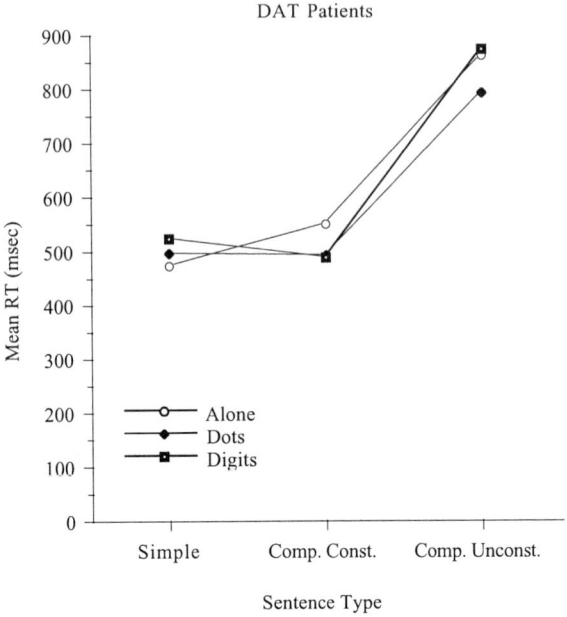
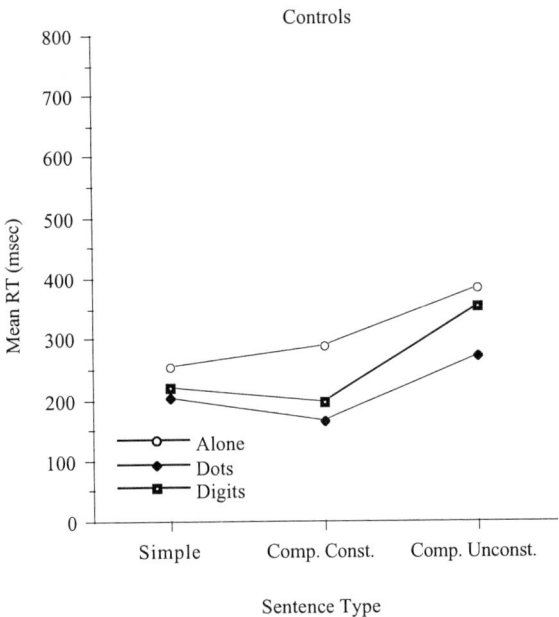

Figure 8. Effect of a Concurrent Load. Sentence-acceptability judgment performances of Alzheimer's patients and controls on sentences containing reflexives under concurrent digit load equal to each subject's span, showing equivalent increases in the effect of syntactic complexity in the two groups under the load condition.

ability to determine the referent for a reflexive pronoun (Waters & Caplan, 1997) (Figure 8). Performance on three different sentence types that differed in terms of syntactic complexity was assessed. Subjects performed the task alone and under two different dual-task conditions that required continuous, externally-paced responses. Alzheimer's patients were more greatly affected than were controls when carrying out the acceptability task under dual-task conditions but were not disproportionately impaired on the more complex sentence types.

Overall, these studies are highly consistent. Relative to their comprehension of syntactically simple structures, patients with Alzheimer's disease have been able to interpret complex syntactic structures as well as controls and have shown similar profiles of on-line sensitivity to local increases in processing load due to syntactic structural complexity. They have shown impairments relative to control subjects in matching propositions to pictures and videos. The pattern suggests that they are largely capable of processing the forms of language at the sentential level and have difficulties with utilizing sentential semantics to perform tasks. The deficit is similar in some ways to that seen at the lexical level, inasmuch as processing of lexical form is often better than processing of lexical meaning in Alzheimer's patients. However, there is evidence from the studies described above that the problems that Alzheimer's patients have with using the propositional content of a sentence to accomplish tasks are related to their working memory limitations. This is not obviously parallel to the lexical semantic problems that have been described in this population. The deficits in Alzheimer's disease at both the lexical and sentential level appear to be similar in affecting semantics more than form, but the extent to which they are due to impairments of the same fundamental underlying cognitive mechanism remains to be investigated.

ACKNOWLEDGMENTS

The research reported here was supported by grant AG09661 from the National Institute of Aging.

REFERENCES

Bayles, K. A. (1982). Language function in senile dementia. *Brain and Language, 16*, 265-280.
Berwick, R. C. & Weinberg, A. (1984). *The grammatical basis of linguistic performance: Language use and acquisition*. Cambridge, MA: MIT Press.
Blanken, G., Dittmar, J., Hass, J. C., & Wallesch, C. W. (1987). Spontaneous speech in senile dementia and aphasia: Implications for a neurolinguistic model of language production. *Cognition, 27*, 247-274.
Case, R., Kurland, M., & Goldberg, J. (1982). Operational efficiency and the growth of short-term memory span. *Journal of Experimental Child Psychology, 33*, 386-404.
Chomsky, N. (1981). *Lectures in government and binding*. Dordrecht, The Netherlands: Foris.
Chomsky, N. (1986). *Knowledge of language* . New York: Praeger.
Chomsky, N. (1994). *The minimalist program*. Camridge, MA: MIT Press.
Emery, O. B. (1985). Language and aging. *Experimental Aging Research* (Monograph), *11*, 3-60.
Frazier, L. & Clifton, C. (1996). *Construal*. Cambridge, MA: MIT Press.
Grober, E. & Bang, S. (1995). Sentence comprehension in Alzheimer's disease. *Developmental Neuropsychology, 11*, 95-107.
Hier, D. B., Hagenlocker, K., & Schindler, A. G. (1985). Language disintegration in dementia: Effects of etiology and severity. *Brain and Language, 25*, 117-133.

Illes, J. (1989). Neurolinguistic features of spontaneous language production dissociate three forms of neurodegenerative disease: Alzheimer's, Huntington's, and Parkinson's. *Brain and Language, 37*, 628-642.

Irigaray, L. (1973). *Le langage des déments*. Hague, The Netherlands: Mouton.

Kemper, S., LaBarge, E., Ferraro, F. R., Cheung, H., Storandt, M. (1993). On the preservation of syntax in Alzheimer's disease: Evidence from written sentences. *Archives of Neurology, 50*, 81-86.

Kemper, S., Anagnopoulos, C., Lyons, K., & Heberlein, W. (1994). Speech accommodations to dementia. *Journal of Gerontology, 49*, 223-229

Kemper, S., Snowdon, D. A., & Greiner, L. H. (1996). *Linguistic abilities across the life span: Findings from The Nun Study*. Cognitive Aging Conference, Atlanta, GA.

Kempler, D., Curtiss, S., & Jackson, C. (1987). Syntactic preservation in Alzheimer's disease. *Journal of Speech and Hearing Research, 30*, 343-350.

Kirshner, H. S. (1982). Language disorders in dementia. In H. S. Kirshner & F. R. Freeman (Eds.), *The neurology of aphasia* (pp. 187-196). Lisse, Holland: Swets and Zeitlinger.

Kontiola, P., Laaksonen, R., Sulkava, R., & Erkinjuntti, T. (1990). Pattern of language impairment is different in Alzheimer's disease and multi-infarct dementia. *Brain and Language, 38*, 364-383.

Lalami, L., Marbelstone, K., Schuster, S., Andersen, E., Kempler, D., Tyler, L., & MacDonald, M. (1996). On-line vs. off-line sentence processing in Alzheimer's disease. Poster presented at the Meeting of Cognitive Aging, Atlanta, GA.

MacDonald, M. C., Pearlmutter, N. J., & Seidenberg, M. S. (1994). Lexical nature of syntactic ambiguity resolution. *Psychological Review, 101*, 676-703.

Rochon, E. & Saffran, E. M. (1995). A semantic contribution to sentence comprehension impairments in Alzheimer's disease. Poster presented at the Academy of Aphasia, San Diego, CA.

Rochon, E., Waters, G. S., & Caplan, D. (1994). Sentence comprehension in patients with Alzheimer's disease. *Brain and Language, 46* (2), 329-349.

Rochon, E., Waters, G. S., & Caplan, D. (under review). The relationship between measures of working memory and sentence comprehension in patients with Alzheimer's disease.

Schwartz, M. F., Marin, O. S. M., & Saffran, E. M. (1979). Dissociations of language function in dementia: A case study. *Brain and Language, 7*, 277-306.

Sherman, J. C., Schweickert, J., Growdon, J., & Corkin, S. (1988). *Sentence comprehension in Alzheimer's disease*. Paper presented at the 18th annual meeting of the Society for Neuroscience, Toronto, CA.

Smith, S. (1989). *Syntactic comprehension in Alzheimer's disease*. Poster session presented at the Academy of Aphasia, Santa Fe, NM.

Snowdon, D. A., Kemper, S. J., Mortimer, J. A., Greiner, L. H., Wekstein, D. R., & Markesbery, W. R. (1996). Linguistic ability in early life and cognitive function and Alzheimer's disease in late life: Findings from the Nun Study. *Journal of the American Medical Association, 275*, 528-532.

Stevens, K., Kempler, D., Andersen, E., & MacDonald, M. C. (1996). Preserved use of semantic and syntactic context in Alzheimer's disease. Poster presented at the Meeting of Cognitive Aging, Atlanta, GA.

Tomoeda, C. K., Bayles, K. A., Boone, D. R., Kaszniak, A. W., & Slauson, T. J. (1990). Speech rate and syntactic complexity effects on the auditory comprehension of Alzheimer's patients. *Journal of Communication Disorders, 23*, 151-161.

Waters, G. S. & Caplan, D. (1997). Working memory and on-line sentence comprehension in patients with Alzheimer's disease. *Journal of Psycholinguistic Research, 26*, 377-400.

Waters, G. S., Caplan, D., & Rochon, E. (1995). Processing capacity and sentence comprehension in patients with Alzheimer's disease. *Cognitive Neuropsychology, 12* (1), 1-30.

Waters, G. S., Rochon, E., & Caplan, D. (1998). Task demands and sentence comprehension in patients with dementia of the Alzheimer's type. *Brain and Language, 62*, 361-397.

Whitaker, H. (1976). A case of the isolation of the language function. In H. Whitaker & H. A. Whitaker (Eds.), *Studies in neurolinguistics* (pp. 1-58). New York: Academic Press.

WRITING IMPAIRMENTS IN ALZHEIMER'S DISEASE

Guila Glosser and Victor W. Henderson

INTRODUCTION

Alzheimer's disease is a common age-associated dementing disorder. Clinical features include pronounced disturbances in episodic memory and in other cognitive domains (McKhann et al., 1984). Well-characterized neuropathological alterations are found in select areas of the cerebrum and the brain stem (Mirra et al., 1991). The extensive loss of synaptic input from other neurons is particularly prominent in limbic and neocortical association areas of the cerebral hemispheres, suggesting that Alzheimer's disease can be conceptualized as an illness of progressive cortical neuronal disconnection (Morrison et al., 1986). Although Alzheimer's disease is variously determined by genetic (Landon, Ashall, & Goate, 1997) and non-genetic factors, etiologically different forms of the illness (with the exception of age at symptom onset) are not distinguishable on the basis of clinical phenotype. For example, the early suggestion that writing impairments might be a clinical marker for heritable forms of Alzheimer's disease (Breitner & Folstein, 1984; Folstein & Breitner, 1981) has not been substantiated (Aarsland, Hoien, Larsen, & Oftedal, 1996; Glosser & Kaplan, 1989; Henderson, Buckwalter, Sobel, Freed, & Diz, 1992; Horner, Heyman, Dawson, & Rogers, 1988; Kumar & Giacobini, 1990).

Language disturbances are frequently described in Alzheimer's patients. Language production is typically fluent and grammatical, but semantic content can be impoverished to the extent that speech is sometimes characterized as *non-informative* (Nicholas, Obler, Albert, & Helm-Estabrooks, 1985). Formal testing typically reveals marked impairments in confrontation naming, category naming, and auditory comprehension beginning in early stages of the disease (Bayles & Kaszniak, 1987; Chertkow & Bub, 1990; Hodges, Salmon, & Butters, 1991; Huff, Corkin, & Growdon, 1986; Williams, Mack, & Henderson, 1989). Despite these impairments in understanding and producing meaningful language, basic syntax is relatively preserved until later in the disease course, as are repetition and oral reading (Cummings, Benson, Hill, & Read, 1985; Cummings, Houlihan, & Hill, 1986; Kempler, Curtiss, & Jackson, 1987).

Agraphia, an acquired disturbance in the written expression of language due to brain damage, is a common feature of Alzheimer's disease. Alois Alzheimer's original descriptions documented writing disturbances in this illness. His first patient was a 51 year-old woman who, "repeated individual syllables several times, left out others, and quickly became stranded" while writing (Alzheimer, 1907). His second patient, a 56 year-old man,

> did not use a pencil but instead took matches and wrote with them.... When [he was later] asked to write his name, he produced a misspelled word, which was different from his name, but he did not try to correct his mistakes (Alzheimer, 1911).

As discussed below, subsequent studies have shown that Alzheimer's patients are impaired on various aspects of writing. For most, writing is affected early in the course of the disease, and it deteriorates progressively.

In patients with brain damage from other causes, agraphia is most often recognized as an accompaniment of a pervasive language disturbance characteristic of aphasia. In aphasic agraphia, a disturbance in oral expression is paralleled by a similar disorder in written expression (Benson & Cummings, 1985). For example, Wernicke's aphasics, who have suffered focal damage to posterior portions of left-hemisphere language areas, commonly produce copious paraphasic speech or written text, both of which are deficient in content words and fail to convey meaning. Similarly, for patients with Broca's aphasia, whose lesions are typically in the more anterior regions of the left-hemisphere, writing tends to be sparse, telegraphic, and marked by grammatical errors, as is the spontaneous speech of these patients. Within the language-dominant left-hemisphere, the inferior parietal lobule is recognized as subserving a critical role in written language (Dejerine, 1892; Roeltgen, 1993).

The presence of impaired writing in Alzheimer patients does not necessarily imply that aphasic disturbances are the primary determinants of agraphia. As emphasized by Albert and colleagues (1981), "writing requires the complex interaction of mechanisms of motor control, or praxis, and of visuospatial and kinesthetic integration in addition to the symbolic basis of a language system." Praxic, visuoconstructive, as well as linguistic disturbances are each common in Alzheimer's disease (McKhann et al., 1984). Moreover, agraphia in the form of letter omissions and substitutions is a salient feature of confusional states characterized by impaired attention (Chédru & Geschwind, 1972), and Alzheimer patients evince difficulties on different aspects of attention (Spinnler, 1991).

Alzheimer's disease offers the challenge not only of delineating the writing disturbance of a common neurodegenerative illness but also the opportunity to discern how widespread neocortical deafferentation affects the neurobehavioral underpinnings of a complex cognitive task such as writing. As summarized below, agraphia in Alzheimer's disease has multiple determinants and differs in substantial ways from that of aphasic patients with focal damage to language areas of the left cerebral hemisphere. These studies have been undertaken at several levels of analysis. The following discussion of agraphia in Alzheimer's disease considers both investigations at the single word level and studies of written discourse.

ANALYSES OF WRITING AT THE SINGLE WORD LEVEL

Much recent research on agraphia in Alzheimer's disease has focused on the writing of single words, where linguistic and nonlinguistic determinants of writing impairments have been explored in considerable detail. A commonly used task is the oral dictation of individual words, but written production is sometimes elicited by other means, such as presenting pictures for written naming. With the elaboration of detailed cognitive neuropsychological models based on information-processing theory (Margolin, 1984; Margolin & Goodman-Schulman, 1994; Morton, 1980; Roeltgen, 1993), it has become possible to assess the integrity of component cognitive processes postulated to be involved in writing. Since writing draws on many of the same central cognitive processes that are involved in oral language comprehension and production, cognitive analyses of writing performances can also shed light on more general aspects of language functioning in Alzheimer's disease. Most single word analyses in Alzheimer patients have been interpreted in terms of these models, and for this reason an overview of a basic, unadorned information-processing model follows. It is recognized, however, that functional modularity presumed by the model does not necessarily indicate that the brain actually processes information in this manner and that other models (e.g., so-called connectionism models based on parallel distributed processing) (Reggia, Berndt, & D'Autrechy, 1994) might also accommodate clinical data.

A Cognitive Model of Writing

Information-processing models of written language typically distinguish *central*, or linguistic, components from non-linguistic processes, most of which are deemed *peripheral* to language processing. In many models, central linguistic components are taken to be common to all language activities regardless of input or output modality.

Within the functional framework of a central language processing system, memory representations of previously encountered word sounds, spellings, and meanings are contained in phonological, orthographic, and semantic lexicons, respectively. Writing a word to dictation begins with the perceptual analysis of the heard word. This peripheral process decomposes the auditory input into phonological units (phonemes), which then can activate and be matched to memory representations of familiar auditory word patterns within the phonological lexicon. This central component is conceptualized to include abstract codes specifying the pronunciations of words. These phonological codes access corresponding orthographic codes, which can be used to spell both familiar words and novel words, provided that the spellings of these novel words are regular (i.e., they follow the usual patterns of sound-to-spelling correspondence in English). The pronunciations and spellings of both real words and pseudowords (pronounceable non-words) are assumed to be derived through the phonological lexicon. Thus, a sound pattern, whether it is a familiar word or a pseudoword, is matched to existing phonological representations, which are combined to compute the spelling of the word. A deficit in decoding, repeating or spelling pseudowords is an important marker for a disturbance in phonological processing (Caplan, 1992).

Once phonological codes are activated, the meanings and the unique spellings associated with particular phoneme patterns can be accessed. The orthographic lexicon consists of representations of the spellings of all previously encountered words. This lexicon is viewed as essential for spellings of exception words, words whose orthographies do not conform to the regular patterns of sound-to-spelling correspondence. Spellings for such words as *plaid* and *girl* cannot be accurately constructed from knowledge of the spellings of other words in the English language. Thus, a reliable indicator of a disturbance in the orthographic lexicon is a spelling deficit for exception words. A second related characteristic of disturbance in orthographic processing is that misspellings often respect regular sound-to-letter(s) correspondence patterns, leading to so-called regularization errors. Exception words, as well as ambiguous words that contain sounds with several possible spellings, tend to be misspelled as phonologically plausible alternatives to the correct spellings (e.g., spelling *plaid* as *plad*, or spelling *girl* as *gurl*). These two characteristics, a disproportionate impairment in the spelling of exception words and the occurrence of regularization errors, are the hallmarks of lexical agraphia (Beauvois & Derouesné, 1981).

When one writes from meaning (as when writing the name of a pictured object), sensory information and ideational concepts first activate lexical semantic representations before associated phonological and orthographic representations can be accessed. The semantic lexicon consists of procedures for computing the meanings of individual words and for relating these meanings to other semantic, conceptual, and factual knowledge in memory. This process can be contrasted with writing to dictation, wherein orthographic representations of word spellings are accessed from the phonological lexicon (regular words and pseudowords) or the orthographic lexicon (any familiar word, but especially exception words). A disproportionate impairment in writing from meaning compared to writing to dictation is an indicator of a disturbance in the semantic lexicon and is characteristic of semantic agraphia (Roeltgen, Rothi, & Heilman, 1986).

Word spellings that are derived from processing in the phonological and orthographic lexicons can be expressed through speech (oral spelling) or through writing. Overt expression requires several peripheral processes to transform the linguistic orthographic information into an oral or written response. Writing involves a graphemic buffer, conceptualized as a working memory device that temporarily maintains the spelling code, while additional peripheral processes are engaged to select the physical (allographic) forms of the written letters (graphemes) (Hillis & Caramazza, 1989). Difficulties maintaining information in the graphemic buffer tend to be manifested as a unique spelling deficit characterized by disproportionate difficulties spelling longer words and errors in letter placement. The latter results in the production of phonemically implausible nonsense words.

The final peripheral components of the writing process involve accessing the allographic codes and the activation of graphic motor patterns for the production of letter shapes corresponding to the orthographic code. Impairment in selecting the appropriate graphic motor pattern results in apraxic agraphia (Friedman &

Alexander, 1989; Roeltgen & Heilman, 1983). This disorder is manifested in illegible spontaneous or dictated writing, poorly formed letters, or the inability to maintain consistent case or script, with or without difficulty copying letters and words (Patterson & Wing, 1989).

WRITING FROM SOUND IN ALZHEIMER'S DISEASE

Writing to sound (dictation) is much better preserved in Alzheimer's disease than writing from meaning, as in written confrontation naming. Based primarily on evidence that Alzheimer patients have difficulty spelling exception words, some investigators suggest that these patients, at least in mild to moderate stages of the illness, have lexical agraphia. Rapcsak, Arthur, Bliklen, and Rubens (1989) reported that subjects with Alzheimer's disease, compared to older control subjects, misspelled significantly more words with irregular spellings; the two groups were similar with respect to spelling regular words and non-words. The authors also noted that Alzheimer patients tend to regularize the spelling of irregular words (e.g., *oner* for *honor*). They interpreted their findings as reflecting selective impairment of lexical orthographic processing. Similar results are reported by others (Croisile et al., 1996; Hughes, Graham, Patterson, & Hodges, 1997; Lambert et al., 1996).

Hughes et al. (1997) conducted comprehensive analyses of agraphia in mildly demented Alzheimer subjects, testing the hypothesis that patients with this disorder have a specific deficit in lexical orthographic processing. Using a carefully chosen set of stimulus words, they found that spelling for both Alzheimer and normal control subjects was affected by word frequency (higher frequency words were spelled more accurately) and by the predictability, or regularity, of the sound-to-spelling correspondence. Further analyses showed that whereas spelling accuracy for controls and very mildly demented patients was slightly reduced only for words with highly unusual spellings (e.g., *yacht*), more demented patients also showed difficulties on words with ambiguous spellings. The authors of this study concluded that mildly demented Alzheimer patients do indeed show mild lexical agraphia.

Platel et al. (1993) conducted a longitudinal study of writing in a small cohort of Alzheimer patients. There was no control group, and spelling was tested for only a small set of dictated items, but findings from this investigation were intriguing. In early stages of the disease, subjects appeared to have difficulties only when spelling exception words. When tested approximately one year later, however, patients showed more errors not only when spelling exception words but also when spelling regular words and pseudowords. Qualitative analyses suggested that the error pattern appeared to progress from predominately phonologically plausible errors, to non-phonologically based spelling errors (letter omissions, insertions, substitutions, transpositions, and distortions), to incomplete or absent responses. Though some patients performed quite well at both sessions, the authors suggested that the writing impairment of Alzheimer's disease evolves from a deficit in lexical orthographic processing, to an impairment in phonological processing, and finally, to a complete breakdown in spelling associated with pervasive impairments in peripheral as well as central processes.

In contrast to the reports just described, other investigators have not found Alzheimer patients to show disproportionate difficulties in spelling exception words (Aarsland et al., 1996; Glosser & Kaplan, 1989). These findings indicate that the advantage shown by patients for writing regular words, as compared to exception words, is similar to that demonstrated by healthy elderly subjects. Glosser, Kohn, Sands, Grugan, and Friedman (1999) examined Alzheimer patients with a broad range of dementia severity. Using a single word spelling test that included carefully selected high and low frequency words with regular, ambiguous, and exceptional spellings, they found that patients performed worse than healthy age-matched controls on each spelling condition. Compared to controls, Alzheimer patients showed a slightly increased advantage for spelling regular words as compared to exception words. However, despite these group differences, performance profiles of patients paralleled those of controls quite closely in most other respects. For example, both groups showed equal facility in writing words with regular and ambiguous spellings, despite slightly worse spelling of exception words; no significant between-group differences were found in the proportions of different kinds of errors (regularization, orthographically related, and unrelated responses). Compared to controls, only 3 of 23 Alzheimer patients showed an abnormally large difference in accuracy for regular versus exception words. These authors concluded that despite overall lower accuracy, spelling performances of most Alzheimer patients did not reflect the types of errors that would be expected from a central deficit in orthographic processing. Rather than representing lexical agraphia, the spelling deficit appeared to emanate from a disturbance in nonlinguistic cognitive functions.

Data regarding the types of misspellings produced by Alzheimer patients have been inconsistent. As noted above, Rapcsak et al. (1989) observed that *most* of the errors made by their Alzheimer patients on irregular words were phonologically accurate, although peripheral writing impairments were also quite prominent (see below). Similarly, phonologically plausible errors were the most common error type among patients of Lambert et al. (1996) and Croisile et al. (1996). Glosser and Kaplan (1989) also noted that the majority of the spelling errors of Alzheimer patients were phonologically plausible, but this pattern was also true for controls. Moreover, Alzheimer and control subjects do not differ in the distribution of regularization or other spelling errors (Glosser et al., 1999).

In sum, the evidence for lexical agraphia in Alzheimer's disease is decidedly mixed. How might discrepancies among studies be explained? First, it is important to consider the types of stimulus words used to assess spelling, as different kinds of words tend to elicit different kinds of errors. For example, regularization errors cannot occur with unambiguous words, which, by definition, contain sounds that have only single invariant spellings. Second, when interpreting the performances of Alzheimer patients, one must also consider the types of errors elicited by the test stimuli in healthy comparison subjects. Not all word spellings are equally difficult for normal persons, so it is possible that some putatively abnormal responses by patients may simply reflect properties of the stimulus list, rather than consequences of their neurological disease. Differences in the composition of the Alzheimer patient group is another possible source for discrepancies among studies of written spelling. Alzheimer's disease is recognized to be heterogeneous in terms of clinical symptoms, disease course, and distribution of neuropathology (Becker, Huff, Nebes, Holland, & Boller, 1988; Chui, Teng, Henderson, & Moy, 1985; Haxby, Raffaelle, Gillette, Schapiro, & Rapoport, 1992; Martin, 1990; Stern & Jacobs, 1995). Heterogeneity is also apparent when single subject analyses of writing are performed (Glosser, Grugan, & Friedman, 1999; Hughes et al., 1997; Platel et al., 1993) or when functional brain imaging is used to evaluate patterns of writing impairment (Penniello et al., 1995). It is easy to overlook the obvious fact that an overall measure of group performance may not reflect the capacities of individual patients within the group. Small differences that have been reported between Alzheimer and control groups on measures of spelling regularity may obscure the existence of patient subgroups with different types of agraphia. Thus, it is likely that some patients do show spelling errors consistent with lexical agraphia, whereas other patients demonstrate deficits suggestive of different agraphic disorders; still others write normally well into the disease.

In Alzheimer's disease, agraphia may sometimes reflect a disturbance in phonological processing, an issue that has been explored using pseudoword spelling. With some exceptions (Rapcsak et al., 1989), Alzheimer subjects seem to have difficulty providing plausible spellings for non-words (Aarsland et al., 1996; Croisile et al., 1996; Hillis, Benzing, & Caramazza, 1996; Lambert et al., 1996; Platel et al., 1993). Glosser et al. (1999) used a large corpus of pseudowords to analyze spelling responses of Alzheimer patients and healthy elderly controls. Alzheimer's disease subjects performed less well than controls and showed a slightly greater difference between real word and pseudoword spelling scores. However, performances of both groups were qualitatively similar. When writing pseudowords containing familiar phoneme sequences, subjects within both groups performed comparably, regardless of whether there was only one, or more than one, possible spelling for the pseudoword. In fact, when spelling ambiguous phoneme sequences (*pern/purn*), both groups showed the same response preferences. In addition, both groups showed equivalent declines when spelling was compared for pseudowords containing unfamiliar phoneme sequences (*fwug*) and those containing familiar sequences (*plock*). The overall pattern of errors was similar between subject groups, except that the errors of Alzheimer subjects more often resulted in real words (lexicalization), perhaps because of difficulties appreciating and maintaining the required response set. Taken together, results of this study suggest that phonological processes underlying spelling are, for the most part, qualitatively similar in Alzheimer patients and normals, with only mild impairments in the former. Only a small minority of patients who perform outside the normal range on pseudoword spelling tasks may have more selective disruption of lexical phonological processing.

Writing From Meaning in Alzheimer's Disease

Cognitive processes involved in writing from sound differ from those involved in writing from meaning. When writing from sound, the phonological representations activate orthographic patterns without involving the semantic lexicon. On the other hand, writing from meaning (as in written picture naming) necessarily involves accessing lexical semantic information prior to retrieval of orthographic information.

The ability to write from meaning is impaired in most Alzheimer patients. In contrast, many patients retain the ability to write to dictation early in the disease course. Difficulty in conveying meaning by writing is not unexpected, given pervasive lexical semantic deficits in Alzheimer's disease. Impaired disruption of, or impaired access to, lexical semantic representations is considered to be a major source of the language impairment in Alzheimer's disease (Chertkow & Bub, 1990; Henderson, Mack, Freed, Kempler, & Anderson, 1990; Hodges, Salmon, & Butters, 1992; Martin & Fedio, 1983; Nebes, 1992). Just as Alzheimer patients have difficulties retrieving and using the meanings of words for speaking and comprehending oral language, they are also impaired in their ability to write meaningfully. Marked reductions in informational content on narrative writing tasks (Henderson et al., 1992) is consistent with this perspective (see below).

Difficulties using semantic-conceptual knowledge to convey meaning in writing have been explored at the single word level with tasks of written picture naming, responsive writing, and homophone writing. Using picture naming and responsive writing (sentence completion) tasks, Glosser and Kaplan (1989) compared Alzheimer patients' writing of single words to their writing of the same words on tasks that did not require semantic mediation (writing to dictation and word copy). Whereas patients were impaired significantly on the former task, they showed only minimal deficits on the latter tasks. When writing from meaning, Alzheimer patients tended to produce words that were either incorrect but were semantically related to the target (e.g., writing *fish* for the picture of an octopus), or were nonspecific or vague. Such errors suggested that patients had difficulties accessing precise semantic representations or suffered from degraded semantic representations, difficulties similar to impairments these patients experience in processing word meanings in spoken language.

Another means of assessing the adequacy of writing from meaning is to test spelling of homophones, such as *son* and *sun*. The correct spelling of homophones requires that different meanings associated with each spelling must be distinguished. Typically, the semantic context is used to determine the particular spelling associated with a homophone. For example, presentation of the sentence "The sun was hot" allows one to determine the correct spelling of *sun*. However, if knowledge about the semantic attributes of a word is degraded or inaccessible, then it may be difficult to determine which particular spelling corresponds to the word in question. Neils, Roeltgen, and Constantinidou (1995) showed that, compared to controls, Alzheimer patients were much more likely to produce errors when asked to spell homophones presented in sentence contexts. Many of the errors on the homophone spelling task consisted of homophone substitutions, such as spelling *doe* when given the context *bake the bread, dough*. Some of the erroneous spellings combined orthographic elements from both members of the homophone pair, as *doue*. The impairment in homophone spelling was associated with impaired performance on visual confrontation naming – a task that also requires semantic processing – and spelling impairments increased over time as patients became more demented. Together, these results were taken to indicate that Alzheimer patients retain considerable knowledge of different spelling patterns, but they have difficulty attaching specific spelling patterns to particular word meanings.

Peripheral Writing Processes in Alzheimer's Disease

Thus far, we have focused on deficits in central language processing components that may contribute to agraphia in Alzheimer patients. Since Alzheimer's disease is not exclusively a disorder of language, it is important also to consider the possible role of deficits in peripheral cognitive processes required for writing.

Neils, Roeltgen, and Greer (1995) systematically investigated the role of attentional impairment in agraphia, concluding that at least some of the spelling difficulties in Alzheimer's disease are the result of a graphemic buffer deficit. Their study specifically considered characteristics associated with impairments in the graphemic working memory component of spelling systems. They found that the effect of word length on spelling accuracy was significantly greater in the patient group (but see Aarsland et al., 1996), a finding consistent with a graphemic buffer deficit. Similarly, this study found that interposing a very brief delay between the visual presentation of a word and writing the same word (delayed copy) disrupted the performance in Alzheimer, but not control, subjects. Finally, a significant correlation was found between spelling accuracy (for both real words and non-words) and psychometric measures of sustained attention (e.g., performance on a letter cancellation task). In a multiple regression analysis, attentional measures better predicted phonemically implausible spelling errors than a language (naming) measure. A similar association between impaired attention and spelling was reported by Croisile et al. (1996), although the relation was significant only for oral, rather than written, spelling.

Finally, other findings suggest that, in at least some Alzheimer patients with more advanced dementia, writing is impaired as a result of a disturbance accessing or producing the actual physical forms of letters. Graphomotor problems in the form of illegible words, letter distortions, letter misplacements, perseverations, and difficulties maintaining letter case are described in group and individual case studies of Alzheimer patients (Henderson et al., 1992; Hughes et al., 1997; Libon et al., 1994; Neils et al., 1995; Neils-Strunjas, Shuren, Roeltgen, & Brown, 1998; Platel et al., 1993). Rapcsak et al. (1989), for example, described apraxic agraphia in almost half of their patients, although others have found prominent graphomotor errors in a smaller proportion of patients (Lambert et al., 1996). Unlike the central forms of agraphia discussed above, the peripheral graphomotor types of agraphia are especially evident in more advanced stages of dementia (Hughes et al., 1997; Platel et al., 1993).

ANALYSES OF WRITTEN DISCOURSE

Several studies have examined writing formulated at the level of sentences or paragraphs. Written discourse draws upon a broad spectrum of cognitive resources, as task demands are usually less structured and constrained than tasks requiring single word production. A common paradigm has been to use a picture description task to elicit a narrative writing sample, but written performance has been examined after simply asking subjects to write a sentence.

Horner et al. (1988) instructed patients with predominantly early-onset Alzheimer's disease to describe in writing, using complete sentences, everything they saw in a standard pictured scene. Writing proficiency – based on ratings of organization, vocabulary, and informational content, grammar, spelling, and writing mechanics – correlated significantly with dementia severity, as well as with oral language abilities as measured by the Wepman Aphasia Screening Test.

Neils, Boller, Gerdeman, and Cole (1989) also used a picture description task to examine narrative writing. Compared to elderly control subjects, mildly-to-moderately impaired Alzheimer patients wrote shorter paragraphs and committed more word errors. Both groups showed perseveration errors (sequentially repeated words), but only the patient group repeated contents of the story. When function words (articles, conjunctions, etc.) and content words (defined as nouns, verbs, adjectives, adverbs, and pronouns) were considered separately, the Alzheimer group made significantly more errors only on the latter. This error category included not only semantic substitutions and neologisms but also other error types less likely to have been linguistically based (incomplete words, word omissions, and sequential or nonsequential repetition of words or phrase). For this reason, it is difficult to discern whether language disturbances in this analysis were a strong determinant of patients' agraphia.

In a large sample of Alzheimer's disease and control subjects, LaBarge, Smith, Dick, and Storandt (1992) and Kemper et al. (1993) examined brief writing samples obtained in response to a request to "write a sentence for me." Patients with severe dementia were excluded, as most such patients were unable to perform the task. Among subject subgroups categorized by global severity (no dementia, questionable dementia, mild dementia, or moderate dementia), the ability to formulate a complete sentence was significantly related to severity, as was the number of errors within a sentence. Syntax was preserved, and subgroups did not differ with regard to sentence type (declarative, imperative, interrogative, and exclamatory), number of words, or frequency of word usage. Informational content was reduced in more demented subjects, however, as defined by the number of propositions in their sentences. In general, mildly-to-moderately demented Alzheimer patients were able to produce complete, grammatically well-formed sentences. Content word errors were infrequent in all groups. The authors also noted that correlations between the total number of errors in the sentence and naming performance or aphasia scores on other tasks were modest; thus there was no convincing evidence for an association between agraphia and aphasia. Correlations between sentence errors and scores on a task requiring the copy of line drawings were similarly modest.

Henderson et al. (1992) examined narrative writing samples from Alzheimer patients and healthy elderly controls. Subjects were asked to "write as much as you can" in describing a pictured scene. As expected, standard narrative writing scores from the Boston Diagnostic Aphasia Examination differed significantly between the two groups, and, within the Alzheimer's disease group, lower scores correlated significantly with disease severity. Quantitatively, both the total number of written words and a measure of informational content (the number of *key categories* mentioned in the narrative) distinguished subject groups. Effects of particular cognitive impairments were considered in multiple regression procedures. Consistent with the hypothesis that the agraphia of Alzheimer's disease is determined by deficits in multiple cognitive domains, measures of praxis, visuoconstructive (drawing) skills, language (naming), and attention (forward and backward digit span) were each significantly associated with writing scores. In stepwise regression procedures that considered all neuropsychological variables, a nonlinguistic measure, viz. visuoconstructive impairment, proved to be the single strongest determinant of narrative writing performance.

In the only study to include an aphasic control group, Glosser and Kaplan (1989) compared Alzheimer patients to patients in various stages of recovery from Wernicke's aphasia due to a single left temporal-parietal infarct. This comparison group was selected because language disturbances in Alzheimer's disease (Cummings et al., 1985; Nicholas et al., 1985), as in Wernicke's aphasia, are typically fluent. The overall severity of the language impairment was similar in the two patient groups. Subjects were instructed to write a sentence in response to pictures depicting one or two people engaged in a familiar action. Pictures were graded on the syntactic complexity of the intended descriptor sentence. Other tasks included writing sentences to dictation and copying sentences. On the picture description task, groups were similar in terms of total words produced. Compared to the aphasics, Alzheimer subjects produced fewer semantic errors and more syntactically complete intelligible sentences. Alzheimer's disease subjects, however, omitted more function words. Unlike fluent aphasics, Alzheimer patients scored better when writing sentences to dictation than when writing sentences spontaneously on the picture description task. Results from the sentence tasks, reinforced by findings from single word tasks in this study, failed to support the contention that the language disorder of Alzheimer's disease is similar to fluent aphasia produced by focal left cerebral damage.

In general, a dearth of information is provided in written narratives of Alzheimer patients. Patients produce significantly fewer words (Henderson et al., 1992; Neils et al., 1989) than older comparison subjects without dementia, and they mention significantly fewer content items or basic ideas (Henderson et al., 1992; Kemper et al., 1993). Methods of analysis have varied considerably, but, in most reports, writing performance has been found to decline as a function of disease severity (Henderson et al., 1992; Horner et al., 1988; Kumar & Giacobini, 1990; LaBarge et al., 1992). Moreover, writing performance effectively discriminates between Alzheimer patients and healthy comparison subjects (Henderson et al., 1992; LaBarge et al., 1992; Neils et al., 1989). As is true for oral discourse (Giles, Patterson, & Hodges, 1996), informational paucity in writing appears to be a key feature in distinguishing patients from controls and mildly demented patients from those with more severe disease (Henderson, Buckwalter, & Diz, 1992).

Overall findings from investigations of written discourse indicate that writing disturbances in Alzheimer's disease have multiple determinants. Semantic impoverishment can be striking, but in many instances central language processing deficits are not otherwise paramount. Although agraphia in Alzheimer's disease is associated with naming errors or other measures of language impairment, the magnitude of the association is not striking (Henderson et al., 1992; Horner et al., 1988; LaBarge et al., 1992). Qualitative analyses of orthographic errors suggest that most misspellings in written discourse are not phonologically plausible (Henderson et al., 1992), reinforcing the importance of peripheral nonlinguistic factors in many patients. Despite observations that oral language deficits of Alzheimer patients resemble those of patients with fluent aphasia, written production differs from that of fluent aphasics with focal left-hemisphere lesions. Thus, written responses often fail to conform to pragmatic constraints of task demands, and Alzheimer patients show less syntactic, phonological, and semantic disruption than aphasics (Glosser & Kaplan, 1989).

CONCLUDING PERSPECTIVE

Throughout this chapter we have stressed that different factors contribute to writing disturbances in Alzheimer's disease. Semantic information, which may be distributed within association neocortex in a widespread manner, is particularly vulnerable to the pathological progression of Alzheimer's disease; and semantic deficits are especially apt to degrade performance on relevant writing tasks (picture naming, homophone writing, and narrative description). Although Alzheimer patients are otherwise heterogeneous with respect to impairments in orthographic, phonological, and peripheral aspects of writing, peripheral impairments are increasing salient for all patients in advanced stages of the illness. Moreover, the functional determinants of agraphia may differ. Disease severity is one cause of clinical heterogeneity, but other clinical subgroups almost certainly reflect variations in the distribution of neuropathological changes within the different language and nonlinguistic processing regions of the cerebrum.

REFERENCES

Aarsland, D., Hoien, T., Larsen, J. P., & Oftedal, M. (1996). Lexical and nonlexical spelling deficits in dementia of the Alzheimer type. *Brain and Language*, *52*, 551-563.

Albert, M. L., Goodglass, H., Helm, N. A., Rubens, A. B., & Alexander, M. P. (1981). *Clinical aspects of dysphasia*. New York: Springer-Verlag.

Alzheimer, A. (1907). Über eine eigenartige Erkrankung der Hirninde. *Allgemeine Zeitschrift für Psychiatrie und Psychisch–Gerichtliche Medizin*, *64*, 146-8.

Alzheimer, A. (1911). Über eigenartige Krankheitsfälle des späteren Alters. *Zeitschrift fuer die Gesamte Neurologie und Psychiatrie*, *4*, 356-385.

Bayles, K. A. & Kaszniak, A. W. (1987). *Communication and cognition in normal aging and dementia*. Boston: College Hill.

Beauvois, M. F. & Derouesné, J. (1981). Lexical or orthographic agraphia. *Brain*, *194*, 21-49.

Becker, J. T., Huff, F. J., Nebes, R. D., Holland, A., & Boller, F. (1988). Neuropsychological function in Alzheimer's disease: Pattern of impairment and rates of progression. *Archives of Neurology*, *45*, 263-268.

Benson, D. F. & Cummings, J. L. (1985). Agraphia. In P. J. Vinken, G. W. Bruyn, H. L. Klawans, & J. A. M. Frederiks (Eds.), *Handbook of clinical neurology* (Vol. 45, pp. 457-472). Amsterdam: Elsevier Science Publishers.

Breitner, J. C. S. & Folstein, M. F. (1984). Familial Alzheimer dementia: A prevalent disorder with specific clinical features. *Psychological Medicine*, *14*, 63-80.

Caplan, D. (1992). *Language: Structure, processing, and disorders*. Cambridge, MA: MIT Press.
Chédru, F. & Geschwind, N. (1972). Writing disturbances in acute confusional states. *Neuropsychologia, 10*, 443-453.
Chertkow, H. & Bub, D. (1990). Semantic memory loss in dementia of Alzheimer's type. What do various measures measure? *Brain, 113*, 397-417.
Chui, H. C., Teng, E. L., Henderson, V. W., & Moy, A. D. (1985). Clinical subtypes of dementia of the Alzheimer's type. *Neurology, 35*, 1544-1550.
Croisile, B., Brabant, M. J., Carmoi, T., Lepage, Y., Aimard, G., & Trillet, M. (1996). Comparison between oral and written spelling in Alzheimer's disease. *Brain and Language, 54*, 361-387.
Cummings, J. L., Benson, D. F., Hill, M. A., & Read, S. (1985). Aphasia in dementia of the Alzheimer type. *Neurology, 35*, 394-397.
Cummings, J. L., Houlihan, J. P., & Hill, M. A. (1986). The pattern of reading deterioration in dementia of the Alzheimer type: Observations and implications. *Brain and Language, 29*, 315-323.
Dejerine, J. (1892). Contribution à l'étude anatomo-pathologique et clinique des différentes variétés de cécité verbale. *Comptes Rendus des Séances de la Société de Biologie, 4*, 61-90.
Folstein, M. F. & Breitner, J. C. S. (1981). Language disorder predicts familial Alzheimer disease. *Johns Hopkins Medical Journal, 149*, 145-147.
Friedman, R. B. & Alexander, M. P. (1989). Written spelling agraphia. *Brain and Language, 36*, 503-517.
Giles, E., Patterson, K., & Hodges, J. R. (1996). Performance on the Boston Cookie Theft picture description task in patients with early dementia of the Alzheimer's type: Missing information. *Aphasiology, 10*, 395-408.
Glosser, G., Grugan, P. K., & Friedman, R. B. (1999). Comparison of reading and spelling in patients with probable Alzheimer's disease. *Neuropsychology, 13*, 1-9.
Glosser, G. & Kaplan, E. (1989). Linguistic and nonlinguistic impairments in writing: a comparison of patients with focal and multifocal CNS disorders. *Brain and Language, 37*, 357-380.
Glosser, G., Kohn, S. E., Sands, L., Grugan, P. K., & Friedman, R. B. (1999). Impaired spelling in Alzheimer's disease: a linguistic deficit? *Neuropsychologia, 37*, 807-815.
Haxby, J. V., Raffaelle, K., Gillette, J., Schapiro, M. B., & Rapoport, S. I. (1992). Individual trajectories of cognitive decline in patients with dementia of the Alzheimer type. *Journal of Clinical and Experimental Neuropsychology, 14*, 575-592.
Henderson, V. W., Buckwalter, J. G., & Diz, M. M. (1992). Agraphia in Alzheimer's disease: Predictors of dementia severity and differentiation of demented from nondemented subjects [abstract]. *Journal of Clinical and Experimental Neuropsychology, 14*, 23.
Henderson, V. W., Buckwalter, J. G., Sobel, E., Freed, D. M., & Diz, M. M. (1992). The agraphia of Alzheimer's disease. *Neurology, 42*, 776-784.
Henderson, V. W., Mack, W., Freed, D. M., Kempler, D., & Anderson, E. S. (1990). Naming consistency in Alzheimer's disease. *Brain and Language, 39*, 530-538.
Hillis, A., Benzing, L., & Caramazza, A. (1996). Dissolution of spelling in a patient with Alzheimer's disease: Evidence for phoneme-to-grapheme correspondence 'rules' [abstract]. *Brain and Language, 55*, 62-65.
Hillis, A. E. & Caramazza, A. (1989). The graphemic buffer and attentional mechanisms. *Brain and Language, 36*, 208-235.
Hodges, J. R., Salmon, D. P., & Butters, N. (1991). The nature of the naming deficit in Alzheimer's and Huntington's disease. *Brain, 114*, 1547-1558.
Hodges, J. S., Salmon, D. P., & Butters, N. (1992). Semantic memory impairment in Alzheimer's disease: Failure of access or degraded knowledge? *Neuropsychologia, 30*, 310-314.
Horner, J., Heyman, A., Dawson, D., & Rogers, H. (1988). The relationship of agraphia to the severity of dementia in Alzheimer's disease. *Archives of Neurology, 45*, 760-763.
Huff, F. J., Corkin, S., & Growdon, J. H. (1986). Semantic impairment and anomia in Alzheimer's disease. *Brain and Language, 28*, 235-249.
Hughes, J. C., Graham, N., Patterson, K., & Hodges, J. R. (1997). Dysgraphia in mild dementia of the Alzheimer's type. *Neuropsychologia, 35*, 533-545.
Kemper, S., LaBarge, E., Ferraro, F. R., Cheung, H., Cheung, H., & Storandt, M. (1993). On the preservation of syntax in Alzheimer's disease: Evidence from written sentences. *Archives of Neurology, 50*, 81-86.
Kempler, D., Curtiss, S., & Jackson, C. (1987). Syntactic preservation in Alzheimer's disease. *Journal of Speech and Hearing Research, 30*, 343-350.

Kumar, V. & Giacobini, E. (1990). Use of agraphia in subtyping Alzheimer's disease. *Archives of Gerontology and Geriatrics, 12,* 155-159.

LaBarge, E., Smith, D. S., Dick, L., & Storandt, M. (1992). Agraphia in dementia of the Alzheimer type. *Archives of Neurology, 49,* 1151-6.

Lambert, J., Eustache, F., Viader, F., Dary, M., Rioux, P., & Lechevalier, B. (1996). Agraphia in Alzheimer's disease: An independent lexical impairment. *Brain and Language, 53,* 222-233.

Landon, C. L., Ashall, F., & Goate, A. M. (1997). Exploring the etiology of Alzheimer disease using molecular genetics. *Journal of the American Medical Association, 277,* 825-31.

Libon, D., Grossman, M., Mickanin, J., Hughes, E., Onishi, K., Biassou, N., D'Esposito, M., Ding, X. S., Alavi, A., & Reivich, M. (1994). Apractic agraphia and ideomotor apraxia for tools: Cognitive and PET studies [abstract]. *Brain and Language, 47,* 446-449.

Margolin, D. I. (1984). The neuropsychology of writing and spelling: Semantic, phonological, motor, and perceptual processes. *Quarterly Journal of Experimental Psychology, 36A,* 459-489.

Margolin, D. I. & Goodman-Schulman, R. (1994). Oral and written spelling impairments. In D. I. Margolin (Ed.), *Cognitive neuropsychology in clinical practice* (pp. 263-297). New York: Oxford University Press.

Martin, A. (1990). Neuropsychology of Alzheimer's disease: The case for subgroups. In M. F. Schwartz (Ed.), *Modular deficits in Alzheimer-type dementia* (pp. 142-176). Cambridge, MA: MIT Press.

Martin, A. & Fedio, P. (1983). Word production and comprehension in Alzheimer's disease: The breakdown of semantic knowledge. *Brain and Language, 19,* 124-141.

McKhann, G., Drachman, D., Folstein, M. F., Katzman, R., Price, D., & Stadlan, E. M. (1984). Clinical diagnosis of Alzheimer's disease: report of the NINCDS-ADRDA Work Group under the auspices of Department of Health and Human Services Task Force on Alzheimer's disease. *Neurology, 34,* 939-944.

Mirra, S. S., Heyman, A., McKeel, D., Sumi, S. M., Crain, B. J., Brownlee, L. M., Vogel, F. S., Hughes, J. P., van Belle, G., Berg, L., & participating CERAD neuropathologists. (1991). Consortium to Establish a Registry for Alzheimer's Disease (CERAD). Part II. Standardization of the neuropathologic assessment of Alzheimer's disease. *Neurology, 41,* 479-486.

Morrison, J. H., Scherr, S., Lewis, D. A., Campbell, M. J., Bloom, F. E., Rogers, J., & Benoit, R. (1986). The laminar and regional distribution of neocortical somatostatin and neuritic plaques: Implications for Alzheimer's disease as a global neocortical disconnection system. In A. B. Scheibel, A. F. Wechsler, & M. A. B. Brazier (Eds.), *The biological substrates of Alzheimer's disease* (pp. 115-131). San Diego: Academic Press.

Morton, J. (1980). The logogen model and orthographic structure. In U. Frith (Ed.), *Cognitive processes in spelling* (pp. 117-133). New York: Academic Press.

Nebes, R. D. (1992). Cognitive dysfunction in Alzheimer's disease. In F. I. M. Craik & T. A. Salthouse (Eds.), *The handbook of aging and cognition* (pp. 373-448). Hillsdale, NJ: Lawrence Erlbaum.

Neils, J., Boller, F., Gerdeman, B., & Cole, M. (1989). Descriptive writing abilities in Alzheimer's disease. *Journal of Clinical and Experimental Neuropsychology, 11,* 692-698.

Neils, J., Roeltgen, D. P., & Constantinidou, F. (1995). Decline in homophone spelling associated with loss of semantic influence on spelling in Alzheimer's disease. *Brain and Language, 49,* 27-49.

Neils, J., Roeltgen, D. P., & Greer, A. (1995). Spelling and attention in early Alzheimer's disease: Evidence for impairment of the graphemic buffer. *Brain and Language, 49,* 241-262.

Neils-Strunjas, J., Shuren, J., Roeltgen, D., & Brown, C. (1998). Perseverative writing errors in a patient with Alzheimer's disease. *Brain and Language, 63,* 303-320.

Nicholas, M., Obler, L. K., Albert, M. L., & Helm-Estabrooks, N. (1985). Empty speech in Alzheimer's disease and fluent aphasia. *Journal of Speech and Hearing Research, 28,* 405-410.

Patterson, K. E. & Wing, A. M. (1989). Processes in handwriting: A case for case. *Cognitive Neuropsychology, 6,* 1-23.

Penniello, M. J., Lambert, J., Eustache, F., Petit-Taboué, M. C., Barré, L., Viader, F., Morin, P., Lechevalier, B., & Baron, J. C. (1995). A PET study of the functional neuroanatomy of writing impairment in Alzheimer's disease: The role of the left supramarginal and left angular gyri. *Brain, 118,* 697-706.

Platel, H., Lambert, J., Eustache, F., Cadet, B., Dary, M., Viader, F., & Lechevalier, B. (1993). Characteristics and evolution of writing impairment in Alzheimer's disease. *Neuropsychologia, 31,* 1147-1158.

Rapcsak, S. Z., Arthur, S. A., Bliklen, D. A., & Rubens, A. B. (1989). Lexical agraphia in Alzheimer's disease. *Archives of Neurology, 46,* 65-68.

Reggia, J. A., Berndt, R. S., & D'Autrechy, C. L. (1994). Connectionist models in neuropsychology. In F. Boller & J. Grafman (Eds.), *Handbook of neuropsychology* (Vol. 9, pp. 297-333). Amsterdam: Elsevier.

Roeltgen, D. P. (1993). Agraphia. In K. Heilman & E. Valenstein (Eds.), *Clinical neuropsychology* (3rd ed., pp. 63-89). New York: Oxford University Press.

Roeltgen, D. P. & Heilman, K. (1983). Apractic agraphia in a patient with normal praxis. *Brain and Language, 18*, 35-46.

Roeltgen, D. P., Rothi, L. G., & Heilman, K. M. (1986). Linguistic semantic agraphia: A dissociation of the lexical spelling system from semantics. *Brain and Language, 27*, 257-280.

Spinnler, H. (1991). The role of attention disorders in the cognitive deficits of dementia. In F. Boller & J. Grafman (Eds.), *Handbook of neuropsychology* (Vol. 5, pp. 79-122). New York: Elsevier.

Stern, Y. & Jacobs, D. M. (1995). Preliminary findings from the predictors study: Utility of clinical signs for predicting disease course. *Alzheimer's Disease and Associated Disorders, 9*, S14-S18.

Williams, B. W., Mack, W., & Henderson, V. W. (1989). Boston Naming Test in Alzheimer's disease. *Neuropsychologia, 27*, 1073-1079.

LANGUAGE IN BRAIN DAMAGE: APHASIA

NEUROBEHAVIORAL MODELS FOR APHASIA REHABILITATION

Nancy Helm-Estabrooks

INTRODUCTION

The history of aphasia rehabilitation begins with the emergence of aphasiology as a discipline for clinical study. Paul Broca himself tried to re-educate a patient with severe word-finding problems and in 1865 stated that he was convinced that, although one could not return to aphasic patients the portion of their intelligence that had been lost, considerable improvement could be obtained.

The first published report of aphasia therapy in the United States was that of Charles Mills, a preeminent American neurologist. In 1880, Mills described the treatment of a patient who had been referred to him by the English neurologist Donald Broadbent. Two years prior to seeing Mills, the patient had an "attack" that left him speechless and unable to write. Mills directed a treatment program that lasted several years, during which time the patient regained sufficient speaking and writing skills to communicate without difficulty. Based on this case and others, Mills concluded that "In aphasia…much (of the recovery) is the result of methodical re-education." (Mills, 1904). To account for this recovery, he theorized that:

(1) If destruction of speech centers is incomplete, part of a certain convolution may learn to do the work of the whole;
(2) If centers on one side are destroyed, corresponding regions in the other hemisphere may take on function;
(3) If channels of communication are cut or blocked, new pathways may be formed (p. 27).

Thus, almost 120 years ago, Mills proposed a neurobehavioral model for aphasia rehabilitation. He continued his efforts to treat his aphasic patients and detailed methods for specific types of aphasia in his 1904 publication.

NEUROBEHAVIORAL MODELS FOR APHASIA THERAPY

Neurobehavioral models for aphasia therapy are based on theories of functional brain mechanisms, spared and impaired brain pathways and functions, and ideas about the nature of the rehabilitation process. In this section, three important neurobehavioral models are reviewed: (1) Luria's model, (2) Albert's application of Laurence and Stein's model, and (3) Rothi's model based on Finger and Stein.

Luria's Model

Nowhere is a neurobehavioral approach to aphasia rehabilitation more manifest than in the work of the Russian aphasiologist Aleksandr Luria. According to Hatfield (1981), Luria stood apart in his ability to integrate theory and practice, combining neuropsychological philosophy with a "veritable immersion" in the practical details of therapy and rehabilitation (p. 338). In the 1970 translation of his 1947 text *Traumatic Aphasia*, Luria describes general principles and specific approaches to restoring disturbed brain functions through reorganization of cortical processes. He stated that "in man almost any cortical area can acquire new functional significance and thus may be incorporated into almost any functional system" (p. 382). Luria described three principles of rehabilitation: *disinhibition*, *intrasystemic reorganization*, and *intersystemic reorganization*.

Luria's principle of disinhibition is based on Pavlov's belief that brain injury may result in inhibition of functions. In some cases, the inhibitory effects of the brain injury may be removed or disinhibited by surgical, pharmacological, or behavioral methods. A current-day example of treating an inhibitory block is the use of bromocriptine, a drug used in Parkinson's disease, to treat the selected feature of impaired speech initiation in transcortical motor aphasia (e.g., Albert, Bachman, Morgan, & Helm-Estabrooks, 1988). The use of drug therapy in aphasia is discussed below in greater detail.

Intrasystemic reorganization involves the use of different elements or levels of activity within the disturbed function. An example of intrasystemic reorganization is the aphasia treatment approach that begins with elicitation of reactive or involuntary speech, which then is brought to a conscious level and rehearsed to improve its use (e.g., Basso, Capitani, & Vignolo, 1979; Helm & Barresi, 1980).

Intersystemic reorganization involves training a different functional system to compensate for a disturbed or destroyed system. One of Luria's examples of this approach was a patient with an occipital lobe lesion who was unable to recognize letters through the visual system but could *read* via the motor/tactile system by tracing the letters with his finger. More recently, Maher, Clayton, Barrett, Schober-Peterson, & Rothi (1998) describe a case of alexia whose treatment involved copying letters with his finger, a method they refer to as a *motor-cross-cueing* strategy.

Albert's Application of Laurence and Stein's Model

In 1989, Martin Albert applied Laurence and Stein's (1978) theories related to recovery of brain mechanisms to the recovery of aphasia. Laurence and Stein describe one physiologically based theory, *diaschisis*, and three anatomically based theories, *redundancy*, *vicarious function*, and *multiple control*.

The theory of diaschisis maintains that brain damage may result in *neuronal shock* which temporarily suppresses metabolic activity in brain regions that are distant, but connected to, the damaged region. During the recovery process, as areas are released from inhibition, normal function would resume in undamaged structures. According to Albert, treatment approaches such as pharmacological manipulations that aid in the release of healthy brain tissue from the effects of diaschisis, might be useful in treating aphasia.

The theory of *redundancy* holds that some behaviors are served by systems of widely distributed and overlapping neural networks that function both in series and in parallel. Damage may occur to only one part of the system so that recovery of a behavior may occur via the undamaged portions of the system. Albert suggests that the mechanism of redundancy might account for the recovery of naming skills in aphasia.

The theory of *vicarious functions* proposes that brain regions other than those that normally carried out a particular function may assume the ability to perform the lost behavior. An example of this theory as applied to recovery from aphasia is the recruitment of the nondominant right hemisphere for language use (Helm-Estabrooks, 1983).

In their theory of *multiple control* Laurence and Stein explain that a specific behavior may be controlled by more than one structure. In the case of language, subcortical structures such as the basal ganglia or thalamus might provide pathways for language processing through their reciprocal connections with cerebral cortex.

Rothi's Model Based on Finger and Stein

Leslie Gonzalez Rothi (1995) proposed a neurobehavioral model for aphasia treatment based on the work of Finger and Stein (1982). In this model, she distinguishes *restitutive* from *substitutive* therapies which are based, in part, on the physiological state of the recovering system.

According to Rothi, restitutive methods are deficit-directed in that they are aimed at restoring impaired abilities using the same functional processes in the ways used premorbidly. She regards the language *stimulation* approaches described in the literature of the 1950s and 1960s as being typical of restitutive methods. A more current example of a restitutive approach to aphasia therapy is the use of cognitive neuropsychological models of normal language functions (e.g., naming) for determining and targeting the level of the language system where impairment resides (e.g., semantic knowledge versus phonological representations). Rothi proposes that such restitutive methods are best applied in early stages post-onset when one might expect the greatest amount of natural, physiological recovery of the damaged neurons and neural systems subserving language.

While restitutive methods may be time-limited, *substitutive* therapies have no temporal limitation. These methods recruit systems or processes not used premorbidly for the target behavior. Rothi describes two types of substitutive methods: *vicariative* and *compensative*. Three explanations are given for recovery of skills through *vicariation*: (1) homologous regions in the opposite hemisphere are now doing the work of the damaged area, (2) a previously *uncommitted* area of the same hemisphere has assumed the skill, (3) a higher- or lower-order structure within the same neuroanatomical system has been recruited. These explanations of vicariative recovery are highly reminiscent of Mills' (1880) hypotheses regarding recovery from aphasia. Rothi considers Melodic Intonation Therapy (Albert, Sparks, & Helm, 1973; Sparks, Helm, & Albert, 1974) to be a good example of a vicariative method because it may recruit the right hemisphere for verbal production.

Rothi's second form of substitutive recovery is based on behavioral compensation. *Compensative* methods alter target tasks so that spared brain areas can be used to accomplish these tasks in a new way. An example of this approach are the symbolic gestures to substitute for verbal naming.

SUMMARY

The neurobehavioral models of recovery from aphasia described above have notable overlap. Luria's theory of *disinhibition* seems to be describing the phenomenon that Laurence and Stein called *diaschisis*. Luria's description of *intersystemic reorganization* appears to be what Rothi calls *vicariative* treatment and Laurence and Stein call *vicarious function*. Rothi's three explanations for vicariative recovery are very close to Mills' much earlier hypotheses regarding the mechanisms for recovery from aphasia with treatment. Luria's *intrasystemic reorganization* seems to encompass Laurence and Stein's theories of *redundancy* and *multiple control*.

Regardless of the labels used, these theories of aphasia recovery meet two of the three criteria for neurobehavioral models for aphasia therapy in that they are based on ideas about: (1) functional brain mechanisms, and (2) spared and impaired brain pathways and functions. Implied, but not explicitly stated in all these theories is the third criterion (i.e., the nature of the rehabilitation process itself). For such a statement we can turn to Basso, Capitani, and Vignolo (1979):

> The hypothesis underlying aphasia rehabilitation is that all intentional verbal behavior, if appropriately reinforced through training, leaves a trace in the cerebral structures that are potentially capable of carrying out linguistic activity, and this trace increases the probability of occurrence of subsequent correct verbal behavior (p. 192).

EXAMINING THE PATIENT: THE BASIS FOR APHASIA THERAPY

Now that we have reviewed neurobehavioral models for aphasia rehabilitation, the next step is to consider how we can use these models in making decisions about modes of treatment. First, a careful and thorough examination of language and other cognitive skills is conducted. Luria (1970) believed that successful treatment of aphasia begins with careful examination of the patient, identification of factors responsible for various symptoms or deficits, and the ways one might compensate for these deficits. This belief is echoed in such statements as that of Weniger and Sarno (1990) who asserted that "Without some detailed knowledge about the pattern of retained and lost skills, it is hardly possible to design a treatment regimen from which the patient can be expected to benefit" (p. 301).

In our 1991 text, Albert and I agree with this concept and maintain further that the *process approach* to examination as described by our colleague Edith Kaplan (1988) is the best way to generate hypotheses for aphasia treatment programs. Kaplan's approach is based on the work of her mentor Hans Werner (1937) who demonstrated that final test scores are not as useful in understanding spared and impaired skills as close observation of an individual's behaviors en route to solutions. In fact, there are many ways to go about any task, and brain-damaged patients may achieve the same score in very different ways. The use of bottom-line test scores often obscures critical information about individual differences in cognitive and communicative styles, strategies, and preserved abilities. It is only by carefully documenting patients' *exact* behaviors that we develop an understanding of: (1) their retained abilities, (2) how to support or compensate for their weaknesses, and (3) how cognitive-linguistic strengths can be used to improve functional skills.

To illustrate this point, we described two patients who received similar scores (27/72 and 26/72) on the Word Discrimination subtest of the Boston Diagnostic Aphasia Examination (BDAE) (Goodglass & Kaplan, 1984). This subtest requires patients to point to 36 items representing six semantic categories (objects, letters, geometric forms, actions, colors, and numbers) as named randomly by the examiner. Two points can be earned for correct item identification in fewer than five seconds. One point can be earned on this subtest for correctly identifying the item in more than five seconds, and half a point is scored for either identifying correct semantic categories (e.g., pointing to another color for *blue*), or for identifying the correct item after the examiner has isolated the target semantic category. Analysis of the actual responses of the two patients showed no overlap in the items identified in less than five seconds (2 points each for full credit). When scores were computed for the semantic categories (possible 12 points each), no overlap in category scores was found for the two subjects. Thus, the similar score earned by these two patients informed us only about the overall *severity* (about the 20th percentile) of their problem in understanding spoken single words. It did not tell us anything about each patient's particular strengths and weaknesses for the six semantic categories.

The process approach also dictates that the examiner record the exact response to each stimulus so that we know the nature of the error responses. Because this was done for these two cases, we were able to analyze responses vis-a-vis the pathological behavior of perseveration (inappropriate repetition of a previous response). Patient A was more perseverative (54% of error responses) than Patient B (34% of error responses). Thus, the process approach to response analysis shows that two aphasic patients who received similar quantitative scores had performed quite differently on a test of single-word comprehension. In designing appropriate treatment programs, the strengths and weaknesses of each patient must be taken into account.

A final example from Helm-Estabrooks and Albert (1991, p. 150) should serve to underscore the value of the process approach. The following responses were attempts by six different patients to name a picture of a *harmonica* on the Boston Naming Test (BNT) (Kaplan, Goodglass, & Weintraub, 1984):

(1) "A musical thing you blow through."
(2) "A marhonika."
(3) "Mon - ka."
(4) "A frelicka."
(5) "I know it, but I can't say it."
(6) "A double-decker bus."

All of these responses received zero credit, but by analyzing the responses according to a neurocognitive model of the naming process used for treating anomia (e.g., that of Nettleson and Lesser, 1991), we glean valuable information. Of the two circumlocutory responses (numbers 1 and 5) only number 1 suggests preservation of semantic knowledge which is basic to naming. Response number 2 indicates difficulty at the higher level of phonological assembly. The patient who produced response number 3, with great articulatory struggle, may have actually retrieved the target word but was unable to speak it. As for the neologistic response of patient number 4, it is impossible to infer the level of break-down without further exploration of the integrity of his semantic knowledge. Finally, response number 6 is not an aphasic error but a visuoperceptual error with the patient seeing the two rows of air holes as the two tiers of windows on a double-decker bus. Thus, only by recording the patients' exact responses can we begin to determine the nature of the problem and target the areas of weaknesses and strengths that allow us to decide upon treatment strategies.

BEYOND LANGUAGE EVALUATION

In 1982, German neurologist Klaus Poeck stated that "the starting point for any scientific approach to aphasia therapy is a precise analysis of the language disorder in a given patient." Albert and I illustrated this point using the two cases reviewed above. In more recent years, however, aphasia has come to be regarded more as a cognitive-communicative deficit than as a strict language disorder. Rothi (1998) speaks of "the cognitive disorder of aphasia", and Peach (1998) defines aphasia as "a disorder involving information processing disturbances at the attentional, memorial, linguistic, and executive levels of the cognitive system for processing language." Language, in fact, is just one aspect of cognition that also includes the domains of attention and concentration, executive functions, memory, and visual spatial functions. As I have said elsewhere (Helm-Estabrooks, 1998), the extent to which cognitive skills (in addition to language) are spared or impaired in aphasic patients is pivotal to their treatment. At the most basic level, response to any therapy depends on attention and concentration, and memory is critical to all learning. Visuoperceptual skills are needed for processing most treatment materials and executive skills are required for patients to generate and implement ways to communicate in unique situations despite aphasia. It is imperative, therefore, to evaluate all aspects of cognition as preparation for aphasia therapy.

Hamsher (1991) reviewed studies of the relation between aphasia and cognition or *intelligence* and concluded that the relation was uncertain. One of the greatest problems we face in resolving this issue is that most intelligence tests are language-based and therefore invalid for use with aphasic patients. According to Hamsher, those studies that have used *nonverbal* tests of various cognitive abilities have produced mixed evidence of a functional relationship between nonverbal intelligence and aphasia. My colleagues at the University of Arizona and I addressed this problem with our own study of 32 non-globally aphasic patients (Helm-Estabrooks, Bayles, Ramage, & Bryant, 1995). Aphasia severity was determined through administration of the Aphasia Diagnostic Profiles (Helm-Estabrooks, 1992). To measure cognitive ability we administered a battery of tests requiring no verbalization: clock drawing/setting, a short version of the Wisconsin Card Sort Test (WCST) (Nelson, 1976), and three subtests of the Wechsler Memory Scale-Revised (WMS-R) (Wechsler, 1987): Visual Paired Associates, Figural Memory, and Visual Memory Span. The highest possible score for the battery was 85 points. No significant relation was found between aphasia severity and cognition as measured by these tests.

The next step in such research may be to compare patients with similar aphasia severity levels but dissimilar levels of cognitive ability to determine the extent to which cognitive scores correlate with functional use of residual communication skills. Clinically, all aphasiologists have observed that two aphasic patients may be equally impaired in language but that one communicates far better. Identification of non-language factors that maximize communication may lead to a different approach to rehabilitation; one that emphasizes treatment of other impaired cognitive skills (such as executive functions) as well as language. From a clinical perspective, however, it has been difficult to evaluate cognitive skills in aphasic patients in the absence of standardized measures that have been normed on aphasic individuals. To address this need, I have developed a short test of attention and concentration, executive functions, memory, language, and visuospatial skills that is currently undergoing standardization by The Psychological Corporation (Helm-Estabrooks, Research Edition).

After patients' strengths and weaknesses in language and other cognitive domains have been determined through careful examination, the treatment-planning process begins. In the next section I review aphasia treatment methods from the perspective of neurobehavioral models.

CLINICAL APPLICATION OF A NEUROBEHAVIORAL MODEL FOR APHASIA THERAPY

In the neurobehavioral models for aphasia therapy reviewed earlier in this chapter we saw substantial overlap among models. Many aphasia therapy approaches used today can fit within Luria's model of disinhibition, intrasystemic, and intersystemic approaches, so we will use this model for discussing certain of the aphasia treatment methods in current use.

Disinhibition Approaches to Aphasia Rehabilitation

Luria (1970) proposed that functional disturbances following brain damage occur secondary to either (1) destruction of the system subserving the function or (2) inhibition of these systems as a result of loss of "the normal conduction of excitation in the areas directly involved" (pg. 374). He recommended the use of pharmacological agents to restore the biochemical processes necessary for normal synaptic conduction to the disturbed function. In particular, he discussed the use of anticholinesterase drugs to combat the inhibiting effect of cholinesterase on acetylcholine, which is essential to synaptic transmission.

The idea that drugs or other ingestible agents might be useful in treating aphasia is very old. Among the earliest suggested treatments are wine, berries, roots and herbs (LaPointe, 1993), and cashews (Mettler, 1947). In the 1940s, intravenous sodium amytal was used to reduce the inhibiting effect of anxiety on language performance in aphasia (e.g., Linn, 1947; Billow, 1949). In the 1970s, Roumanian aphasiologists such as Voinescu and Gheorghita (1973; 1978) reported on use of the antidepressants imipramine and pyrithioxine. The latter drug was said to have the greatest effect on repetition and naming and a lesser effect on reading, comprehension, and writing.

More recent attempts to disinhibit language in aphasic patients concentrated on use of dopminergic agents. This work was motivated by clinical and anatomicochemical evidence that dopamine mediates verbal fluency (for a fuller explanation see Mimura, Albert, & McNamara, 1995). In 1988, my colleagues and I (Albert, Bachman, Morgan, & Helm-Estabrooks) described a patient with moderate transcortical motor aphasia of 3½ years duration. His primary symptoms were impaired ability to initiate speech, long response latencies, and word-finding difficulties. Auditory comprehension and repetition were relatively spared. The dopamine agonist bromocriptine was administered using an open-label, test-retest design. While taking the drug, the patient showed a reduced number of pauses between and within utterances, improved naming, and decreased paraphasias. However, the drug was discontinued because it caused the patient to experience a feeling of vertigo.

Subsequent to our 1988 study, Bachman and Morgan (1988) and other investigators such as Gupta and Mlcoch (1992), and Sabe, Leiguarda, and Starkstein (1992) described beneficial effects of bromocriptine on speech fluency in aphasia. In reviewing these studies Mimura and colleagues (1995) caution that these studies were methodologically weak and uncontrolled. Few subjects were sampled, drug trials were unblinded, and no placebos were used. A placebo was used by MacLennan, Nicholas, Morley, and Brookshire (1991), and they found improvement only in the number of words produced by their subjects during the bromocriptine phase. Meaningful speech and language functions were not affected by this drug. Mimura et al. (1995) recommend that future studies of the effect of dopamine therapy for aphasia employ placebos, consider the type and severity of aphasia being treated, the type of dopaminergic agent chosen, its optimal dose, and its side effects.

In Europe, the central nervous system stimulant known as piracetam is being used to treat aphasia. Piracetam (Nootropyl) is a gamma-aminobutyric acid (GABA)-derivative "that improves cognitive functions such as learning and memory through faciliation of cholinergic and excitatory amine neuortransmission" (Huber, Willmes, Poeck, Van Vleyman, & Deberdt, 1997). Studies of the effect of piracetam on recovery from aphasia have been well-controlled using a double-blind, placebo-controlled, two parallel groups, randomized design. Results indicate that patients treated with piracetam after stroke demonstrate better recovery from aphasia (Enderby, Broeckx, Hospers, Schildermans, & Deberdt, 1994; Huber et al., 1997; Poeck, 1998; Orgogozo, 1998).

At the initiation of these studies the piracetam and placebo groups were comparable with respect to age, sex, type, severity and duration of aphasia, and number of hours of language therapy. Enderby et al. studied 68 patients with recent aphasia (five to nine weeks post onset), while Huber and colleagues studied 66 patients with chronic aphasia. Unlike patients who received a placebo, patients who received piracetam showed a significant overall improvement in aphasia severity. The 373 acute patients seen by Poeck and Orgogozo were treated within 12 hours of stroke. Again, results favored piracetam. In her review of the results of these studies, Van Vleymen (1998) concluded that "piracetam has an effect on the recovery of aphasia irrespective of the time of onset of treatment, but that this therapeutic effect is higher when treatment is started early after the stroke."

Thus, there continues to be great interest in the use of pharmacological agents to facilitate recovery from aphasia. As new drugs are developed, pharmacotherapy may have great impact on this devastating disorder.

Intrasystemic Approaches to Aphasia Rehabilitation

Intrasystemic approaches to rehabilitation involve the use of different elements, or levels of activity, within the disturbed function (Luria, 1970). A behavior may be shifted to a lower level so that it is carried out in a more automatic, primitive way or to a higher level where it is implemented as a conscious, cortical activity. In the case of aphasia, the disturbed function is language. Language has not only several modalities (e.g., speaking, understanding, and writing) but several levels ranging from reactive, emotional speech such as the automatic use of expletives ("ouch!") to highly intentional assertions such as those I am formulating and stating in this chapter. The commonly used clinical task of confrontation naming lies somewhere between those two extremes. Hughlings Jackson (1878) was the first to observe that some aphasic patients can utter appropriate words in an automatic, involuntary way but are unable to use the same words intentionally. He described a patient who had never been heard to speak a meaningful word until a fire occurred on the ward and he cried "Fire! Fire!" Jackson came to regard aphasia as a disorder of propositional use of language and stated that the higher the propositional value of a task, the less likely the patient is to perform it correctly. Much later, Vignolo (1964) described how he used this characteristic of aphasia for rehabilitative purposes: "First an automatic way to elicit a correct response is found, and the response is then tentatively elicited in more and more voluntary ways." Vignolo did not provide detail as to how this was accomplished, but in 1980 Barresi and I presented a paper on a method we called *Voluntary Control of Involuntary Utterances* (VCIU) which did detail this intrasystemic approach. We used VCIU with three patients whose attempts at intentional speech had been limited to a few stereotypic expressions such as "real good" and "I don't know" for two months to three years. All three had shown poor response to other therapy programs. One area of strength for each was the ability to understand, but not speak, written single words as demonstrated by BDAE word-picture matching. They were, however, able to read aloud some words such as their stereotypic expressions and some emotionally-laden words such as *kiss* and *die*. We used this ability as a springboard for treatment, using written emotional words as primes and following each patient's lead when real-word errors were made. An example follows.

Stimulus word: *father*
Response: "mother"
New stimulus word: *mother*
Response: "Mama"
New stimulus word: *Mama*
Response: "Mama"

Once a word was read correctly and consistently, it was written on a 3" x 5" card and a pictorial representation was drawn on the back side for confrontation naming. In the final steps of VCIU, patients were given conversational opportunities to use these words.

Another intrasystemic approach to aphasia treatment is one that is commonly used in remediating aphasic naming problems. This involves the use of cueing hierarchies in which verbal cues are ordered from those that are most likely to elicit the target response in an automatic manner to those that place more and more burden of intentionality on the patient. For example, a cue such as "You sweep the floor with a br..." may elicit the target word *broom* in a very automatic way. A slightly less helpful cue might be to omit the target word phonemes (i.e., "You sweep the floor with a...." The next step might be to replace the semantically informative sentence with a neutral sentence ending with initial phonemes of the target word (i.e., "This is a br..."). The goal of such cueing hierarchies is for the patient to produce the target word in response to weaker and weaker cues and finally in a confrontation naming task. Many studies have shown that sentence completion and phonemic cues are quite successful in eliciting target words from aphasic patients (e.g., Pondraza & Darley, 1977; Pease & Goodglass, 1978), but unfortunately, effects of cueing may be quite transitory (e.g., Patterson, Purell, & Morton, 1983).

A common problem that occurs when aphasic patients are confronted with the task of intentionally naming items is the phenomenon of recurrent perseveration in which all or part of a previous response is inappropriately repeated (e.g., "scissors" for *scissors* and then again "scissors" for *whistle* or "sissle" for *whistle*). Such perseverative errors may be the result of persistent semantic or motor-speech memory traces (Hotz & Helm-Estabrooks, 1995). Luria (1972) considered them to be after-effects of excitation that persist for abnormally long periods, thus making plastic changes needed for different responses impossible. Regardless of the mechanism(s) responsible for recurrent perseveration, it occurs in practically every form of aphasia. According to Albert and Sandson (1986) perseveration may be an integral part of aphasia. This opinion was supported by results of a study conducted by Emery and Helm-Estabrooks (1989) who analyzed the naming responses of 15 fluent and 15 nonfluent aphasic patients given the BDAE confrontation naming subtest. We found that for 26 patients, at least 35% of their errors were perseverative in nature and that severity of perseveration was not related to time post-onset or the fluent/nonfluent status of the aphasia.

The therapy program we called TAP, for Treatment of Aphasic Perseveration (Helm-Estabrooks, Emery, & Albert, 1987), specifically addresses the problem of perseveration for confrontation naming. The goals of TAP are to bring perseverative responses to patients' level of awareness, to help them suppress these perseverative responses, and to encourage them to ask for cues, if needed, to produce correct, non-perseverative responses (for a fuller description, see Helm-Estabrooks & Albert, 1991). Thus, TAP also may be regarded as an intrasystemic approach to aphasia rehabilitation in that it helps bring an unconscious verbal behavior to a conscious level where it can be brought under voluntary control.

Intersystemic Approaches to Aphasia Rehabilitation

According to Luria (1970), intersystemic reorganization involves training a different functional system to compensate for a disturbed or destroyed system as opposed to working at different levels within the disturbed process. Maher and colleagues (1998) contrasted an intersystemic (*substitutive*) approach with an intrasystemic (*restitutive*) approach in treating a patient with pure alexia of 14 months duration. For the intersystemic approach, they used a *motor cross-cueing* strategy in which the patient used his finger to pretend to copy letters in words and sentences. His reading aloud with this method was 100% accurate and his reading speed was doubled after four weeks of this therapy. This intersystemic (substitutive) method was contrasted with an intrasystemic approach based on a cognitive neuorpsychological model for word recognition and reading aloud. The goal of this approach was to help the patient gain access to the lexical-semantic representations for words. Target words were presented subthreshold for recognition (under one second) to prevent the patient from using letter-by-letter analysis. The patient was asked to make a semantic decision regarding the target (e.g., target word *apple*: Is it edible or nonedible?). This intrasystemic (restitutive) method was unsuccessful in improving reading.

Another method widely regarded as being intersystemic is that of Melodic Intonation Therapy (Albert, Sparks, & Helm, 1973; Helm-Estabrooks & Albert, 1991; Sparks, Helm, & Albert, 1974). This hierarchically structured program, in which functionally communicative sentences (e.g., "Open the door") are intoned slowly with continuous voicing, emerged from the long-standing clinical observation that some aphasic patients can produce words only in song (e.g., Mills, 1904). In the 1960s and 1970s, several studies showed that the right hemisphere plays an important role in mediating music and intonational contours (for a review see Helm-Estabrooks, 1983). The results of these studies lend credence to the notion that melodic intonation therapy (MIT) taps right hemisphere functions in facilitating recovery of speech. In fact, it would appear, based on the 1985 CT-scan study conducted by Naeser and Helm-Estabrooks, that the right hemisphere must be intact for MIT to be effective. That is not to say that patients who respond well to melodic intonation therapy learn to speak with the right hemisphere but rather that the right hemisphere *assists* in deblocking language. To this point, Albert, Sparks, and I (1973) stated in our discussion of the first three patients treated with MIT that "neither spontaneous recovery nor development of new language areas in the right hemisphere can account for the improvements noted, since the recovery of grammatical structure and vocabulary was too rapid following the beginning of melodic intonation therapy" (p. 131).

SUMMARY AND CONCLUSIONS

Neurobehavioral models for aphasia rehabilitation appear to have their roots in Mills' (1904) ideas about processes responsible for improvement of language with treatment. The more recent theories of Luria (1970) and Albert's (1989) application of the Laurence and Stein model, as well as Rothi's (1995) application of Finger and Stein's model, show a great deal of overlap with one another and with Mills' much earlier hypotheses. Because of this overlap, Luria's model for recovery seemed as useful a framework as any for discussing some of the aphasia treatment methods in current use and was adopted in the chapter.

The choice of therapy methods depends to a great extent on identification of spared and impaired functional systems and skills. Careful patient evaluation using a *process approach* as advocated by Kaplan (1988) is required before specific treatments can be selected and applied.

Treatment examples were discussed within the framework of Luria's concepts of disinhibition, intrasystemic, and intersystemic reorganization. Only a few methods were chosen to illustrate the three rehabilitation processes. Many other effective aphasia therapy methods exist (see, for example, Helm-Estabrooks & Holland, 1998). As to the future of aphasia rehabilitation, a quote from Martin Albert seems to point the way.

> Contemporary research in basic neuroscience, cognitive neuroscience, and neuorimaging is expanding our therapeutic options for treatment of aphasia in ways that might not have been considered possible just a few years ago (p. 1417).

ACKNOWLEDGMENTS

The author of this chapter thanks Dr. Marjorie Nicholas for her helpful editorial comments.

REFERENCES

Albert, M. L. (1989). Experimental approaches to aphasia therapy. *Journal of Neurolinguistics, 4* (3), 427-434.

Albert, M. L. (1998). Treatment of aphasia. (Neurological Review). *Archives of Neurology, 55*, 1417-1419.

Albert, M. L., Sparks, R. W., & Helm, N. A. (1973). Melodic Intonation Therapy for aphasia. *Archives of Neurology, 29*, 130-131.

Albert, M. L. & Sandson, J. (1986). Perseveration in aphasia. *Cortex, 22*, 103-115.

Albert, M. L., Bachman, D. L., Morgan, A., & Helm-Estabrooks, N. (1988). Pharmacotherapy for aphasia. *Neurology, 38*, 877-879.

Bachman, D. L. & Morgan, A. (1988). The role of pharmacotherapy in the treatment of aphasia: Preliminary results. *Aphasiology, 2*, 225-228.

Basso, A., Capitani, E., & Vignolo, L. A. (1979). Influence of rehabilitation on language skills in aphasia patients: A controlled study. *Archives of Neurology, 36*, 190-196.

Billow, B. W. (1949). Observations on the use of sodium amytal in the treatment of aphasia. *Medical Records, 162*, 12-13.

Broca, P. (1865). Sur le siège de la faculté du langage articulé. *Bulletin de la Société d'Anthropologie de Paris, 6*, 337-393.

Emery, P. & Helm-Estabrooks, N. (1989). The role of perseveration in confrontation naming performance. In T. Prescott (Ed.), *Proceedings of the conference of clinical aphasiology* (pp. 271-280). Austin, TX: Pro-Ed.

W., Schildermans, F., & Deberdt, W. (1994). Effect of piracetam on recovery and rehabilitation after stroke: A double-blind, placebo-controlled study. *Clinical Neuropharmacology, 17* (4), 320-331.

Finger, S & Stein, D. G. (1982). *Brain damage and recovery: Research and clinical perspectives.* New York: Academic Press.

Goodglass, H. & Kaplan, E. (1984). *Boston diagnostic aphasia examination.* Philadelphia: Lea & Febiger.

Gupta, S. & Mlcoch, A. (1992). Bromocriptine treatment of nonfluent aphasia. *Archives of Physical and Medical Rehabilitation, 73,* 373-376.

Hamsher, K. (1991). Intelligence and aphasia. In M. T. Sarno (Ed.), *Acquired aphasia* (pp. 339-372). New York: Academic Press.

Hatfield, F. M. (1981). Analysis and remediation of aphasia in the U.S.S.R: The contribution of A. R. Luria. *Journal of Speech and Hearing Disorders, 46,* 338-347.

Helm, N. A. & Barresi, B. (1980). Voluntary control of involuntary utterances: A treatment approach for severe aphasia. In R. Brookshire (Ed), *Clinical aphasiology conference proceedings.* Minneapolis, MN: BRK.

Helm-Estabrooks, N. (1983). Exploiting the right hemisphere for language rehabilitation: Melodic intontation therapy. In E. Perecman (Ed.), *Cognitve processing in the right hemisphere.* New York: Academic Press.

Helm-Estabrooks, N. (1992). *Aphasia diagnostic profiles.* Austin, TX: Pro-Ed.

Helm-Estabrooks, N. (1998). A "cognitive" approach to treatment of an aphasic patient. In N. Helm-Estabrooks & A. L. Holland (Eds.), *Approaches to the treatment of aphasia.* San Diego, CA: Singuler Publishing Group, Inc.

Helm-Estabrooks, N. (Research Edition). *Cognitive-linguistic quick test.* San Antonio, TX: The Psychological Corporation.

Helm-Estabrooks, N., Emery, P., & Albert, M. L. (1987). Treatment of Aphasic Perseveration (TAP) program. *Archives of Neurology, 44,* 1253-1255.

Helm-Estabrooks, N. & Albert, M. (1991). *Manual of aphasia therapy.* Austin, TX: Pro-Ed.

Helm-Estabrooks, N., Bayles, K., Ramage, A., & Bryant, S. (1995). The relationship between cognitive performance and aphasia severity, age and education: Females versus males. *Brain and Language, 51* (1) 139-141.

Helm-Estabrooks, N. & Holland, A. L. (1998). *Approaches to the treatment of aphasia.* San Diego: Singular Publishing Group, Inc.

Hotz, G. & Helm-Estabrooks, N. (1995). Perseveration. Part I: A review. *Brain Injury, 9* (2), 151-159.

Huber, W., Wilmes, K., Poeck, K., Van Vleymen, B., & Deberdt, W. (1997). Piracetam as an adjuvant to language therapy for aphasia: A randomized, double-blind placebo-controlled pilot study. *Archives of Physical Medicine and Rehabilitation, 78,* 245-250.

Hughlings Jackson, J. (1878). On the affections of speech from disease of the brain. *Brain, 1,* 304-330, 19-41.

Kaplan, E. (1988). A process approach to neuropsychological assessment. In T. Boll & B. K. Bryant (Eds.), *Clinical neuropsychological and brain function: Research, measurement, and practice.* Washington, D.C.: American Psychological Association.

Kaplan, E., Goodglass, H., & Weintraub, S. (1984). *The Boston naming test.* Philadelphia: Lea & Febiger.

LaPointe, L. L. (1983). Aphasia intervention in adults: Historical, present, and future approaches. In J. Miller, D. Yodel, & R. Schiefieldbusch (Eds.), *Contemporary issues in language intervention. ASHA Reports 12* (pp. 127-136). Rockville, MD: American Speech-Language-Hearing Association.

Laurence, S. & Stein, D. G. (1978). *Recovery from brain damage.* New York: Plenum Press.

Linn, L. (1947). Sodium amytal in treatment of aphasia. *Archives of Neurology and Psychiatry, 58,* 357-358.

Luria, A. R. (1970). *Traumatic aphasia.* The Hague: Mouton (Original work published 1947).

Luria, A. R. (1972). Aphasia reconsidered. *Cortex, 8,* 34-40.

MacLennan, D. L., Nicholas, L. E., Morley, G. K., & Brookshire, R. H. (1991). The effects of bromocriptine on speech and language function in a man with transcortical motor aphasia. In T. E. Prescott (Ed.), *Clinical aphasiology* (Vol. 20, pp. 145-156).Austin, TX: Pro-Ed.

Maher, L., Clayton, M., Barrett, A., Schober-Peterson, D., & Rothi, L. (1998). Rehabilitation of a case of pure alexia: Exploiting residual abilities. *Journal of International Neuropsychological Society, 4,* 36-647.

Mettler, C. C. (1947). *History of medicine.* Philadelphia: Blakiston.

Mills, C. K. (1904). Treatment of aphasia by training. *Journal of the American Medical Association, 43,* 1940-1949.

Mimura, M., Albert, M. L., & McNamara, P. (1995). Toward a pharmacotherapy for aphasia. In H. S. Kirshner (Ed.), *Handbook of neurological speech and language disorders* (pp. 465 482). New York: Marcel Dekker.

Naeser, M. & Helm-Estabrooks, N. (1985). CT scan lesion localization and response to Melodic Intonation Therapy with nonfluent aphasia cases. *Cortex, 21,* 203-223.

Nelson, H. E. (1976). A modified card sorting test sensitive to frontal lobe defects. *Cortex, 12,* 313-324.

Nettleson, J. & Lesser, R. (1991). Therapy for naming difficulties in aphasia: Application of a cognitive neuropsychological model. *Journal of Neurolingistics, 6* (2), 139-157.

Orgogozo, J. M. (1998). Piracetam in the treatment of acute stroke. *CNS Drugs Supplement, 1,* 41-49.

Patterson, K., Purell, C., & Morton, J. (1983). Facilitation of word retrieval in aphasia. In C. Code & D. J. Muller (Eds.), *Aphasia therapy: Studies in language disabilities and remediation* (pp. 76-87). London: Edward Arnold.

Peach, R. (1998). *Diagnostic considerations for aphasia.* 19th Health South and Braintree Hospital Annual Conference on Head Injury and Stroke, Boston, MA.

Pease, D. M. & Goodglass, H. (1978). The effects of cueing on picture naming in aphasia. *Cortex, 14,* 178-189.

Poeck, K. (1982, May). *Modern methods of aphasia therapy.* Paper presented at the 7th Annual Meeting of the Japanese CVD society, Hirosaki, Japan.

Pondraza, B. L. & Darley, F. L. (1977). Effects of auditory prestimulation on naming in aphasia. *Journal of Speech and Hearing Research, 20,* 669-683.

Poeck, K. (1998). Piracetam treatment in post-stroke aphasia. *CNS Drugs, 1,* 51-56.

Rothi, L. J. G. (1998). Cognitive disorders. Searching for the circumstances of effective treatment: Introduction by the symposium organizer. *Journal of the International Neuropsychological Society, 4,* 593-594.

Rothi, L. J. G. (1995). Behavioral compensation in the case of treatment of acquired language disorders resulting from brain damage. In R. A. Dixon & L. Backman (Eds.), *Compensating for psychological deficits and declines.* Mahwah, NJ: Lawrence Erlbaum Associates.

Sabe, L., Leiguarda, R., & Starkstein, S. E. (1992). An open-label trial of bromocriptine in nonfluent aphasia. *Neurology, 42,* 1637-1638.

Sparks, R., Helm, N., & Albert, M. (1974). Aphasia rehabilitation resulting from Melodic Intonation Therapy. *Cortex, 10,* 303-316.

Van Vleymen, R. (1998, August). *The role of piracetam in post stroke aphasia.* Paper presented at the 8th International Aphasia Rehabilitation Conference, Kwa Maritane, Pilanesburg National Park, South Africa.

Vignolo, L. A. (1964). Evolution of aphasia and language rehabilitation: A retrospective exploratory study. *Cortex, 1,* 344-367.

Voinescu, I. & Gheorghita, N. (1973). Tratamentul afaziel cu imipramina. *Neurologia Psihiatria Neurochirurgia, 18,* 423-430.

Voinescu, I. & Gheorghita, N. (1978). Adjuvant drug therapy with psychologopedic rehabilitation of aphasic patients, *Revue Romaine de Medecine, 16* (3), 155-161.

Wechsler, D. (1987). *Wechsler memory scale - revised.* New York: The Psychological Corporation.

Weniger, D. & Sarno, M. T. (1990). The future of aphasia therapy: More than just new wine in old bottles? *Aphasiology, 4* (4), 301-306.

Werner, H. (1937). Process and achievement: A basic problem of education and developmental psychology. *Harvard Educational Review, 7,* 353-368.

SELF-DETERMINATION AND SELF-ADVOCACY: NEW CONCEPTS FOR APHASIC INDIVIDUALS AND THEIR PARTNERS

Audrey L. Holland

INTRODUCTION

Most people understand that some disorders are chronic. For example, once an individual develops diabetes or arthritis, then lifestyle changes, medications, and adjustments of various types become part of daily life. However, current medical practice does not appear to believe that stroke is a chronic condition. That is, rehabilitative efforts immediately following stroke are assumed to achieve the best that can be accomplished. Yet difficulties with walking, using one's hand, and particularly with speaking, understanding, reading and writing typically linger after rehabilitation has done its work. These problems are largely ignored by medical practice, or accepted as inevitable. Just as other chronic conditions, however, the aftereffects of stroke should mandate continual management. The notion of aphasia as a chronic condition that follows stroke underlies the concepts of self-determination and advocacy explored in this paper.

In the "good old days", persons with aphasia had far greater access to clinical service, far longer into the course of their aphasia. Under these circumstances, the chronicity of their residual language disabilities was perhaps obscured. But health care has become more limited and time-bound, and the chronic needs of aphasic individuals have become more apparent. Simultaneous with decrying the need for continued services, aphasic people, their partners, and some professionals, have begun seeking and creating alternatives to managing aphasia's long-term consequences. A number of new approaches to the therapeutic process are appearing. They are based on social, rather than medical models. (See Jordan and Kaiser, 1996 for a comprehensive report on social models of aphasia.)

The social model of disability was first articulated in Great Britain by Oliver in 1983. The model influenced the terminology initially adopted by both the World Health Organization (WHO) and the Institute of Medicine (IOM). These medically-oriented concepts of *disability* and *handicap* have since come under attack by the disability movement itself, as connoting powerlessness on part of individuals with impairments. For simplicity, however, the term *disability* will be used in this paper to cover the limitations of activity – a joint process involving both society and the individual with impairments – which result from conditions such as stroke.

Two general features distinguish the social model of disability. First is the notion that the true experts are those who have experienced the disorder firsthand. Thus, in the case of aphasia, the reactions and experiences of aphasic people and their partners and families are central to understanding what living with aphasia is all about. Second, the barriers faced by those with "disabling" conditions do not simply result from impairments themselves; society also plays a role by imposing physical and psychological barriers to full societal participation. These two features form the basis for reconsidering decision-making and control in disabling conditions. The social model of disability seeks to increase self-determination, personal responsibility, and self-advocacy for individuals with impairments as they attempt to regain their former active places in society.

A number of factors have traditionally coalesced to limit self-determination for individuals with aphasia. First, there is the language impairment itself. Difficulty in speaking creates special problems in advancing one's causes and beliefs. Society's uneasiness with brain damage also compounds the problem. Third, until recently, there has been a lack of advocacy for stroke victims generally, much less for those with aphasia. The result has been both public apathy and public ignorance. One of the few bright spots in the continuing crisis in health care is that, as aphasic individuals and their caretakers have faced curtailment in their services, they and the professionals who work with them have begun to make noise about it. Advocacy for and by aphasic persons is increasing worldwide. Jordan and Kaiser (1996) document growing empowerment of aphasic individuals and their families in the United Kingdom; organizations for aphasic persons are flourishing in the rest of Europe as well. Australia, South Africa and Canada all have growing programs and activities for chronic aphasic individuals. In 1998, the first United States conference of aphasic individuals, their partners and families, was held in Chicago under the auspices of the increasingly more visible National Aphasia Association.

The following comments are made in this context. They reflect the vantage point of a clinician who has been listening to aphasic people and their families for many years, and who has a lifelong concern with the effects of aphasia and its treatment on everyday life post stroke. Here, I will share some ideas that I believe are important for aphasic persons, their partners and their families as they increase their efforts to take back their own lives and choose to live them, rather than to be victims of aphasia.

UNDERSTANDING ONE'S OWN APHASIC CONDITION

It has been stated previously that the real experts on aphasia are aphasic persons themselves. Probably because of the language deficit itself, however, many individuals with aphasia have notable difficulty in understanding why and how some aspects of this very perplexing problem affect them. Unlike individuals with other, more obvious and well-publicized impairments such as amputations or spinal cord injuries, aphasic people usually had limited knowledge of aphasia before becoming aphasic themselves. Further, although all impairments have unique manifestations, aphasia comes in almost infinite variations. These variations are related to the location and extent of a given person's brain damage, as well as to former language use and style, education, literacy, age, temperament, to name a few. Thus, even when aphasic speakers have previous experience with aphasia, the personal details of the problems may be very different. Perhaps guided by a skilled clinician, aphasic persons need to learn about both aphasia in general and their own particular problems using language. Experience dictates that the more that one knows about aphasia and its effects, the better one is prepared to cope with it.

Answers to questions such as the following should increase aphasic speaker's self-knowledge, and help them to help themselves: What circumstances make it difficult to understand what other people say? What changes might facilitate understanding? If speakers slow down?; If they talk louder?; When there are fewer distractions?; When they seem to be really listening? What things make it easier to talk to some people? How can others be instructed to do things that help? What happens to speech and understanding when the aphasic speaker is tired? How can fatigue be controlled? What happens to speech and understanding in the presence of depression? What can be done about it?

There are many more such questions about speaking and comprehending, as well as similar questions about reading and writing. There is a great advantage in considering them and in knowing details such as these about one's own language problems. Once known, aphasic individuals can take responsibility for working within and around their strengths and limitations.

Such questions can also instruct other, non-aphasic persons about how they might help. Families and friends of aphasic individuals are also likely to be strangers to the general problem of aphasia and certainly at its outset, to this particular aphasia. They too can be shown how to observe details such as those listed above, and to take responsibility for working within and around them.

USING GROUPS TO MANAGE CHRONIC APHASIA

Information about the increasing importance of aphasia groups is burgeoning (cf., Elman, 1998; Marshall, 1998; Avent, 1997). Most writers stress the economic advantages of groups, but more importantly acknowledge the importance of social contact in recovery from aphasia. Fundamental to the success of groups is the fact that members share the aphasic situation. Holland and Ross (1998) comment:

> Clinicians may have read about aphasia, language and communication or interacted with aphasic talkers in clinical encounters. But the fact is that very few of us have actually been there. The essence of aphasia is its uniqueness. Few other problems that humans encounter are quite so exotic, so pervasive, so unexpected, so baffling in their variability.

Holland and Ross go on to point out that empathy is likely to be greater among group members than between aphasic persons and either their families or their clinicians. Mutual experiences have given them a basic understanding of the complex problems that result from aphasia. This understanding probably transcends differences in types of aphasia, levels of severity, or even the length of time one has been aphasic. This high degree of understanding constitutes empathy. Here is what an aphasic man, Kiran, has to say:

> When I looked at them... there was... We can understand each other, quite simply. That we are on the same boat – The important thing was... you didn't have to say a word. It was brilliant. I don't know why I felt so wonderful... I suppose it's because of that. I know that she... he were the same as me (Parr, Byng, Gilpin, & Ireland, 1997).

Aphasia groups are not just empathetic. Group members also share solutions to problems, and permit a kind of toughness that only those who have been through such an experience can provide. Holland and Ross (1998) give an example:

> The youngest member of this group, Herb, was going for a job interview, and the other group members decided to help him practice for it. (In fact, every member of this group except Herb had previous experience in hiring other people.) My (i.e., Holland's) role was to watch and comment. I watched the interviews and the subsequent criticisms with growing horror, for Herb's questioners were very hard on him, and the feedback was particularly forceful and direct. Herb did not seem disturbed by it, but appeared to be taking it very well. I intervened nonetheless. And the group told me quite pointedly that if Herb expected to get the job, he was going to have to be far surer of himself. Particularly because he had a language problem, they argued, he had to demonstrate his ability to handle this job in a strong and forthright manner. Herb clearly understood the support that underlay the group's remarks, and I did not. Are you surprised to find out that Herb got the job?

At the University of Arizona, we have had almost ten years of experience in conducting therapy groups for persons with aphasia. Almost from the outset, our experience has been positive. Aphasic people, their partners, families and clinicians all shared that recognition. It has shaped in all of us a commitment to aphasia groups. Indeed, we view such groups as a central component in effective management of chronic aphasia, not as an adjunct to individual treatment.

INCLUDING APHASIA IN ONE'S SELF-DEFINITION

Both clinicians and aphasic people themselves have historically focused their energies on "getting over" aphasia. However, even people who have made excellent recoveries from aphasia still have some sticky, residual problems that continue to bother them long past stroke, suggesting that accommodating to aphasic residuals, that is, fitting them in, might be a more appropriate way to view speech and language problems. Here is Donald Moore, as he explains an aspect of his chronic problem:

> A mild stroke, indeed, but I cannot today do any two things simultaneously. If you ask me a question, I have to turn off the television, figuratively speaking at least. In an interview, I can't write anything down, while listening to you because if I do try to write, I can't hear a word of what you say. If there is a

group of people in a room, if there are two or more conversations at the same time, and if the people talk loud, the event is pure torture. And it takes several hours of sleep for me to recover. Noise is brutality, every aphasic will tell you. And truly there should be a law against it (Moore, 1994).

Given the current brevity of reimbursed treatment time, many aphasic speakers are even less well recovered when they leave acute treatment than they were previously. Holland and Beeson (1993) have argued that taking the aphasia into account is an extremely important part of learning to cope. It is not simply a matter of "overcoming" the problem – some part of it will probably always be there. To "await" a return to life as it was before – or even to approach individual or group therapy experiences with that as a goal is very likely to be a discouraging path.

However, once aphasia is entered into one's personal equation, a number of approaches to living with aphasia, developing a more decisive role in its management, and advocating for oneself begin to open up. Here are a few examples:

(1) Accepting aphasia means that aphasic speakers can begin using strategies that *compensate* for their language problems. The most natural thing in the world for both aphasic patients and their families to do in response to aphasia is to dig in and work on language that seems to be lost or inaccessible. But it is not as simple as it sounds, and represents only one, sometimes unreachable, goal. Knowing one's individual aphasia and incorporating it into one's self definition permits one to consider ways to make "end runs" around some aphasic problems. For example, when having difficulty in retrieving a word, an aphasic individual might alternatively provide listeners with related words or near synonyms, superordinates, or subordinates, which permit listeners to retrieve the exact word for themselves. Although this circumlocutory behavior is imprecise, it is an effective way to communicate in many instances, and a decided improvement over a potential communicative impasse. There are countless examples of such alternative strategies, not only for word-retrieval, but for increasing auditory comprehension as well.

(2) Accepting aphasia increases recognition of the need for group involvement. Many people in the aphasia groups conducted at the University of Arizona are committed to the notion that coming to an aphasia group is what has started them on the road to "recovery". Further, to stay on this road includes the group support described earlier in this paper. One member of our aphasia group, Claudia, made this extremely obvious to Andrew, a new member who was eager to be done with the group, and to have his aphasia long behind him. Claudia looked Andrew in the eye and pointedly noted: "Get used to it. You're here for life!" (Both of them are still regular attendees.)

(3) Accepting aphasia initiates the process by which self-confidence is rebuilt. Claudia's comment serves as excellent example of the acceptance that can be developed, as well as the growth of self-confidence. Here are a few more, from other aphasic speakers:

> I have had to fight for that self-respect. That I'm fed up of saying 'I'm sorry,' I'm sorry. I do not want to say that any more. I'm NOT sorry (unidentified aphasic speaker in Parr, Byng, Gilpin, & Ireland, 1997).

> It's confidence, it's all about confidence – When I first... embarrassed about everything, you know. Perhaps the years seem to have gone by and my aphasia.... I mean I am still aphasic, obviously, but it doesn't seem to matter anymore. My loss isn't so great anymore. So if I miss a few words, it doesn't really matter anymore. I'm one of the world's listeners now. I'm not one of the talkers (Judith in Parr, Byng, Gilpin, & Ireland, 1997).

These are not necessarily representative or ideal attitudes regarding aphasia. Nevertheless, they take aphasia into account, and in the process reflect a self-confidence often compromised with the onset of aphasia. And self-confidence is the cornerstone of self-determination and self-advocacy.

(4) Accepting aphasia diminishes passivity. Re-establishing a sense of personal responsibility is crucial for self-determination. It is also crucial for taking a more proactive role in treatment, and probably more important, assuring a more active role in society. In self-confident aphasic people, a range of everyday lifestyles obviously related to pre-aphasic personality and preferences can be seen. Some of our aphasic group members have remarkable self-discipline and motivation. For example, Roger spends at least an hour a day reading self-selected books and articles, with the expectation that it will improve his reading skills. (This expectation is being fulfilled.) Conversely, Laura has "settled" in the sense of having no interest in working on language skills at all. She comes to group to socialize, and achieves self-fulfillment in solitary gardening. The point, however, is that both Roger and Laura have decided for themselves how to cope. Self-determination should not end with the onset of aphasia.

CHANGING THE ROLE OF FAMILIES

Just as chronic aphasia is undergoing re-definition in relation to the social approach to its management, so is the role of the family. There is growing interest in helping families of aphasic patients to function as *communication ramps*, a term coined by Kagan (1995). Kagan noted that although ramps and wheelchairs and the like provide access for many stroke patients with physical disabilities, there is nothing like them in terms of communication access. She suggested that families and clinicians must play a supportive role by becoming appropriate communication ramps for aphasic individuals. The essence of *ramping* is to learn how to talk with aphasic persons by making adjustments to typical communication. Learning simple approaches such as speaking more slowly, confirming what you think the aphasic person is attempting to communicate, or perhaps taking a disproportionate share of the burden of communicating are all pertinent examples. Other techniques include accompanying speech with drawings and writing that clarify ones messages to aphasic speakers. Aphasic people themselves can be encouraged to draw, write, or gesture in order to facilitate their communicative success. A fairly recent development is specific training (for families, volunteers, and for other professionals) in the use of such methods. Kagan (1998) has described one such program in detail. Conversational coaching (Holland, 1991) represents an approach to train both families and aphasic patients in more effective interpersonal communication.

SELF-ADVOCACY AT WORK

All of the above can culminate in a many forms of advocacy by aphasic persons and their families. Three examples follow:

(1) Pound (1998) has recently described two approaches to aphasia groups that have self-advocacy as their main goals. The first group was co-facilitated by an aphasic person and a speech-language pathologist. Group activities involved identifying and then challenging barriers in the social environment, as well as engaging in tasks that addressed personal change and *renegotiation of self-identity*. The second group developed personal portfolios related to their history, current functioning and future plans. These portfolios enabled "aphasic people to define themselves in relation to their past, present and future" (Pound, 1998). Pound reports great success in both approaches in terms of improved quality of life with longstanding aphasia.

(2) Community advocacy projects are also appearing. Jordan and Kaiser (1996), for example, describe a *Shop Sign* project involving businesses and public services in Bury, Lancashire, UK. Establishments were given instructions about aphasia and its aftermath, then provided with written information about aphasia and how to assist aphasic speakers, along with simple picture touch cards designed to facilitate communication. Then they were given well-designed signs with logos identifying them as knowledgeable about aphasia to display in their windows. Thus, they became *user friendly* to aphasic individuals, who carried wallet cards identifying themselves to shopkeepers as needing extra help. Jordan and Kaiser (1996) report that this project is being successfully replicated elsewhere in the United Kingdom.

(3) Finally, spouses and families are increasingly more visible in the aphasia self-advocacy arena. Families are providing new and durable voices for their aphasic family members. They also have become increasingly involved in advocating for themselves, and the problems that aphasia imposes on the family unit as a whole. Spouse groups are increasing, and families, like aphasic individuals themselves, are learning that one of the major sources of support lies in individuals whose problems are similar to one's own.

CONCLUSIONS

Even though there is a discouraging shortage of services available for individuals with chronic aphasia and their families, there has been a recent, quite exciting response to this shortage. A growing awareness of the importance of self-determination and advocacy has begun to infuse aphasic people with a new and somewhat differently slanted hope for improved quality of life. This paper has attempted to outline some of the changes and benefits that should influence aphasia treatment in the future.

ACKNOWLEDGMENTS

The author thanks members of the University of Arizona Aphasia Groups and their partners and families for the insights they have provided. National Multipurpose Research and Training Center Grant DC 01409 from the National Institute on Deafness and Other Communication Disorders supported this work in part.

REFERENCES

Avent, J. (1997). *Manual of cooperative group treatment for aphasia*. Woburn, MA: Butterworth.
Elman, R. (Ed.). (1998). *Group treatment of neurogenic communication disorders*. Woburn, MA: Butterworth.
Holland, A. (1991). Pragmatic aspects of intervention in aphasia. *Journal of Neurolinguistics*, 6, 197-211.
Holland, A. & Beeson, P. (1993). Finding oneself following stroke: A reply to Brumfitt's *Losing one's sense of self following stroke*. *Aphasiology*, 7, 581-583.
Holland, A. & Ross, R. (1998). The power of aphasia groups. In R. Elman (Ed.), *Group treatment of neurogenic communication disorders*. Woburn, MA: Butterworth.
Jordan, L. & Kaiser, W. (1996). *Aphasia – A social approach*. London: Chapman and Hall.
Kagan, A. (1995). Revealing the competence of aphasic adults through conversation: A challenge to health professionals. *Topics in Stroke Rehabilitation*, 2, 15-28.
Kagan, A. (1998). *Training volunteers as conversational partners using "supported conversation for adults with aphasia": An efficacy study*. Paper presented at the 8th International Aphasia Rehabilitation Conference, Kwa Maritane, South Africa.
Marshall, R. (1998). *Introduction to group treatment for aphasia: Design and management*. Woburn, MA: Butterworth.
Moore, D. (1994). A second start. *Topics in Stroke Rehabilitation*, 2, 100-103.
Parr, S., Byng, S., Gilpin, S., & Ireland, C. (1997). *Talking about aphasia*. Buckingham, UK: Open University Press.
Pound, C. (1998). *Power, partnership and perspectives: Social model approaches to long term therapy and support*. Paper presented at the 8th International Aphasia Rehabilitation Conference, Kwa Maritane, South Africa.

NEUROIMAGING IN SEVERE APHASIA AND OUTCOME FOLLOWING TREATMENT WITH THE NONVERBAL, COMPUTER-ASSISTED VISUAL COMMUNICATION PROGRAM, C-VIC

Margaret A. Naeser, Errol H. Baker,
Carole L. Palumbo, Marjorie Nicholas,
Michael P. Alexander, Ranji Samaraweera,
Malee N. Prete, Steven M. Hodge,
and Tamily Weissman

INTRODUCTION

   The topic of this paper is treatment of severe aphasia patients with no recovery of meaningful spontaneous speech. This paper reports on a recent study on whether CT scan lesion site patterns in chronic, severe aphasia patients who have no meaningful spontaneous speech may be useful to predict outcome level following treatment with a nonverbal, icon-based, Computer-assisted Visual Communication program (Naeser, Baker, Palumbo, Nicholas, Alexander, Samaraweera, Prete, Hodge, & Weissman, 1998a).
   Treatment of stroke patients with severe aphasia, including patients with no meaningful spontaneous speech, has generally been ineffective (Collins, 1986). Most treatments have been designed to compensate for the severely reduced speech output and writing through the use of gesture, pantomime, drawing, or picture manipulation; success has been limited (Heilman, Rothi, Campanella, & Wolfson, 1979; Helm-Estabrooks, Fitzpatrick, & Barresi, 1982; Johannsen-Horbach, Cegla, Mager, Schempp, & Wallesch, 1985; Morgan & Helm-Estabrooks, 1987; Rao & Horner, 1980; Skelly, 1979; Velletri-Glass, Gazzaniga, & Premack, 1973).
   Over 20 years ago, the first systematic attempts to utilize a nonverbal substituted language based on pictures and icons (Visual Communication, ViC) were reported (Baker, Berry, Gardner, Zurif, Davis, & Veroff, 1975; Gardner, Zurif, Berry, & Baker, 1976). These early reports demonstrated that some patients did have the capacity to learn and implement these nonverbal languages, but functional improvement was limited, in part, because of the awkwardness of manipulating the large deck of cards necessary for all of the icons.

More recently, this early attempt (ViC) was extended to a nonverbal iconic language that can be manipulated with a computer (Computer-assisted Visual Communication, C-ViC) (Steele, Weinrich, Wertz, Kleczewska, & Carlson, 1989; Weinrich, Steele, Kleczewska, Carlson, Baker, & Wertz, 1989; Weinrich, Steele, Carlson, Kleczewska, Wertz, & Baker, 1989). These investigators demonstrated that severely aphasic patients could manipulate the mouse and button-click necessary for operation and could learn rules of lexical organization. The patients learned to construct and comprehend sentences in the nonverbal, pictorial C-ViC language. Not all apparently equally severe aphasia patients, however, have been able to completely grasp the lexical and syntactic rules of the C-ViC language and use them to independently initiate communication.

Lesion sites that might underlie this difference in response to treatment with C-ViC were reported in our pilot investigation of seven cases (Naeser, Palumbo, Baker, & Nicholas, 1994). Those results suggested that there was a specific left-hemisphere lesion site pattern associated with ability to use C-ViC to initiate communication (Best Response). A different lesion site pattern was associated with an inability to use C-ViC to initiate communication, but an intact ability to use C-ViC to answer questions posed by others (Moderate Response). Patients with Best Response had either no lesion in, or extensive lesion in, only one of the following two left-hemisphere areas: Area 1-temporal lobe structures (Wernicke's cortical area, or the subcortical, anterior temporal isthmus area, containing afferent auditory projections from medial geniculate body to Heschl's gyrus); or Area 2-supraventricular frontal lobe structures (supplementary motor area [SMA]/cingulate gyrus area 24; cortical or white matter). Patients with Moderate Response had extensive lesion in both Areas 1 and 2.

In the present study, the lesion site patterns from the smaller pilot study were applied to predict C-ViC outcome level for 17 new patients with severe aphasia. This was a retrospective study in which lesion site analysis was performed after the patients had completed a series of C-ViC training sessions.

The primary objective of the present study was to test the validity of the original hypothesis that patients with Best Response would have either no lesion in, or extensive lesion in either Area 1 or Area 2; and patients with only Moderate Response would have either no lesion in, or extensive lesion in, both Areas 1 and 2. The study had two secondary objectives: (1) To examine the relationship between lesion sites and absence of recovery of meaningful spontaneous speech – that is, to define lesion sites associated with candidacy for C-ViC, and (2) to examine the relationship between C-ViC outcome and test scores on the Boston Assessment of Severe Aphasia (BASA) exam (Helm-Estabrooks, Ramsberger, Morgan, & Nicholas, 1989) prior to C-ViC training.

METHOD

Subjects

Data for 17 chronic, severely aphasic stroke patients treated with C-ViC were reviewed (Table 1). All patients had suffered a single left-hemisphere cerebrovascular accident (CVA). Four patients also had a silent right-hemisphere

Table 1. Patient Data. Patients are rank ordered according to their Phase II C-ViC performance rating.

C-ViC Outcome Group	Patient Id.	Age Entering C-ViC Treatment	Post-stroke Onset Time Entering C-ViC Treatment	Pre C-ViC BASA, Auditory Comprehension Raw Score (Max. = 16)	Pre C-ViC BASA, Oral/Gestural Raw Score (Max. = 21)	Pre C-ViC Overall BASA Score (Max. = 61)	Phase II C-ViC Performance Rating (VICA Rating) (Max. = 7)
Best Response	JH	44	10 Yr.	15	1	39	6.50
	PS	42	10 Yr.	14	7	44	6.20
	AC	77	46 Mo.	10	6	39	5.77
	FM	53	21 Mo.	13	5	42	5.43
	BM	49	10 Mo.	16	12	49	4.93
	JC	69	19 Mo.	12	12	41	4.59
	LM	60	25 Mo.	-*	-*	-*	-*
Moderate Response	RR	47	43 Mo.	12	12	43	4.40
	AP	69	77 Mo.	12	7	36	3.76
	RP	59	28 Mo.	12	11	36	3.59
	TS	56	7 Mo.	5	2	15	3.44
	ND	59	9 Mo.	7	2	27	3.03
	WT	64	26 Mo.	9	6	30	2.73
No Response	BG	73	3 Mo.	-*	-*	-*	CND
	DM	70	14 Mo.	8	6	30	CND
	HR	75	7 Mo.	8	2	20	CND
	DT	65	13 Mo.	12	7	41	CND

C-ViC - Computer-Assisted Visual Communication treatment program.
BASA - Boston Assessment of Severe Aphasia test.
VICA - Visual Index of Communicative Ability.
* No data available.
CND - Could Not Do C-ViC

CVA which was first documented on the CT scan performed at the time of the left-hemisphere CVA. The age at onset of left-hemisphere stroke ranged from 33 to 74 years (M = 57.8, SD = 12.6). All patients were right-handed. All patients except two (cases FM and JC) had severe right hemiplegia; none had left hemiplegia.

Prior to treatment with C-ViC, the patients had been tested with the BASA exam (Helm-Estabrooks, Ramsberger, Morgan, & Nicholas, 1989). All patients met the major criterion for entry into the study – that is, severe limitation in speech output, with little or no meaningful spontaneous speech (or writing) in conversation or in picture description. Auditory comprehension was also impaired in all cases. However, there was variability among the patients in severity of auditory comprehension; not all patients were globally aphasic. Table 1 summarizes language capacity as tested with the BASA. Prior to treatment with C-ViC, most patients had been treated with one or more traditional treatment programs without success.

The decision to recommend a patient for treatment with C-ViC was made by the speech/language pathologist administering the BASA prior to C-ViC treatment. No lesion site information was used in determining whether a patient would be treated with C-ViC.

All patients began treatment with C-ViC during the chronic phase post-stroke, ranging from three months post-stroke onset (MPO) to ten years post-stroke onset (see Table 1). All patients were able to control the computer mouse with the non-paralyzed hand. The participants were seen as outpatients for one-hour treatment sessions, usually twice per week for about one year.

The C-ViC Treatment Program

Patients were pre-screened to determine whether they could match eight icons on the computer screen to the same eight real objects. Four patients could not perform this icon-to-object matching task, despite two to four weeks of training; they were classified as *No Response*. The C-ViC training consists of two phases (Baker & Nicholas, submitted). In Phase I, patients are trained to use the computer mouse to carry out commands given to them in C-ViC (comprehension), to answer simple questions, and, finally, to compose descriptions of simple acts (production). Patients learn to use three verb action icons (lift, turn, and give), pictures of objects (16 to 24 icons), and pictures of people (minimum of three). For these icons of people, faces from photographs are scanned into the computer including those of the patient and therapist. Patients learn to arrange person, action, and object icons in a left-to-right grammatically correct order. Phase I is completed when a patient can describe events without error and without guidance, utilizing two grammatical constructions: (1) subject-predicate-object and (2) subject-predicate-indirect object-direct object. (See top of Figure 1.)

Phase II training focuses on real-life communicative acts, including describing simple acts, expressing needs, asking questions, and making requests (giving commands). (See bottom of Figure 1.) Patients learn to use up to 23 verb action icons, up to 160 pictures of objects, and five to ten pictures of people, conjunctions, and modifiers for a maximum vocabulary of 240 icons. Criterion for mastery of each verb action icon is reached at 75% (or better) correct use without guidance over two consecutive treatment sessions. Phase II is completed when up to seven different grammatical constructions have been mastered.

The quality of the communications generated by patients using C-ViC in Phase II was rated by the clinician administering the program (EB) using a rating scale based on, but different from, the Porch Index of Communicative Ability (PICA) (Porch, 1967). This eight-point rating scale (VICA, Visual Index of Communicative Ability) ranged from 0 to 7. (See Appendix A.) Phase II VICA ratings greater than 4.5 were considered good C-ViC productions; scores less than 4.5 were considered poor.

CT Scan Acquisition

We have observed that acute CT scans performed less than 3 MPO do not adequately reveal the complete borders of an area of infarction, especially in white matter adjacent to a ventricle (Palumbo, Naeser, Samaraweera, Hodge, & Prete, submitted). These areas are important to examine in relationship to potential for recovery of speech (Naeser, Palumbo, Helm-Estabrooks, Stiassny-Eder, & Albert, 1989). Therefore, all patients underwent non-contrast CT scanning at 3 MPO or later. (See Figure 2.)

CT Scan Analysis Methods

The lesion areas on the CT scan were analyzed using two methods: (1) lesion site analysis and (2) total brain lesion size analysis. Lesion site analysis included visual assessment of each neuroanatomical area (e.g., Broca's area, Wernicke's area, etc.), where presence or absence of lesion, and extent of lesion within that area were determined. The neuroanatomical areas examined were those previously observed to be relevant to outcome with C-ViC (Naeser, Palumbo, Baker, & Nicholas, 1994) and to recovery of speech and comprehension (Alexander, Naeser, & Palumbo, 1987; Naeser, Palumbo, Helm-Estabrooks, Stiassny-Eder, & Albert, 1989; Naeser, Alexander, Helm-Estabrooks, Levine, Laughlin, & Geschwind, 1982; Naeser, Helm-Estabrooks, Haas, Auerbach, & Srinivasan, 1987; Naeser, Gaddie, Palumbo, Stiassny-Eder, 1990). Lesion size analysis included calculation of the percent lesion size across the whole brain.

Lesion Site Analysis

The specific neuroanatomical areas examined for presence or absence of lesion and extent of lesion are diagrammed in Figure 2. The extent of lesion within each area was visually assessed using a 0 to 5 point rating scale where 0 = no lesion, 1 = equivocal lesion, 2 = small, patchy or partial lesion, 3 = lesion in half of that area, 4 = lesion in more than half of that area, and 5 = lesion in that entire area. Lesion extent values greater than 3 (indicating lesion in greater than half of a specific area) are considered to be extensive lesions and have been observed to be associated with more severe language deficits (Naeser et al., 1987; 1989; 1990).

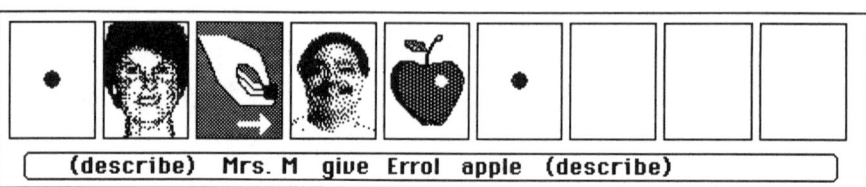

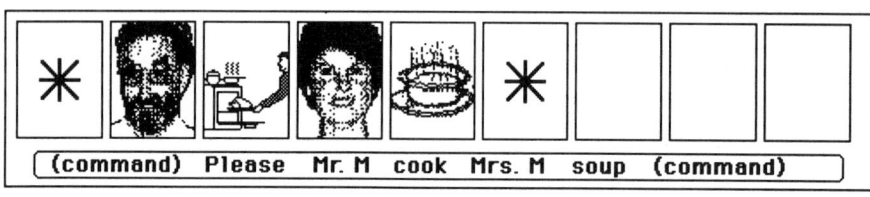

Figure 1. Top: Example of C-ViC communication generated by a severe, nonverbal aphasia patient in Phase I of the C-ViC program. The patient has just given the therapist an apple. The therapist then asked the patient to use C-ViC to compose a description of this simple act. This C-ViC description required the patient to correctly sequence the icons for a sentence requiring subject-verb-indirect object-direct object. The patient's photo, as well as that of the therapist, have been scanned into the computer. Note, the written English is not usually provided below each picture or icon because this tends to confuse the patient who cannot read or write. The written English is provided here only for purposes of illustration. Bottom: Example of C-ViC communication generated by a severe nonverbal aphasia patient in Phase II of the C-ViC program, where real-life communicative acts are taught. In this sentence, the patient is asking her husband to prepare some soup for her. The C-ViC program is customized to individual patient needs, including photographs of family members, pets, hospital staff, etc.

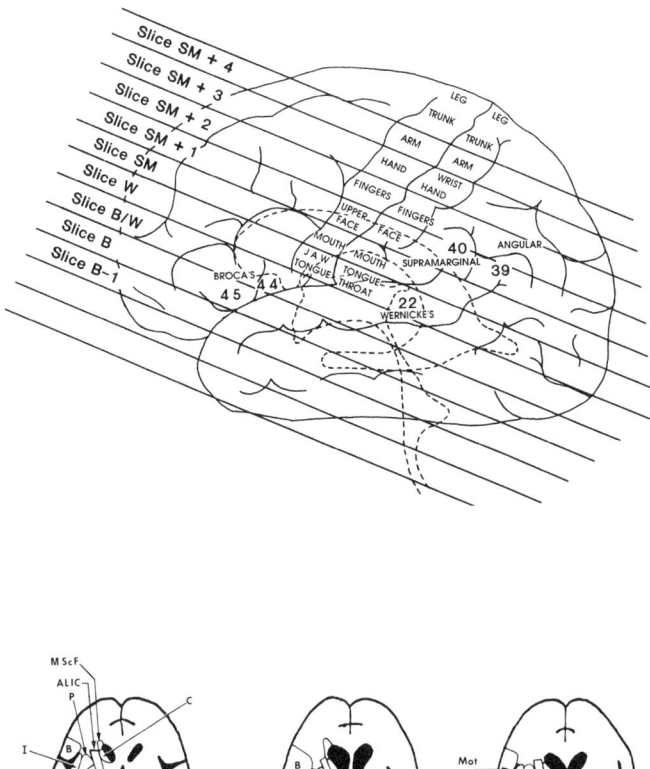
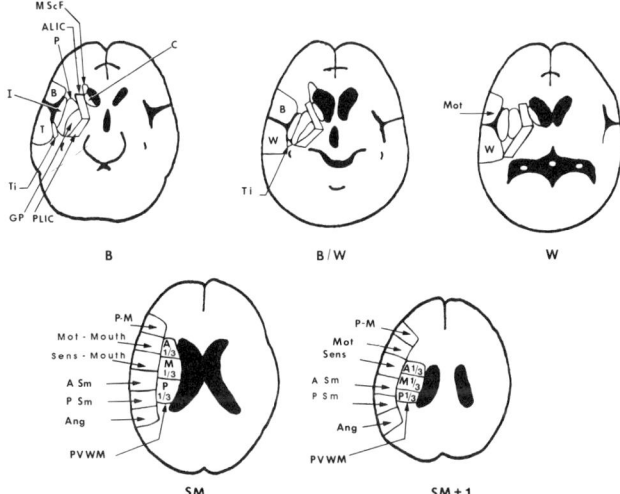

Figure 2. Location of specific neuroanatomical areas on CT scan that were examined for presence or absence of lesion and extent of lesion within that area. Top: lateral view. Bottom: axial view (15 degrees to canthomeatal line) for slices B, B/W, W, SM and SM+1 (Naeser, Palumbo, Helm-Estabrooks, Stiassny-Eder, & Albert, 1989). The CT scan slices are labeled with reference to specific cortical areas present on each slice: B = Broca's; B/W = Broca's and Wernicke's; W = Wernicke's; SM = supramarginal gyrus. Each neuroanatomical area on each slice was visually assessed for extent of lesion using the 0 to 5 point rating scale (0 = no lesion; 3 = half of area has lesion; 5 = entire area has lesion, see text). The areas most relevant to this paper were the following: W = Wernicke's area; Ti = subcortical, anterior temporal isthmus area; MScF = medial subcallosal fasciculus area; M 1/3 PVWM = middle 1/3 periventricular white matter area. See text for additional explanation of these areas.

The CT scans were rated by two experienced raters (MN and CP) and conferenced data were used. Inter-rater reliability coefficients ranged from +0.93 ($p < 0.001$) to +0.97 ($p < 0.001$) (Borod, Carper, Goodglass, & Naeser, 1984; Palumbo, Naeser, Samaraweera, Hodge, & Prete, submitted). CT scan analyses were performed in a blinded manner, without information regarding C-ViC outcome.

Within Area 1, each structure (Wernicke's cortical area and the subcortical temporal isthmus area) was examined separately for extent of lesion using the 0 to 5 point rating scale. Area 2, however, the supraventricular frontal lobe structures (SMA/cingulate gyrus area 24), was assessed only for presence or absence of lesion. The location of white matter pathways originating from these cortical areas is not known, thus, it was not possible to know if lesion was present in greater than, or less than, half of these structures. A plus indicated that visible lesion was present in either the SMA, the supraventricular cingulate gyrus area 24, or white matter deep to them; a minus indicated no visible lesion.

One secondary objective was to define a lesion site pattern which could be identified with candidacy appropriate for C-ViC training – that is, lesion sites compatible with no recovery of meaningful spontaneous speech. Patients who do not recover speech have extensive lesion in two subcortical white matter pathway areas (Naeser, Palumbo, Helm-Estabrooks, Stiassny-Eder, & Albert, 1989): (1) the medial subcallosal fasciculus area (located deep to Broca's area, antero-lateral and adjacent to the left frontal horn), and (2) the middle 1/3 periventricular white matter (PVWM) area (located deep to the motor/sensory cortex area for mouth, lateral and adjacent to the body of the left lateral ventricle).

The medial subcallosal fasciculus area contains, in part, white matter pathways from the SMA and supraventricular cingulate gyrus area 24 to the head of the caudate, and is believed to be important, in part, for initiation of speech. The middle 1/3 PVWM area contains efferent and afferent white matter pathways for the mouth as well as other thalamo-cortical, intra- and interhemispheric pathways believed to be important, in part, for motor/sensory aspects of speech (Naeser, Palumbo, Helm-Estabrooks, Stiassny-Eder, & Albert, 1989). Each of these two areas was visually assessed for extent of lesion using the 0 to 5 point rating scale. The extent-of-lesion rating for the medial subcallosal fasciculus area was assessed at slice B and at slice B/W (Figure 2), and a mean across the two slices was computed. This mean was added to the single extent-of-lesion rating for the middle 1/3 PVWM area at slice SM. Maximum possible summed extent-of-lesion rating for these two areas combined is 10.

Most aphasia patients who have a summed extent-of-lesion rating greater than 7 for these two areas have no recovery of meaningful spontaneous speech (Naeser, Palumbo, Helm-Estabrooks, Stiassny-Eder, & Albert, 1989) – that is, they are likely candidates for C-ViC. Most aphasia patients who have a summed extent-of-lesion rating less than 7 for these two areas have some recovery of meaningful non-fluent speech (Naeser, Palumbo, Helm-Estabrooks, Stiassny-Eder, & Albert, 1989); these patients are candidates for verbal treatment programs (Albert, Sparks, & Helm, 1973; Frumkin, Palumbo, & Naeser, 1994; Sparks & Holland, 1976).

Additional left perisylvian areas examined included frontal operculum (Broca's area), supramarginal gyrus, angular gyrus, and additional areas shown in Figure 2.

Total Lesion Size Analysis

The borders of a lesion (lesion size) were defined as areas of visible low-density signal which were separate from ventricles and fissures. The size of the area of infarction on CT scan was computed in percent of the whole brain for each patient using a program developed by the National Institutes of Health (NIH Image, version 1.57). A MacTablet Summagraphics board was interfaced with a Macintosh IIsi computer and used as follows: (1) The borders of the lesion were manually traced onto the Summagraphics board for each CT scan slice where lesion was present, beginning at the first slice above the suprasellar cistern and continuing, if necessary, to the vertex. These lesion area values were summed for each CT scan. (2) The borders of the inner table of the skull for the whole brain were also manually traced for each CT scan slice beginning at the first slice above the suprasellar cistern and continuing to the vertex. These whole brain area values were summed for each CT scan. (3) The total lesion area value was divided by the total brain area value to yield an approximate percent lesion size in relation to the whole brain. This is a methodology which has been used in our laboratory in previous studies (Naeser et al., 1998b).

If a lesion was also present in the right hemisphere, the borders of that lesion were also traced and recorded. The size of the right-hemisphere lesion was then combined with the size of the left-hemisphere lesion to compute a total percent brain lesion size.

Hemispheric Asymmetries

The CT scan occipital length asymmetries were measured using the method of Pieniadz et al. (Pieniadz, Naeser, Koff, & Levine, 1983). The asymmetries were measured because some global aphasia patients with atypical occipital asymmetry on CT scan (equal or increased right asymmetry) have been observed in the chronic phase post-stroke (after eight months or later post-stroke) to have better recovery at the single word level in comprehension, repetition, or naming compared to global aphasia patients with typical asymmetry on CT scan (left asymmetry) (Pieniadz, Naeser, Koff, & Levine, 1983).

RESULTS

C-ViC Outcome Levels

The outcome levels following Phase II C-ViC training are summarized in the last column in Table 1 (Phase II C-ViC Performance Rating, VICA Rating). Seven patients were able to use C-ViC to initiate communication (Best Response Group). Six patients were not able to use C-ViC to initiate communication, but they were able to use C-ViC to respond to questions posed by others (Moderate Response Group). Four patients were unable to learn to match eight icons on the computer screen to the same eight real objects, skills essential to mastering C-ViC. Therefore, these patients could not enter Phase I of the C-ViC treatment program (No Response Group). Subsequent statistical analyses were performed between the Best and Moderate Response Groups.

Table 2 shows that there were no significant differences between the Best and Moderate Response Groups regarding age at entering C-ViC training, MPO at entering C-ViC training, or in the total number of weeks the patients received C-ViC training. There was a trend for the No Response cases to be older than the other two groups regarding age at stroke onset ($p = 0.06$).

Table 3 summarizes statistical comparisons between the two groups during C-ViC training. There was variability among subjects and a tendency for the data to be skewed, therefore, medians were computed and comparisons were carried out using the Mann-Whitney U-test. The Best Response Group required significantly fewer sessions to complete Phase I (median = 7.5 sessions) than the Moderate Response group did (median = 18.5 sessions, $p = 0.004$). The two groups were nearly identical in number of sessions in Phase II. However, Best Response cases mastered an average of 20.8 verb action icons, while Moderate Response cases mastered only 12 verb action icons ($p = 0.02$). The number of sessions necessary to reach a common criterion point (12 verb action icons, a number reached by 12/13 of the subjects) was a median of 28 sessions for the Best Response Group and 69 for the Moderate Response Group ($p = 0.004$).

Table 4 shows that all Best and Moderate Response cases had only a unilateral left-hemisphere lesion while the four patients with No Response had bilateral lesions. Subsequent testing on lesion site patterns was performed only between the Best and Moderate Response cases.

Discriminant Function Analyses

Hypotheses were tested utilizing discriminant function analysis. Resulting group identification decision matrices were tested for significance by means of the Odds Ratio method. The first hypothesis tested the validity of our original neuroanatomical model where Areas 1 and 2 were included. Because the extent-of-lesion data for Area 2 were always in a categorical format (plus or minus), the extent-of-lesion data for Area 1 were converted to a plus or minus. If the extent-of-lesion rating was greater than 3 (lesion in greater than half), for either Wernicke's area or the temporal isthmus area, then Area 1 was rated a plus; less than 3 or equal was rated a minus. (See Table 4 *Summary Area 1*.)

Testing of the Original Hypothesis

The first discriminant analysis was carried out by forcing in the categorical data for Areas 1 and 2. While 7/7 subjects with Best Response were correctly identified, 3/6 subjects with Moderate Response (RP, ND, WT) were mis-classified

Table 2. Unpaired *t*-Test Results: Two-tailed for Best Response Group versus Moderate Response Group regarding C-ViC treatment time, and BASA scores prior to entering C-ViC treatment.

	Best Response Group		Moderate Response Group		*t*-Value	*p*-Level
	Mean (SD)	Range	Mean (SD)	Range		
Age Entering C-ViC	56.3 (13.1)	42-77	59.0 (7.5)	47-69	0.45	0.66
Months Post-stroke Onset Entering C-ViC *	25	10-120	27	7-77	z = 0.57	0.57
Total Weeks in C-ViC Treatment	42.1 (38.5)	4-99	45.7 (33.5)	17-104	0.18	0.86
Pre C-ViC, BASA Scores:						
Auditory Comprehension	13.3 (2.2)	10-16	9.5 (3.0)	5-12	2.53	0.03
Oral/Gestural	7.2 (4.3)	1-12	6.7 (4.3)	2-12	0.20	0.84
Overall Score	42.3 (3.8)	39-49	31.2 (9.7)	15-43	2.66	0.02

*The average reported here is a median; and the Mann–Whitney U-Test is reported.

Table 3. Mann-Whitney U-Test Results for Best Response Group versus Moderate Response Group regarding Phase I and Phase II C-ViC Training.

	Best Response Group		Moderate Response Group		z-Score	p-Level
	Median	Range	Median	Range		
Total Sessions to Complete Phase I C-ViC Training	7.5	3-14	18.5	11-22	2.86	0.004
Total Sessions to Complete Phase II C-ViC Training	66	13-126	78	47-94	0.245	0.81
Total Number of Verb Action Icons Learned in C-ViC Training	20.8	15-23	12	12-20	2.36	0.02
Number of Sessions to Learn 12 Verb Action Icons in Phase II	28	9-37	69	42-82	2.88	0.004

Table 4. Lesion site data (extent-of-lesion ratings, 0 = no lesion, 5 = entire area has lesion) for 17 severe aphasia patients treated with the C-ViC program.

C-ViC Outcome group	Patient Id.	CT Scan MPO	Right-Hemisphere Lesion	Area 1 Wernicke's Area	(Temporal Lobe) Temporal Isthmus Area	Summary Area 1	Area 2 SMA/Cing. G. Area 24	Original Hypothesis, Correct Outcome Predicted?	Med. Subc. Fasc. Area	Middle 1/3 PVWM Area	Summed Lesion, Med. Subc. Fasc. + Middle 1/3 PVWM	Total Brain Lesion Size, Percent	Occip. Length Asymn.
Best Response	JH	21	-	1.5	5	+	-	Yes	5	4.9	9.9	5.0	R
	PS	9y9m	-	1	1.75	-	+	Yes	5	4.75	9.75	15.2	L
	AC	17	-	4.55	5	+	-	Yes	4.3	4.9	9.27	15.4	L
	FM	23	-	0	4	+	-	Yes	4.38	4.25	8.63	11.9	L
	BM	14	-	4.63	3.88	+	-	Yes	0	4.99	4.99	8.5	L
	JC	17	-	3.67	5	+	-	Yes	0	3.5	3.5	6.8	L
	LM	25	-	2	4.75	+	-	Yes	3.75	3.75	7.5	7.4	L
Moderate Response	RR	43	-	3.87	4	+	+	Yes	5*	4	9.0	11.8	L
	AP	89	-	5	5	+	+	Yes	4.95	4.95	9.9	32.5	=
	RP	18	-	4	5	+	-	No (BR)[a]	4	4	8.0	13.4	L
	TS	11	-	4.67	5	+	+	Yes	5*	4.95	9.95	19.7	L
	ND	9	-	2.37	5	+	-	No (BR)[b]	2.25	4.85	7.1	8.4	L
	WT	28	-	4.63	3.88	+	-	No (BR)[c]	3.63	4	7.63	15.8	L
No Response	BG	3	+[d]	2	5	+	+	Bi-lateral	5	4.5	9.5	14.0	L
	DM	13	+[e]	4.92	5	+	-	Bi-lateral	2.38	4.95	7.33	12.7	L
	HR	8	+[f]	4.87	5	+	-	Bi-lateral	5	4.9	9.9	20.2	L
	DT	12.5	+[g]	1	3.5	+	-	Bi-lateral	3.5	4	7.5	11.9	L

a L occipital lesion, not present in other cases. (BR = Best Response predicted)
b Flat affect, severe depression, not present in other cases, never showed emotional improvement following mastery of Phase I C-ViC training.
c Medically ill, multiple infections; died a few months after discharge from Phase II C-ViC training.
d Small R frontal, small R parietal.
e R lower motor cortex, R lacune, anterolateral to the frontal horn.
f R frontal lacune, R extreme capsule and claustrum.
g R occipital.
* No lesion in the medial subcallosal fasciculus area, however extensive lesion was present at the origin of this pathway (SMA/Cingulate G. Area 24) Thus, the lesion extent rating of 5 was used here.

as Best Response (Odds Ratio = 8, p = 0.205, two-tailed). (See column in Table 4 *Original Hypothesis, Correct Outcome Predicted?*) All seven Best Response cases had extensive lesion in only one of the two critical areas. (See Figures 3 and 4.) The 3/6 Moderate Response cases who were correctly identified each had extensive lesion in both Areas 1 and 2. (See Figure 5.) Although there may be post-hoc explanations for the three Moderate Response cases mis-classified as Best Response (RP, ND, WT, Notes, Table 4), these results prompted additional discriminant analyses.

Testing of Additional Neuroanatomical Hypotheses

There were two concerns with the results from the first discriminant analysis based on the original hypothesis. First, the procedure weighted Wernicke's cortical area and the subcortical temporal isthmus area equally. Second, the extent-of-lesion ratings for these two temporal lobe structures (Wernicke's area and the temporal isthmus area) were treated as categorical, although extent-of-lesion data were available for each area. Therefore, a second discriminant analysis was carried out using three variables: Wernicke's area and the temporal isthmus area as two separate quantitative variables, and the SMA/cingulate gyrus area 24 as one categorical variable. When these three structures were each considered, one patient with Best Response was mis-classified (AC), and two patients with Moderate Response were mis-classified (ND, WT) (Odds Ratio = 12, p = 0.10, two-tailed).

Two additional discriminant analyses were carried out with the latter three variables plus one additional extent-of-lesion variable. When lesion for the middle 1/3 PVWM area was added to the three variables, the discriminant analysis became less reliable, mis-classifying four subjects: two with Best Response (JC, AC) and two with Moderate Response (ND, WT) (Odds Ratio = 6, p = 0.22). However, when lesion for the medial subcallosal fasciculus area was forced in with the three variables (Wernicke's area, temporal isthmus area, and SMA/cingulate gyrus area 24), the prediction rate became highly significant, mis-classifying only two subjects: one with Best Response (AC) and one with Moderate Response (ND) (Odds Ratio = 30, p = 0.029).

Each No Response case had bilateral lesions. Analysis of the left-hemisphere lesion alone would have predicted Best Response for cases DM, HR, and DT (extensive lesion only in Area 1), and Moderate Response for case BG (Areas 1 and 2). With additional right-hemisphere lesion, the predicted effect of the left-hemisphere lesion site patterns alone was not valid.

Lesion Site Patterns in Relationship to Absence of Recovery of Speech

Patients who have no recovery of meaningful spontaneous speech usually have summed extent-of-lesion rating greater than 7 for the medial subcallosal fasciculus area plus the middle 1/3 PVWM area (Naeser, Palumbo, Helm-Estabrooks, Stiassny, & Albert, 1989). Table 4 shows that 15 of the 17 cases in the present study (88.2%) had summed extent-of-lesion ratings greater than 7.0 (range 7.1 to 9.9). The two cases who had ratings less than 7.0, compatible with recovery of non-fluent speech, were cases BM (4.99) and JC (3.5). Case BM recovered to a phrase

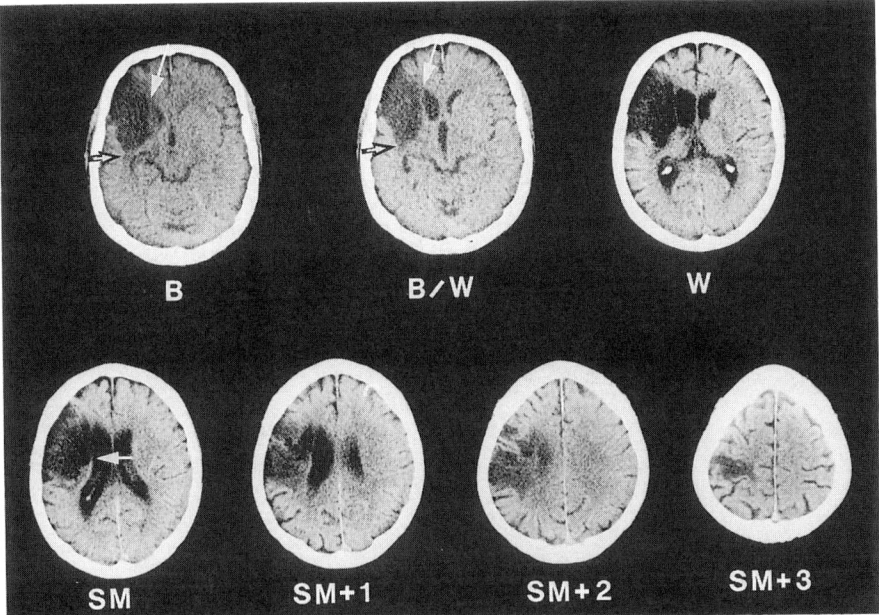

Figure 3. CT scan for Best Response case FM who entered the C-ViC program at 21 MPO. Extensive lesion was present only in one of the two areas relevant to outcome level with C-ViC training. Extensive lesion was present in Area 1 (temporal lobe structures). Black and white arrows on slices B and B/W indicate extensive lesion in the temporal isthmus area. No lesion was present in Wernicke's cortical area, located lateral to the third ventricle (slices B/W and W). No lesion was present in Area 2 (supraventricular frontal lobe structures, SMA/cingulate gyrus area 24). See slice SM+3. The lesion site pattern associated with no recovery of spontaneous speech and appropriate candidacy for C-ViC training was present – that is, extensive lesion in the MScF area, adjacent and antero-lateral to the left frontal horn, on slices B and B/W (white arrows), and in the M 1/3 PVWM area, adjacent and lateral to the body of the lateral ventricle, on slice SM (white arrow). CT scan is 23 MPO.

132 Neurobehavior of Language and Cognition

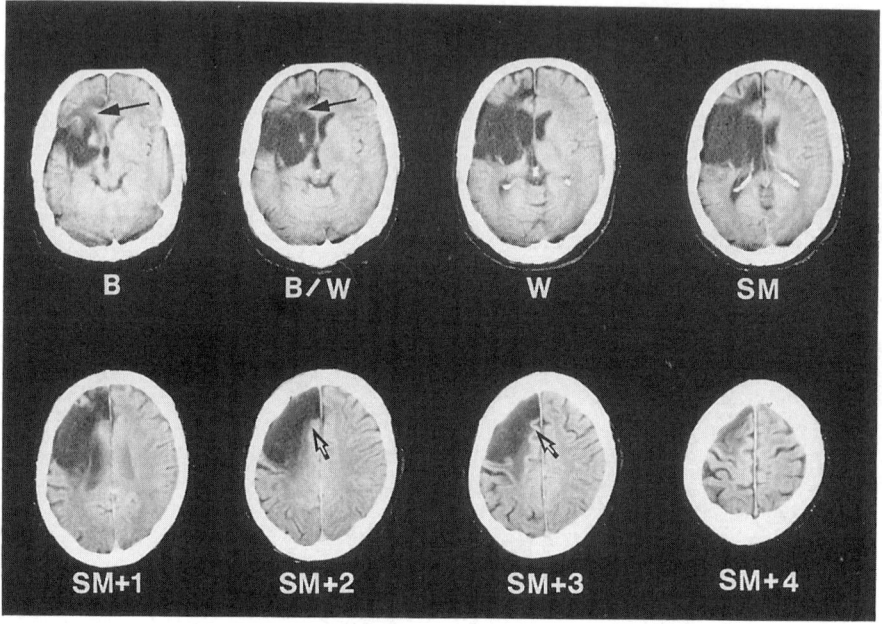

Figure 4. CT scan for Best Response case PS who entered the C-ViC program at 10 years post-stroke. Extensive lesion was present only in one of the two areas relevant to outcome level with C-ViC training. Extensive lesion was present in Area 2 (supraventricular frontal lobe structures, SMA/cingulate gyrus area 24, deep white matter). See slices SM+2 and SM+3 (black and white arrows). In Area 1 (temporal lobe structures) only small, patchy lesion was present in the temporal isthmus on slice B. Only minimal, equivocal lesion was present in Wernicke's cortical area, located lateral to the third ventricle (slices B/W and W). The lesion site pattern associated with no recovery of spontaneous speech and appropriate candidacy for C-ViC training was present, extensive lesion in the MScF area, adjacent and antero-lateral to the left frontal horn, on slices B and B/W (black arrows), and in the M 1/3 PVWM area, adjacent and lateral to the body of the lateral ventricle, on slice SM (black arrow). CT scan is 9 years, 9 months post-stroke onset.

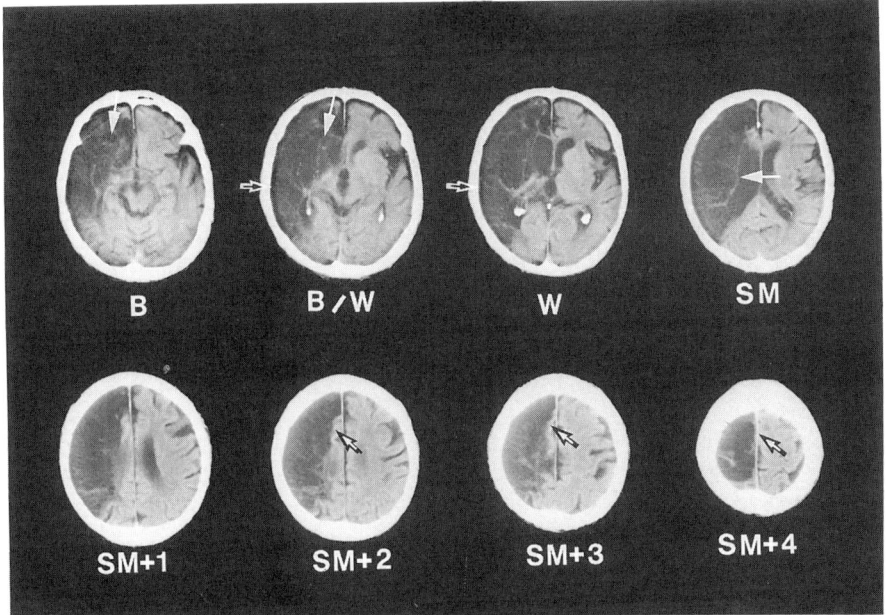

Figure 5. CT scan for Moderate Response case AP who entered the C-ViC program at 6.5 years post-stroke. Extensive lesion was present in both of the two areas relevant to outcome level with C-ViC training. Extensive lesion was present in Area 1 (temporal lobe structures). Black and white arrows on slices B/W and W indicate extensive lesion in Wernicke's cortical area, located lateral to the third ventricle. Extensive lesion was also present in the temporal isthmus. Extensive lesion was also present in Area 2 (supraventricular frontal lobe structures, SMA/cingulate gyrus area 24, cortical and deep white matter). See slices SM+2, SM+3, and SM+4 (black and white arrows). The lesion site pattern associated with no recovery of spontaneous speech and appropriate candidacy for C-ViC training was present – that is, extensive lesion in the MScF area on slices B and B/W, adjacent and antero-lateral to the left frontal horn (white arrows), and in the M 1/3 PVWM area on slice SM, adjacent and lateral to the body of the lateral ventricle (white arrow). CT scan is 7.4 years post-stroke onset.

length of three words (he received some therapy focusing on improving verbal expression concurrently with C-ViC); case JC had no recovery of speech.

Unexpectedly, two other cases did recover some speech, despite summed extent-of-lesion ratings greater than 7.0, compatible with no recovery of speech (JH, 9.9; AC, 9.27). Case JH was transferred to a verbal treatment program and has a phrase length of five to six words; case AC has a phrase length of three words.

Overall, 14 of the 17 cases (82.3%) had the level of speech expected from their lesion site patterns. The majority of cases (15/17, 88.2%) had summed extent-of-lesion ratings compatible with absence of recovery of speech, and the majority of these latter cases (13/15, 86.6%) were appropriate candidates for nonverbal C-ViC training.

Total Lesion Size

Analysis of variance showed no significant difference in lesion size between the Best Response ($M = 10.0\%$, $SD = 4.2$), Moderate Response ($M = 16.9\%$, $SD = 8.5$), and No Response ($M = 14.7\%$, $SD = 3.8$) groups, $F(2, 14) = 2.21$, $p = 0.15$. In addition, a post hoc Scheffé comparison showed no significant difference between the Best Response and Moderate Response groups ($p = 0.16$).

Hemispheric Asymmetries

The majority of cases had typical left occipital length asymmetry (15/17 cases). The single case with atypical right occipital length asymmetry (JH) had an unexpected recovery of nonfluent speech, despite a lesion site pattern compatible with no recovery of meaningful speech.

BASA Scores Prior to C-ViC Treatment

BASA scores prior to C-ViC training were available for six Best, six Moderate, and three No Response cases (Table 1). The Best Response Group had significantly better BASA auditory comprehension subscores ($p = 0.03$) and overall BASA scores ($p = 0.02$) than the Moderate Response Group (Table 2). There were too few subjects in the No Response Group for statistical comparisons.

The BASA scores were subjected to discriminant function analyses for Best Response and Moderate Response to determine whether they could be used to predict C-ViC outcome. When the auditory comprehension subscore was entered, four subjects were mis-classified: one Best Response (AC) and three Moderate Response (RR, AP, RP; Odds Ratio = 5, $p = 0.545$). When the oral-gestural communication subscore was entered, six subjects were mis-classified: three Best Response (JH, AC, BM) and three Moderate Response (RR, AP, RP; Odds Ratio = 1, $p = 0.99$). When the overall BASA score was entered, however, only one subject was mis-classified, case RR from the Moderate Response Group (Odds Ratio = 25, $p = 0.04$).

The median cut-off overall BASA score for Best Response was 38 (range 39 to 49 out of a possible 61). Five of the six Moderate Response cases had overall

BASA scores of less than 38 (range 15 to 36; one patient had a score of 43, case RR). (See Table 1.)

The three No Response cases had overall BASA scores which fell within the range of both Best and Moderate Response. Case DT had a BASA score of 41 (Best Response, greater than 38), and cases DM and HR each had overall BASA scores of 20 and 30 (5/6 Moderate Response cases, 15 to 36).

DISCUSSION

This study tested the validity of a previously identified lesion site hypothesis to predict outcome level following C-ViC training. When the original lesion site hypothesis was modified to include not only the two original areas, Area 1, temporal lobe structures (Wernicke's area and the temporal isthmus area) and Area 2, supraventricular frontal lobe structures (SMA/cingulate gyrus area 24), but also the medial subcallosal fasciculus area, 6/7 of the Best Response cases and 5/6 of the Moderate Response cases were correctly classified with discriminant function analysis. Most Best Response cases had extensive lesion in only one of the two original critical areas, whereas most Moderate Response cases had extensive lesion in both of the two original areas.

The effect of the additional factor, extent of lesion within the medial subcallosal fasciculus area, is not completely understood in relationship to outcome level with C-ViC. For example, 5/7 Best Response cases and 5/6 Moderate Response cases had extensive lesion in the medial subcallosal fasciculus area. However, two Best Response cases had no lesion in the medial subcallosal fasciculus area and this factor may have been considered to be important in the discriminant function analysis when it was included. Lesion in the medial subcallosal fasciculus area could have an additive effect to interruption of the initiation/limbic pathways from the SMA/cingulate gyrus area 24, to the head of the caudate, deep to Broca's area. However, since five cases with extensive lesion in the medial subcallosal fasciculus area had Best Response with C-ViC, it would be difficult to apply this additional lesion factor in a practical manner in the clinic when predicting outcome level with C-ViC.

The original lesion site pattern associated with Best Response to C-ViC (ability to initiate communication with C-ViC) is one which spares large portions of either the posterior systems or the anterior systems involved in language recovery. Sparing of posterior systems, including Area 1 (Wernicke's cortical area or the temporal isthmus area), may allow enough preservation of structures in the left hemisphere that pictorial representations used in C-ViC can gain access to semantic meaning. Sparing of anterior systems, including Area 2 (SMA/cingulate gyrus area 24), may allow enough frontal callosal pathways to be preserved that the overall frontal capacity to learn and execute a novel system is possible (Petrides & Milner, 1982).

It is also possible that sparing of anterior systems has a specific initiation/limbic effect (Jurgens, 1984). If enough frontal medial limbic structures (including the SMA) are preserved, then the patients can probably initiate access to a semantic system if they have one that is intact (perhaps either in the left posterior temporo-parietal area or in the right hemisphere). That the patients with Moderate Response could use C-ViC to respond to questions, but not to initiate interaction, suggests that Moderate Response was related more to initiation and utilization rather than to semantic production capacity. This would be compatible with an initiation/limbic explanation, not a frontal capacity account. In summary, extensive lesion in both anterior systems and posterior systems is compatible with only Moderate Response to C-ViC.

The pre-C-ViC overall BASA score also showed significance in predicting outcome level with C-ViC, where 6/6 Best Response cases and 5/6 Moderate Response cases were correctly predicted. The incorrect prediction involved Moderate Response case RR, whose overall BASA score was 43 (a score greater than 38, and therefore compatible with Best Response to C-ViC) although only Moderate Response was observed. This Moderate Response outcome in case RR was correctly predicted, however, from the CT scan lesion site data using the original hypothesis. The original hypothesis lesion site data had mis-classified three Moderate Response cases as Best Response, however, their BASA scores were less than 38 (RP, 36; ND, 27; and WT, 30), thus, compatible with the observed Moderate Response.

A practical clinical method of predicting C-ViC outcome is proposed from these two data sets combined. If both BASA data (overall score greater than 38) and lesion site data (extensive lesion, in Area 1 or 2) are compatible with Best Response, then Best Response is likely. If both BASA data (overall score less than 38) and lesion site data (extensive lesion, in Areas 1 and 2) are compatible with only Moderate Response, then Moderate Response is likely. However, if either one of these data sets (lesion site data or overall BASA score) is compatible with only Moderate Response, then Moderate Response is likely. Both neuroanatomical and behavioral data appear to be necessary for optimal prediction.

This study also examined lesion site patterns in relationship to absence of recovery of speech, thus, likely candidacy for entry into C-ViC training. The basic lesion site pattern associated with absence of recovery of speech (extent-of-lesion ratings which total greater than 7.0 for the medial subcallosal fasciculus area plus the middle 1/3 PVWM area) was observed in 88% of the 17 cases referred for C-ViC in this study; and 87% of patients in this latter group did not recover meaningful spontaneous speech. Hence, the lesion site pattern associated with absence of recovery of meaningful spontaneous speech is also appropriate for candidacy for C-ViC training.

Most patients without speech who have bilateral lesions, however, do not appear to be good candidates for C-ViC training, although some exceptions will occur.

In addition, the issue of hemispheric asymmetries (potential for anomalous dominance for language) was examined. One patient in the present study had atypical right occipital length asymmetry (case JH). He had recovery of some non-fluent speech, which was otherwise not expected from his lesion site pattern. This phenomenon was also observed in our previous study (Naeser, Palumbo, Baker, & Nicholas, 1994), where one case recovered nonfluent speech, despite a lesion site pattern compatible with no recovery of speech. That patient (BJ) was left-handed, aphasic from a left-hemisphere lesion and had equal occipital length on CT scan. Each of these two cases, however, was also young at the time of stroke onset, age 34 for case JH, and age 43 for case BJ. Each of these two cases also had a lesion site pattern which was compatible with Best Response to C-ViC. Hence, there may have been multiple factors that contributed to excellent response with C-ViC, and some speech recovery.

This unusual recovery of some speech may be related to a gradual involvement of the right hemisphere. Recovery of word comprehension in global aphasia may continue for years (Sarno & Levita, 1981) and it has been hypothesized that this recovery may reflect the gradual involvement of right-hemisphere semantic systems in comprehension in chronic aphasia patients (Gazzaniga & Hillyard, 1971; Zaidel, 1976; 1977). A gradual pattern of improvement in naming ability (despite left-hemisphere lesion size expansion) after five to 15 years post-stroke has also been observed (Fitzpatrick, Glosser, & Helm-Estabrooks, 1988; Naeser et al., 1998b). The systems involved in this long-term recovery are not known. A recent PET study with recovery in Wernicke's aphasia has observed a bilateral network to be important in functional reorganization of the language system after stroke (Weiller, et al., 1995).

Nonverbal aphasia patients with severe deficits at one month post-onset have a bleak prognosis for recovery of useful language output (Alexander & LoVerso, 1991). The results from the present study suggest that if a severe aphasia patient has had no recovery of meaningful spontaneous speech by three months post-stroke, a non-contrast CT scan plus a speech/language evaluation with the BASA are likely to provide predictive information that may be useful for long-term treatment planning. However, it has been our clinical experience with over 30 severe nonverbal aphasia patients that many are not ready for C-ViC training until approximately nine months post-stroke. Thus, CT scan and BASA could be obtained at that later time.

CT scans are currently our first choice for structural imaging in chronic aphasia patients where lesion site analysis regarding potential for long-term recovery and treatment planning will be performed. We have attempted to apply our lesion site analysis to MR scans. However, the T1-weighted MR images tend to underestimate the extent of the lesion near ventricle, and the T2-weighted MR images tend to overestimate the extent of the lesion near ventricle as compared to CT (Naeser & Palumbo, 1990). The lesion site analysis used in this research requires analysis of white matter areas adjacent to ventricle (at the frontal horn and body of the lateral ventricle). Therefore, specific lesion site analysis on CT scans is preferred at this time.

A study on the cost-effectiveness of the C-ViC treatment program and its impact on functional communication for severe aphasia patients is in progress. There are currently five patients using the C-ViC system outside the therapy setting. The C-ViC computer program is in the public domain and available through EB. The cost of a personal computer (less than $2,000) and the cost of twice-weekly treatment sessions for a 6 to 12 month period, comprise the major costs. The refinement provided in the present study (C-ViC candidacy and predicted outcome level) suggests that future cost-savings could be appreciated with severe nonverbal aphasia patients, in part, through timely intervention with an appropriate nonverbal treatment program likely to promote increased communication ability, versus long-term intervention with inappropriate verbal treatment programs where no increased communication ability is likely to be observed. The role of augmentative and alternative communication devices in rehabilitation of severe aphasia patients has been reviewed by Kraat (1990). She suggests that these devices show promise, but direct application needs refinement. The present study is one approach toward that refinement.

ACKNOWLEDGMENTS

The authors would like to acknowledge the invaluable assistance of Patricia Fitzpatrick, Ph.D. for assistance in data collection. We also thank the Radiology Service of the Boston V. A. Medical Center including Drs. M. E. Gale and A. Robbins, and the Medical Media Service, Boston V. A. Medical Center for photography and illustrations (John Dyke and Kathleen Burns).

This research was supported in part by the Medical Research Service of the Department of Veterans Affairs and by NIDCD Grant DC00081.

APPENDIX A

The VICA (Visual Index of Communicative Ability) Rating Scale used to assess the quality of C-ViC sentences generated by the nonverbal patient using icons on a personal computer.

7 Accurate; reliable; confident (quick); no feedback
6 Accurate (some guidance); confident; minimal on-line feedback
5 Accurate (some guidance); slow; minimal on-line feedback
4 Correct with guidance and cueing; mostly semantic errors (e.g., choose incorrect icon in correct category); reduced on-line feedback
3 Some guessing and/or perseveration; some guidance or cueing provided; mostly semantic but some syntactic errors (e.g., wrong icon order, wrong action icon resulting in syntactic error); reduced on-line feedback
2 Some guessing and/or perseveration; strong guidance or cueing provided; syntactic errors as frequent as semantic errors; reliance on constant on-line feedback (positive and negative)
1 Considerable guessing and/or perseveration; strong guidance or cueing provided; constant repetition of target item required; rote behavior; mostly syntax errors; heavy reliance on on-line feedback, especially negative
No response at all; unable to perform at all on own; constant guidance or overt demonstration for each movement required

REFERENCES

Albert, M. L., Sparks, R., & Helm N. (1973). Melodic intonation therapy for aphasia. *Archives of Neurology, 29*, 130-131.

Alexander, M. P. & LoVerso, F. (1991). *A specific treatment for global aphasia.* Paper presented at the Clinical Aphasiology Conference, Sandestin, FL.

Alexander, M. P., Naeser, M. A., & Palumbo, C. L. (1987). Correlations of subcortical CT lesion sites and aphasia profiles. *Brain, 110,* 961-991.

Baker, E. H., Berry, T., Gardner, H., Zurif, E., Davis, L., & Veroff, A. (1975). Can linguistic competence be dissociated from natural language functions? *Nature, 254,* 609-619.

Baker, E. H. & Nicholas, M. Method: Computer assisted Visual Communication (C-ViC) treatment program for severe nonverbal aphasia patients. Submitted for publication.

Borod, J. C., Carper, M., Goodglass, H., & Naeser, M. A. (1984). Aphasic performance on a battery of constructional, visuospatial, and quantitative tasks: Factorial structure and CT scan localization. *Journal of Clinical Neuropsychology, 6,* 189-204.

Collins, M. (1986). *Diagnosis and treatment of global aphasia.* San Diego: College Hill Press.

Fitzpatrick, P., Glosser, G., & Helm-Estabrooks, N. (1988). Long term recovery of linguistic and nonlinguistic functions in aphasia. Poster presented at the Academy of Aphasia, Montreal, Canada.

Frumkin, N. L., Palumbo, C. L., & Naeser, M. A. (1994). Brain imaging and its application to aphasia rehabilitation: CT and MRI. In R. Chapey (Ed.), *Language intervention strategies in adult aphasia* (3rd ed., pp. 47-79). Baltimore: Williams & Wilkins.

Gardner, H., Zurif, E. B., Berry, T., & Baker, E. H. (1976). Visual communication in aphasia. *Neuropsychologia, 14,* 275-292.

Gazzaniga, M. S. & Hillyard, S. A. (1971). Language and speech capacity of the right hemisphere. *Neuropsychologia, 9,* 273.

Heilman, K. M., Rothi, L., Campanella, D., & Wolfson, S. (1979). Wernicke's and global aphasia without alexia. *Archives of Neurology, 36,* 129-133.

Helm-Estabrooks, N., Fitzpatrick, P., & Barresi, B. (1982). Visual action therapy for global aphasia. *Journal of Speech and Hearing Disorders, 47,* 385-389.

Helm-Estabrooks, N., Ramsberger, G., Morgan, A., & Nicholas, M. (1989). *Boston Assessment of Severe Aphasia.* San Antonio, TX: Special Press.

Johannsen-Horbach, H., Cegla, B., Mager, U., Schempp, B., & Wallesch, C. (1985). Treatment of chronic global aphasia with a nonverbal communication system. *Brain and Language, 24,* 74-82.

Jurgens, U. (1984). The efferent and afferent connections of the supplementary motor area. *Brain Research, 300,* 63-81.

Kraat, A. W. (1990). Augmentative and alternative communication: Does it have a future in aphasia rehabilitation? *Aphasiology, 4,* 321-338.

Morgan, A. & Helm-Estabrooks, N. (1987). Back to the drawing board: A treatment program for nonverbal aphasic patients. In R. H. Brookshire (Ed.), *Clinical aphasiology conference proceedings* (pp. 64-72). Minneapolis: BRK Publishers.

Naeser, M. A., Alexander, M., Helm-Estabrooks, N., Levine, H. L., Laughlin, S. A., & Geschwind, N. (1982). Aphasia with predominantly subcortical lesion sites: Description of three capsular/putaminal aphasia syndromes. *Archives of Neurology, 39,* 2-14.

Naeser, M. A., Baker, E. H., Palumbo, C. L., Nicholas, M., Alexander, M., Samaraweera, R., Prete, M. N., Hodge, S. M., & Weissman, T. (1998a). Lesion site patterns in severe, nonverbal aphasia to predict outcome with a computer-assisted treatment program. *Archives of Neurology, 55,* 1438-1448.

Naeser, M. A., Gaddie, A., Palumbo, C. L., & Stiassny-Eder, D. (1990). Late recovery of auditory comprehension in global aphasia: Improved recovery observed with subcortical temporal isthmus lesion versus Wernicke's cortical area lesion. *Archives of Neurology, 47,* 425-432.

Naeser, M. A., Helm-Estabrooks, N., Haas, G., Auerbach, S., & Srinivasan, M. (1987). Relationship between lesion extent in "Wernicke's Area" on CT scan and predicting recovery of comprehension in Wernicke's aphasia. *Archives of Neurology, 44,* 73-82.

Naeser, M. A. & Palumbo, C. L. (1990). Neuroimaging and language recovery in stroke. *Journal of Clinical Neurophysiology, 11* (2), 150-174.

Naeser, M.A., Palumbo, C. L., Baker, E. H., & Nicholas, M. L. (1994). CT scan lesion site analysis in severe aphasia: Relationship to no recovery of speech and treatment with the nonverbal Computer-Assisted Visual Communication program (C-ViC). *Seminars in Speech and Language, 15,* 53-70.

Naeser, M. A., Palumbo, C. L., Helm-Estabrooks, N., Stiassny-Eder, D., & Albert, M. L. (1989). Severe non-fluency in aphasia: Role of the medial subcallosal fasciculus plus other white matter pathways in recovery of spontaneous speech. *Brain, 112,* 1-38.

Naeser, M. A., Palumbo, C. L., Prete, M. N., Fitzpatrick, P. M., Mimura, M., Samaraweera, R., & Albert, M. L. (1998b). Visible changes in lesion borders on CT scan after five years poststroke, and long-term recovery in aphasia. *Brain and Language, 62* (1), 1-28.

Palumbo C. L. , Naeser, M. A., Samaraweera, R., Hodge, S. M., Prete, M. N. (submitted for publication). Predicting outcome in aphasia with CT scans performed before two months poststroke versus two-to-six months poststroke. Ph.D. Dissertation, Department of Behavioral Neuroscience, Boston University School of Medicine and Graduate School.

Pieniadz, J. M., Naeser, M. A., Koff, E., & Levine, H. L. (1983). CT scan cerebral hemispheric asymmetry measurements in stroke cases with global aphasia: Atypical asymmetries associated with improved recovery. *Cortex, 19*, 371-391.

Petrides, M. & Milner, B. (1982). Deficits on subject-ordered tasks after frontal- and temporal- lobe lesions in man. *Neuropsychology, 20* (3), 249-262.

Porch, B. E. (1967). *Porch index of communicative ability*. Palo Alto, CA: Consulting Psychologists Press.

Rao, P. & Horner, J. (1980). Non-verbal strategies for functional communication by aphasic adults. In M. Burns & J. Andrews (Eds.), *Neuropathologies of speech and language diagnosis and treatment: Selected papers*. Evanston, IL: Institute for Continuing Professional Education.

Sarno, M. T. & Levita, E. (1981). Some observations on the nature of recovery in global aphasia after stroke. *Brain and Language, 13*, 1-12.

Skelly, M. (1979). *American-Indian gestural code based on universal American Indian hand talk*. New York: Elsevier.

Sparks, R. & Holland A. L. (1976). Method: Melodic intonation therapy for aphasia. *Journal of Speech and Hearing Disorders, 41*, 287-297.

Steele, R. D., Weinrich, M., Wertz, R. T., Kleczewska, M. K., & Carlson, G. S. (1989). Computer- based visual communication in aphasia. *Neuropsychologia, 27*, 409-426.

Velletri-Glass, A., Gazzaniga, M., & Premack, D. (1973). Artificial language training in global aphasics. *Neuropsychologia, 11*, 95-103.

Weiller, C., Isensee, C., Rijntjes, M., Huber, W., Muller, S., Dier, S., Dutschka, K., Woods, R. P., Noth, J., & Diener, H. C. (1995). Recovery from Wernicke's aphasia: A positron emission tomographic study. *Annals of Neurology, 37*, 723-732.

Weinrich, M., Steele, R., Kleczewska, M., Carlson, G. S., Baker, E. H., & Wertz, R. T. (1989). Representation of "verbs" in a computerized visual communication system. *Aphasiology, 3*, 501-512.

Weinrich, M., Steele, R., Carlson, G. S., Kleczewska, M., Wertz, R. T., & Baker, E. H. (1989). Processing of visual syntax in a globally aphasic patient. *Brain and Language, 36*, 391-405.

Zaidel, E. (1976). Auditory vocabulary of the right hemisphere following brain bisection or hemidecortication. *Cortex, 12* (3), 191-211.

COMBINATORIAL OPERATIONS IN SENTENCE COMPREHENSION

Edgar Zurif and Maria Piñango

INTRODUCTION

Our contribution has to do with the neurological organization of some features of language capacity. With respect to the brain part of this characterization, we capitalize quite conventionally on the lesion localizing value of the traditional syndromes from which we gather our linguistic data. Specifically, we focus on the performance differences observed in Broca's and Wernicke's aphasia (Goodglass & Kaplan, 1972); and we use these differences to infer the functional commitments of the different brain regions implicated in these aphasias. Thus, while there is considerable variation in lesion extent for Broca's aphasia, which is associated with large superficial and deep lesions often including but certainly not limited to the frontal operculum (Broca's area), the fact is that the modal lesion site for this form of aphasia is different from the modal posterior region associated with Wernicke's aphasia. (For details see, e.g., Alexander et al., 1990; Benson, 1985; Naeser et al., 1989; Vignolo, 1988.) Moreover, the brain-language correspondences based on the study of lesion effects converge with recent neuroimaging data – with roughly the same grain size and degree of coherence.

As for our linguistic analyses, we focus on the contrast between syntactic and semantic processing; this much is standard. Less standard, however, is the fact that we examine semantics not at the single word level, but rather, at the less studied sentential level. That is, just as with the syntactic system, we study the semantic system within its proper ecological niche (in terms of the operations involved in combining word meanings into contextualized interpretations within sentence boundaries).

Another feature of our work that warrants highlighting has to do with the way in which we distinguish syntactic and semantic operations. We do not rely simply on the fact that the representational formats of these two components are different – that syntax is a system built up out of a hierarchical arrangement of nouns, verbs, adjectives and the like, and semantics, a system based on lexical information about such entities as conceptualized objects, events, properties, times, and quantities. Of course, we start by acknowledging this difference. But we then seek evidence for the uniqueness of syntactic and semantic processing constituents in terms of each of their real-time fixed and mandatory operating characteristics. In effect, we try to reveal the nature of each of these processing systems by taking measurements during the brief course of their operation. Moreover, our analyses of functional lesions in the aphasias are framed in the form of alterations to these real-time operations.

In what follows, we very briefly review some of this work – syntax first, then semantics.

SYNTAX

The first point to emphasize here is that at the level of sentence comprehension, Broca's aphasic patients show a very clear pattern: They understand canonical structures (i.e., structures in which the noun phrase preceding the verb is mapped as the agent, as in active-voice sentences), but they have considerable difficulty understanding non-canonical structures in which the noun phrase preceding the verb is linked, not as the agent of the action, but rather as the entity acted upon or undergoing the action (e.g., as in passive-voice sentences). To be sure, not all Broca's patients show this pattern – no more so than ten coin tosses always yield five heads and five tails. But just as a large set or series of ten coin tosses yields a binomial distribution around five heads and five tails thereby revealing the true nature of the coin, so, too, do the many published reports of comprehension in Broca's aphasia attest to this canonical-noncanonical contrast.

We write confidently about his matter, having just surveyed the literature dealing with comprehension in Broca's aphasia (Grodzinsky, Piñango, & Zurif, in press). In that review, we find that the Broca's patients' comprehension for canonical structures clusters tightly around a performance level that is well above chance (85% out of 42 cases), whereas their comprehension for noncanonical structures clusters tightly around the 50% or chance level of performance. It appears, therefore, that Broca's patients who do not show this canonical-noncanonical contrast must, at least for the present, be considered outliers.[1]

Grodzinsky (1990) and others in our lab and elsewhere (Hickok et al., 1993; Mauner et al., 1993; Piñango, 1998) have captured this contrast in syntactic terms. To be sure, these various efforts do not agree on the precise source of the deficit. So, without entering the matter in detail, one claim is that the problem involves access to information in argument traces (Grodzinsky, 1990; Hickok et al., 1993); another is that it involves the formation of argument chains (Mauner et al., 1993) (both accounts turning on features of syntactic dependencies); and a third proposes that the problem has to do with temporally unconstrained correspondence between argument structure and syntactic functions (Piñango, 1998). What must be

---

[1] This finding is at odds with a so-called meta-analysis recently presented by Berndt, Mitchum, and Haendiges (1996) and for good reason: Berndt et al. failed to restrict subject selection to Broca's aphasics. (Only half of the subjects they selected for their analysis were reported as Broca's patients.) Because of this, they ended up with scattered data (and doubtlessly also, a collection of scattered lesion sites). In addition, the analysis itself was methodologically flawed: Whenever a subject participated in two or more studies, even though the same constructions were used in these studies, Berndt et al. entered that subject as an independent case for each of the studies. Also, all the studies reviewed were given the same weight despite noticeable differences in sample size (trials per construction) and no statistical analyses were carried out beyond binomial tests on each patient's performance on each construction. In short, Berndt et al. did not carry out a meta-analysis, but rather an incomplete analysis on aphasic patients of different diagnoses.

emphasized, however, is that all these generalizations agree that the deficit is both minimal and syntactic in nature.

Building on this insight, a number of us have taken the syntactic pattern a step further by linking it to a real-time processing disruption that manifests itself as an inability to establish dependency relations (Swinney et al., 1996; Zurif et al., 1993). A dependency relation can be conceived as a connection between the position where a constituent (a noun phrase) is heard in a sentence and the position where it is interpreted, such as in the following sentence: (1) This is the cat_i that Tom, still in his pajamas, chased (*the cat*)$_i$ last night. In (1) the noun phrase, "the cat" is heard at the beginning of the sentence, but its interpretation, that is, its thematic role as *chasee*, is only obtained further down the sentence, where the verb "chased" is realized. We signal where "the cat" is putatively interpreted by recopying "the cat" in italics. (But, of course, this copy is a hypothetical construct; "the cat" is only heard once.) We call the relation between the noun phrase "the cat" and the position following the verb (i.e., the gap), a dependency relation because of the necessary connection that must exist between this gap position (where interpretation takes place) and the noun phrase (also called the *antecedent*) for the sentence to be semantically well-formed.[2]

Research on real-time comprehension has shown – via the investigation of the processes that take place in the moment-by-moment unfolding of the comprehension of an utterance – that, whereas neurologically intact subjects readily form this kind of dependency relation, Broca's patients are not able to do so. By contrast, Wernicke's patients, quite surprisingly, do seem able to form this linking operation in real-time (Zurif et al., 1993; Swinney et al., 1996).

How has this been shown? By the use of *priming* – a low-tech, but highly reliable method for charting word activation (e.g., Neely, 1977). So, if the word *cat* is followed by a related word *dog* in one instance and an unrelated work *bank* in another, the processing of *dog* will be seen to be facilitated relative to *bank* – it will take less time, for example, to decide that *dog* is a word than that *bank* is a word. And this result has been taken to indicate that the meaning of the preceding word *cat* has been activated to facilitate the processing of all words (including *dog*) within its semantic/associative network.

Consider now the case of *cat* embedded in our earlier sentence, "This is the cat_i (1) that Tom, still in his pajamas (2) chased (cat_i) (3) last night." Again, the subscript *i* shows the syntactic dependency existing between *cat* and the gap. The superscripts here show the locations of the probe sites – i.e., the sites at which the experimenter examines whether the word *cat* has been activated. And when this sentence is spoken in a normal fashion, what routinely happens is that lexical decisions for *dog* are faster than for *bank* at positions (1) and (3), but not at position (2). In the normal case then, the meaning of *cat* is active just after it is heard in the sentence; it is no longer active several seconds after it is heard; and it is active again at the gap – i.e., it has been reactivated at the gap. To state the matter simply, the

---

[2] Contrast (1) with (2): This is the cat_i that Tom, still in his pajamas, chased the dog last night. Sentence (2) is ungrammatical precisely because "the cat" cannot be interpreted as the object of chase as there is another noun phrase in that position, "the dog." As a result, "the cat" is left without a thematic role – it is uninterpretable in the context of the sentence – thus rendering the sentence ungrammatical.

gap has been "filled" – the syntactic dependency has been formed on-line, and we thereby isolate an evanescent syntactic operation (e.g., Swinney & Fodor, 1989).

It is this fleeting operation that Wernicke's patients carry out but that Broca's patients do not. And note, the success of this operation cannot be inferred just by examining comprehension end-points. Wernicke's patients link antecedents and gaps both for canonical and noncanonical structures, even though they have problems understanding both. Broca's patients, by contrast, do not show gap-filling, even for sentences that they do routinely understand (e.g., actives and subject relatives) (Swinney et al., 1996; Zurif et al., 1993).

It appears then that the description given to the comprehension deficit in Broca's aphasia does not seem to apply to the comprehension limitations of Wernicke's aphasic patients. This is also because, in addition to showing an impaired performance across-the-board, Wernicke's patients often choose semantically inappropriate foils in picture matching tasks, unlike Broca's patients who choose only syntactically inappropriate foils (e.g., Caramazza & Zurif, 1976; Heilman & Scholes, 1976). In effect, it would appear that whatever syntactic limitations Wernicke's patients exhibit in their comprehension, their problem seems also to require a consideration of semantic factors.

From a functional localization perspective, this contrast in performance between Broca's and Wernicke's aphasic patients suggests that damage to the left anterior region of the brain associated with Broca's aphasia disrupts syntactic processing in a way that posterior damage associated with Wernicke's aphasia does not. But this should not be taken to mean that the brain area implicated in Broca's aphasia is necessarily devoted to syntactic competence or knowledge. Rather, it seems to be committed to the syntactic reflex of gap-filling only to the extent that it provides some of the resources that sustain this fast-acting, evanescent stage of sentence processing. There exists independent evidence that quite apart from sentence processing, Broca's patients generally show slower-than-normal processing of words (Prather et al., 1992; Prather et al., 1997). And given their inability to activate lexical information in the normal time frame, it is natural to suppose that gap-filling – with its heavy temporal imperatives – is especially vulnerable.

SEMANTICS

Since semantic operations are temporally less demanding than syntactic operations (McElree & Griffith, 1995), a delay in the availability of lexical information sufficient to disrupt syntactic gap-filling need not also affect semantic processing. And this is borne out: Broca's patients do not have problems at the semantic level. In particular, they do not have problems carrying out compositional semantic work. Wernicke's patients, by contrast, do have such problems (Piñango & Zurif, 1998).

We have focused, in this respect, on a combinatorial lexical-semantic operation termed aspectual coercion – an operation known to be locally compositional, mandatory, and purpose specific (Jackendoff, 1997; Pustejovsky, 1995). Briefly, this semantically-based operation enables us to obtain a sense of repetition in sentences such as "The girl jumped until dawn," even though the repetition sense does not come from the meaning of any of the individual lexical items in the sentence or from any morpho-syntactic element. Yet, it is indispensable to the proper interpretation of the sentence. (Compare this to a syntactically transparent sentence such as, "The girl rested until dawn," where the interpretation of the sentence comes directly from the meaning of the lexical items in the sentence put together solely by syntactic processes – where no extra meaning has to be pasted in.)

Our first step was to determine if semantic composition of the aspectual coercion sort could be isolated during the course of normal sentence processing, and we observed that it could. Specifically, using a dual-task interference paradigm, we found that the time to carry out an independent secondary task was significantly greater when the primary task was to listen to and understand a sentence requiring semantic composition (the pasting in of the sense of *repetition*) than when the primary task was to listen to and understand a sentence whose word meanings could be composed entirely by syntactic means. Also the temporal parameter of this operation was different from that of a syntactic operation: Whereas the syntactic operation of gap-filling is reflexive, occurring as soon as it is structurally licensed, we observed the *cost* of the semantic compositional operation 250 msecs. downstream from the point at which it was licensed (Piñango, Zurif, & Jackendoff, in press).

We have not yet carried out a comparable on-line study with aphasic patients. We do, however, have some data from a task that requires patients to answer binary-choice questions following sentence presentations. So, for the sentence "The tiger jumped for an hour" we contrast "Did the tiger jump only one time?" (the incorrect choice) versus "Did the tiger jump time and time again?" (the correct choice). This, of course, is an example of a sentence requiring semantic composition over and above syntactic composition. Its syntactically transparent counterpart is "The tiger jumped over the fence" and the same binary choice is offered.

So far we have tested three Broca's patients and two Wernicke's patients, and the contrast between the two different kinds of aphasic patients is clear. The Broca's patients performed well on both the syntactically transparent sentences and the non-transparent sentences requiring the semantic combinatorial operation of aspectual coercion. The Wernicke's patients, however, did well only on the transparent ones. For the sentences requiring the extra step of semantic combination they had double the number of errors that they did for the transparent sentences (Piñango & Zurif, 1998).

FUNCTIONAL NEUROANATOMY

At the outset we stated our connection to functional neuroanatomy in terms of the lesion localizing value of the classical syndromes of Broca's and Wernicke's aphasia. And in these terms there seems to be clear functional differentiation within the language region of the left hemisphere. Thus, the anterior brain region associated with Broca's aphasia, but not the posterior region associated with Wernicke's aphasia, appears crucial at least for the syntactic operation of gap-filling. Indeed, many of the sentence-level comprehension problems found in

Broca's aphasia can be seen as reflections of the failure to form syntactically governed linkages in real time.

By contrast, the system of semantic inference seems not to depend on Broca's area, but on the integrity of the posterior area of the brain associated with Wernicke's aphasia. And so we have a double dissociation – a specific compositional role at the semantic level for the left-posterior region that can be set against the role of syntactic composition charted for the left-anterior region.

ACKNOWLEDGMENTS

One of us (MP) is a brand new member of the Aphasia Research Center; the other (EZ) has benefited very many times over the course of almost 30 years from Marty Albert's advice and personal kindness. Both of us salute him as the head of the Boston Aphasia Research Center – as the successor to Norman Geschwind and Harold Goodglass. And we are pleased to have been asked to participate in this festschrift.

The preparation of this manuscript and some of the research reported in it were supported by NIH grants DC 02984 and DC 00081. (Thanks, Marty.)

REFERENCES

Alexander, M., Naeser, M. A., & Palumbo, C. L. (1990). Broca's area aphasias: Aphasia after lesions including the frontal operculum. *Neurology, 40*, 353-362.

Beeman, M., Friedman, R., Grafman, J., Perz, E., Diamond, S., & Lindsay, M. (1994). Summation priming and coarse semantic coding in the right hemisphere. *Journal of Cognitive Neuroscience, 6*, 26-45.

Benson, F. (1985). Aphasia. In K. Heilman & E. Valenstein (Eds.), *Clinical neuropsychology*. New York: Oxford University Press.

Berndt, R. S., Mitchum, C. C., & Haendiges, A. N. (1996). Comprehension of reversible sentences in "agrammatism": A meta-analysis. *Cognition, 58*, 289-308.

Caramazza, A. & Zurif, E. (1976). Dissociation of algorithmic and heuristic processes in language comprehension: Evidence from aphasia. *Brain and Language, 3*, 572-582.

Francis, W. N. & Kucera, H. (1982). *Frequency analysis of English usage: Lexicon and grammar*. Boston: Houghton Mifflin Company.

Goodglass, H. & Kaplan, E. (1972). *The assessment of aphasia and related disorders*. Philadelphia, PA: Lea and Febiger

Grodzinsky, Y. (1990). *Theoretical perspectives on language deficits*. Cambridge, MA: MIT Press.

Grodzinsky, Y., Piñango, M., & Zurif, E. (in press). The constrained nature of Broca's aphasia comprehension.

Heilman, K. & Scholes, R. J. (1976). The nature of comprehension errors in Broca's, conduction and Wernicke's aphasics. *Cortex, 12*, 258-395.

Hickok, G., Zurif, E., & Canseco-Gonzalez, E. (1993). Structural description of agrammatic comprehension. *Brain and Language, 45* (3), 371-395.

Jackendoff, R. (1997). *The architecture of the language faculty. Linguistic inquiry monograph*. Cambridge, MA: MIT Press.

Mauner, G., Fromkin, V., & Cornell, T. L. (1993). Comprehension and acceptability judgments in agrammatism: Disruptions in the syntax of referential dependency. *Brain and Language, 45*, 340-370.

McElree, B. & Griffith, T. (1995). Syntactic and thematic processing in sentence comprehension: Evidence for a temporal dissociation. *Journal of Experimental Psychology: Learning, Memory, and Cognition, 21*, 134-157.

Naeser, M. A., Palumbo, C., Helm-Estabrooks, N., Stiassny-Eder, D., & Albert, M. L. (1989). Severe nonfluency in aphasia: Role of the medial subcallosal fasciculus and other white matter pathways in recovery of spontaneous speech. *Brain, 112*, 1-38.

Neely, J. H. (1977). Semantic priming and retrieval from lexical memory: Roles of inhibitionless spreading activation and limited capacity attention. *Journal of Experimental Psychology: General, 106*, 226-254.

Piñango M. & Zurif, E. (1998). Semantic composition: Processing parameters and neuroanatomical considerations. In R. Bastiaanse & Y. Grodzinsky (Eds.), *Grammatical disorders in aphasia: A neurolinguistic perspective*. London: Whurr.

Prather, P., Zurif, E., & Love, T. (1992). The time course of lexical access in aphasia. Toronto, CA: Academy of Aphasia.

Prather, P., Zurif, E., Love, T., & Brownell, H. (1997). Speed of lexical activation in nonfluent Broca's aphasia and fluent Wernicke's aphasia. *Brain and Language, 59*, 391-411.

Pustejovsky, J. (1995). *The generative lexicon*. Cambridge, MA: MIT Press.

Swinney, D. & Fodor, J. D. (1989). Special issue on sentence processing: Introduction. *Journal of Psycholinguistic Research, 18* (1), 1-3.

Swinney, D., Zurif, E., Prather, P., & Love, T. (1996). Neurological distribution of processing resources underlying language comprehension. *Journal of Cognitive Neuroscience, 8*, 174-184.

Vignolo, L. (1988) The anatomical and pathological basis of aphasia. In F. C. Rose, R. Whurr, & M. A. Wyke (Eds.), *Aphasia*. London: Whurr.

Zurif, E., Swinney, D., Prather, P., Solomon, J., & Bushell, C. (1993). An on-line analysis of syntactic processing in Broca's and Wernicke's aphasia. *Brain and Language, 45*, 44

PRIMARY PROGRESSIVE APHASIA: DISSOCIATION OF THE LOSS OF SYNTAX AND SEMANTICS IN A BIOLOGICALLY DETERMINED BRAIN DEGENERATION

Andrew Kertesz

INTRODUCTION

Obler and Albert (1980) stimulated the recent upsurge in the interest of language disorders in aging and in dementia (Obler et al., 1980). However, the appearance of language disturbance has been part of the descriptions of dementia for a long time. Both Pick (1892) and Alzheimer (1907) described their original patients as being significantly aphasic. Pick's conclusion was "a more or less circumscribed type of aphasia could result from a single circumscribed atrophic process." Caron (1934), in his review of Pick's disease (PiD), stated the most common form is characterized by early development of aphasia, and others also emphasized early speech disturbance or aphasia in PiD (Ohashi, 1983; Lüers, 1947; Kosaka, 1976). Many authors, however, ignored the prominence of aphasic deficits and textbooks emphasized the personality changes in early PiD, and some state that aphasia is rarely a presenting feature. Mutism, however, is often mentioned, and it is used as a shorthand form for nonfluent aphasia, or simply describes the final outcome.

As to Alzheimer's disease (AD), we standardized our aphasia test, the Western Aphasia Battery, on a population of Alzheimer patients (Appell et al., 1982). We found all of the hospitalized AD patients aphasic, predominantly fluent, anomic, and Wernicke's type and compared their deficit to stroke aphasics. Subsequently, we found that approximately 10% of the patients presenting to a dementia clinic appeared to have primary aphasia (Kertesz et al., 1986). This was around the same time when Mesulam (1982) collected his cases of slowly progressive aphasia and subsequently named it primary progressive aphasia (PPA) (Mesulam, 1987).

The relation among PPA and the language changes of Pick's disease and Alzheimer's disease remains unclear. The purpose of this paper is to discuss major current issues of PPA such as definition, taxonomy, linguistic and clinical features, and biology. I will highlight the three major varieties of PPA (logopenic, apractic, and semantic) and attempt to place them in the context of language disorders in other degenerative diseases. Finally, the relationship between PPA, and the behaviour and movement disorders of PiD will be discussed with the genetic evidence to support their cohesion.

DEFINITION: TAXONOMIC ISSUES

In the initial stages of the illness, the progressive aphasia can be a unitary symptom and Weintraub et al. (1990) originally suggested two years of primary aphasia for the definition of illness. However, in many instances the behavioral and personality disorder of frontotemporal dementia (FTD) also appear, and extrapyramidal symptomatology and even motor neuron disease may be superimposed. The converse is also true: cases of FTD often develop a progressive aphasia or logopenia and a mutism that is indistinguishable from PPA, although it is not primary in those instances (Kertesz & Munoz, 1998). The overlap between PPA and the behavioral syndrome of FTD is so substantial that we suggested the term "Pick complex" to describe the spectrum clinically and pathologically (Kertesz et al., 1994).

A number of varieties of progressive aphasia have been identified using different terminology such as progressive nonfluent aphasia (Turner et al., 1996), pure progressive aphemia (Cohen et al., 1993), and semantic dementia (Snowden et al., 1989) or primary progressive semantic aphasia (Kertesz et al., 1998). The differences between these clinical syndromes appear considerable, but some of the differences are related to the stage of the illness. Patients examined at different stages may have a clinical picture of initially fluent aphasia with anomia and then subsequently developed a nonfluent aphasia which is similar to verbal apraxia or Broca's aphasia. Eventually the picture of mutism with relatively preserved comprehension supervenes. The syndrome of semantic dementia or semantic aphasia appears distinctive, although the extent of overlap between fluent and nonfluent progressive aphasia is still unknown. There are cases of FTD that develop fluent aphasia later and even features of semantic dementia can occur. In many cases of semantic dementia eventual frontal type of disinhibition occurs with stereotypic compulsive behaviours, hoarding, food fads, etc. (Snowden et al., 1996).

LINGUISTIC FEATURES OF PPA

The initial presentation of PPA is often with word finding difficulty, or anomia. In this respect, PPA patients are not much different from Alzheimer patients, except they have relatively preserved memory and non-verbal cognition. Typical AD presentation is loss of episodic memory with relative preservation of semantic memory and language. The initial two years of the disease symptomatology distinguishes the two groups of patients. The more typical clinical picture progresses from anomia to a non-fluent type of aphasia with increasing word finding difficulty. Sometimes patients are called logopenic, yet fluent when the word finding difficulty is prominent but the phrase length is longer than four words and syntax is preserved (Mesulam et al., 1992).

We have now seen 50 cases of primary progressive aphasics in our cognitive neurology clinic. In 13 patients not enough information could be obtained concerning the onset of the illness, and these are considered as possible PPA patients. Of the 37 with definite language presentation, 24 patients had anomia or word finding difficulty initially and they later developed logopenia with progressive decrease of speech output and in some eventual mutism. Most of these patients at one time of their course have nonfluent speech output and good comprehension, although not the agrammatism and the phonological impairment of Broca's aphasics due to stroke. Decreasing speech output involves spontaneous speech and repetition to a lesser extent initially (Karbe et al., 1993). Comprehension remains relatively preserved until late in the course of the illness.

Other patients present with stuttering or slow, dysprosodic speech and verbal apraxia including articulatory difficulty and phonological paraphasias. These patients are less likely to be mistaken for AD. However the unexplained progressive articulatory disturbance in a younger, middle-aged person is often ignored as functional or hysterical. Aphemia or pure motor aphasia, are not appropriate terms to describe these phenomena since writing is also impaired. The articulatory involvement is characterised by particular difficulty with initial consonants, such as omission, repetition, and substitution, described as verbal apraxia. This occurs with or without buccofacial limb apraxia. We have seen five of these stuttering presentations. Two of them had classical PiD pathology. Sometimes the evolving aphasic disturbance is more like Broca's aphasia with grammatical errors.

Mutism used to be considered characteristic of Pick's disease as well, and it tends to be the end-stage of all forms of frontotemporal dementia, who survive long enough even in those who start with behavioral abnormalities rather than language disturbance initially (Gustafson et al., 1990; Neary et al., 1988). Logopenia and mutism are prevalent symptoms in the description of frontal lobe dementia (FLD), and there is a great deal of overlap between the descriptions of language deficit in FLD, PPA, and PiD. End-stage mutism also occurs in AD, but usually in a patient who already has a global dementia with loss of comprehension and basic functions of daily living (Appell et al., 1982).

LINGUISTIC FEATURES OF SEMANTIC APHASIA (DEMENTIA)

Another form of PPA that is different from the more common non-fluent variety was described as *semantic dementia* by Snowden et al. (1989). These patients progressively lost the meaning of words, but retained fluency and were able to carry out a conversation. Subsequent descriptions of this entity adopted this term (Hodges et al., 1992), although the patients were arguably more aphasic than demented. The picture is similar to *transcortical sensory aphasia* in which articulation, phonology and syntax remain intact but the patient does not comprehend well and has word finding difficulty. In other reports of fluent progressive aphasia the semantic deficit is not emphasized or less clearly evaluated (Parkin, 1993; Harasty et al., 1996). We had five cases of typical progressive semantic aphasia (semantic dementia) where the meaning of the words are lost primarily and syntax and phonology are preserved. One of them has been published with documentation of several clinical features including the item consistency and transmodal nature of the semantic loss, the preservation of autobiographical memory and contextual speech (Kertesz et al., 1998). This condition contrasts with nonfluent PPA in the specific loss of semantic field and preservation of syntax. This dissociation is so striking that the diagnosis of hysteria is often made in both types of patients. Most stroke aphasics have a loss of semantic processing but this occurs in association with problems in articulation, phonological and syntactic processing and the difficulty is often in accessing semantic concepts rather than a loss of semantic field.

The loss of meaning occurred throughout all categories, although personalized items appeared better named and comprehended by the patient in our publication, similar to the observations of Snowden et al. (1996). Although these patients can distinguish categories of objects and preserve some visuosemantic processing at the superordinate level, detailed knowledge of attributes are not available to identify the object at a base level. Although the semantic loss appears to be frequency dependent, there was a particular preservation of the animals category. The patient could always identify verbally that the stimulus in the auditory modality was an animal but could not specify which one (could not describe or choose attributes, etc.). On the other hand, she could not identify other categories verbally, even though sorting of the drawings of each category such as fruits, clothes, furniture, and vehicles remained intact.

We also observed the preservation of verbs versus the loss of nouns in a test of polysemous words where she typically gave the verb meaning of the stimuli, in contrast to controls which tend to find the noun meaning in most instances if there are no grammatical clues as to the meaning of the stimulus. In addition to verbs, colours and numbers were relatively preserved. Furthermore, this patient retained the use of abstract concepts, verb phrases, nominalized verbs, and closed class words, in contrast to the loss of nouns and proper names. She could continue to discuss visiting relatives, shopping, travelling to her birth place at the same time when she could not define the word "steak" nor name it from a picture. She also developed a striking surface alexia and surface agraphia where she could not handle irregular written words when she did not know their meaning.

CLINICAL FEATURES OF PPA

The age of onset of PPA is usually presenile (under 65), although there are numerous exceptions. A careful history is needed to determine the initial symptoms. When the patients are seen later in the illness, the time from onset is difficult to determine and is often underestimated. The course is variable, eight to ten years, but sometimes patients who develop pathology in the basal ganglia or motor neurons progress quickly to mutism and develop difficulty with swallowing and choking, and the course may be as little as two years from onset to death (Kertesz et al., 1994). It is yet to be determined whether the rapid progression represents a different pathology. However, most patients, whose illness remains mainly in the cortical regions at least as far as symptoms are concerned, progress very gradually, six or seven years, before they develop severe aphasia, mutism or extrapyramidal disease. Several patients, well after ten years of illness, continue to function normally at home even though they are completely mute. In these striking cases, a considerable amount of comprehension, memory, visuospatial, and motor function are retained. These patients can get around independently and even carry out complex tasks even though they are unable to talk. One of our younger patients, who managed to take care of her children and her household, was considered hysterical by the psychologist, speech pathologist and neurologist before finally neuroimaging showed severe frontal atrophy and the patient was diagnosed as having probable PiD (Kertesz et al., 1994).

BEHAVIORAL AND MOTOR SYMPTOMS OF PPA

Behaviour changes that are related to frontal lobe involvement often occur later on in the illness, although at times simultaneously or shortly after the language presentation. Apathy, irritability, and lack of insight occur commonly and may be misinterpreted as depression. One of our pathologically examined PPA cases received psychiatric treatment for depression and uncharacteristic aggression towards his wife (Kertesz et al., 1994). We have followed 36 patients with PPA for more than three years and 17 (47%) have developed the behavioral and personality disorder of FLD such as hyperorality, utilization behaviour, aggressiveness, emotional flatness, and bizarre obsessive behaviour. An additional 12 patients (33%) developed corticobasal degeneration (CBD) as the secondary syndrome. A further 7 patients (19%) of the total PPA population developed FLD as a tertiary syndrome later on the course of their illness. The average duration of follow up of these patients was six to eight years.

Patients with PPA may develop extrapyramidal symptoms which are often unilateral and associated with severe apraxia and *alien hand*, a motor phenomenon of levitation, uselessness, and rigidity. This syndrome is referred to as corticonigral (Rebeiz et al., 1968) or *corticobasal degeneration* (CBD) (Gibb et al., 1989; Thompson et al., 1992). The pathology appeared distinct but even the original description noted a significant overlap between the pathology of CBD and PiD (Rebeiz et al., 1968). Sporadic cases of PPA with CBD have been published (Lang et al., 1992; Sakurai et al., 1996). There are also patients with PPA with motor neuron disease. In addition to the pathological overlap, there is a substantial clinical overlap with 12 cases of CBD (33%) and 7 cases of FLD (30%) developing corticobasal degeneration syndrome (CBDS) as a secondary and tertiary syndrome. The overlap exists in a reverse fashion and 8 out of 15 (63%) CBDS patients develop progressive aphasia and 7 out of 15 (47%) with FLD. In these cases, the term *primary* is not appropriate as the progressive aphasia follows the other two major presentations.

NEUROIMAGING OF PPA

Neuroimaging abnormalities, such as left sided ventricular or sulcal atrophy, were relatively common in PPA, occurring in 65% of the published cases in the review of Mesulam and Weintraub (1992). Focal hypometabolism on PET in the left temporal and parietal lobes (Chawluk et al., 1986; Tyrell et al., 1990; Yamamoto et al., 1990; Croisile et al., 1990) and various other patterns, including asymmetrical temporal, frontal, and bifrontal hypometabolism on single photon emission computerized tomography (SPECT), were present (McDaniel et al., 1991; Sakurai et al., 1996; Snowden et al., 1992; Caselli et al., 1993). Frontal opercular atrophy, anterior and superior temporal atrophy, and bifrontal and left temporoparietal atrophy were shown on the MRI in three patients with PPA by Caselli et al. (1992). They also commented that hypoprofusion with SPECT seemed to be even more extensive than atrophy on MRI.

The role of neuroimaging in focal atrophies is clearly important. There are several issues, however, that require clarification, such as the extent of atrophy, the structures commonly affected, the best modality to document it and its correlation with the clinical manifestations. We had neuroimaging in patients with the presumptive diagnosis of PPA in 34 patients. We have further divided this group into 19 probable PPA patients, who fulfil the stricter criteria of PPA, on the basis of relatively preserved memory and visuospatial function historically for two years, and in some documented neuropsychologically on the initial examination and on follow-up. The other group of 15 patients had a history in which it was either doubtful if the initial symptom was memory loss or forgetting proper names and dates as the feature of early anomia, or fluent aphasia was the major clinical feature for years. This group was designated as possible PPA. A comparison for each of the anatomical structures between the probable and the possible PPA group showed no significant differences, except there was a trend for a difference for more atrophy in the probable group in all the structures. These results suggested that the possible group also has focal, asymmetrical atrophy. Focal atrophy on MRI or CT, affecting the left temporal and parietal lobes, is a hallmark of PPA and it was seen in all of the probable cases (Kertesz, 1998).

NEUROPATHOLOGY AND GENETICS

The neuropathology of PPA was initially considered heterogenous and some authors still do not seem to recognize the connection between the varieties of focal atrophy that underlie PPA and other clinical manifestations of Pick complex. The heterogeneity of the pathology has been over-emphasized because of the failure to recognize the commonalities. The initial reports emphasized non-specific findings, such as lipofuscinois (Mesulam, 1982) and spongiform change. The latter is common to all forms of the Pick complex and also seen in other conditions. Not everyone is sympathetic to the view that it constitutes the characteristic alteration of PPA (Kirshner et al., 1987), although it is seen in virtually all cases. Confusion of this superficial linear spongiosis, restricted to the upper cortical layers, with the transcortical spongiosis characteristic of the transmissible encephalopathies is the most likely explanation of the reports of PPA due to Creutzfeldt-Jakob disease. The spongiosis of the latter disease involves the basal ganglia, whereas the spongiosis in PPA is restricted to the cortex. Prion proteins are absent in PPA, as determined by immunohistochemistry and Western blotting.

Others, including our group, described Alzheimer's pathology in PPA (Pogacar et al., 1984; Benson et al., 1991; Karbe et al., 1993). Some of these cases, however, appear to represent the coexistence of Pick complex abnormalities with minor Alzheimer-type pathology, similar to that seen in many non-demented elderly individuals. Characteristically, the Alzheimer-type pathology, consisting of abundant senile plaques, and rare neurofibrillary tangles, spread throughout the cortex, contrasting with the focal distribution of the Pick complex type abnormalities. In other patients, the language disturbance came later, not much different from AD with prominent aphasia. In these cases, the initial history of memory loss may have been overlooked or under-estimated. They were probably mislabeled as PPA. Pathological descriptions of focal AD have appeared sporadically but the clinical correlation with PPA is not a convincing one.

Many cases of PPA turned out to have PiD with classical silver staining globose Pick bodies and ballooned achromatic neurons called Pick cells (Wechsler et al., 1982; Malamud, 1940; Holland et al., 1985; Graff-Radford et al., 1990; Kertesz et al., 1994). In addition to the cases published as PPA, this category includes patients in whom such a diagnosis can be made retrospectively. For example, one of the two cases with partial atrophy of the brain presented by Rosenfeld (1909) had characteristic PPA, with relatively well-preserved mentation in other domains, and PiD established on autopsy. Wechsler (1977) published the first modern case of presenile dementia presenting with aphasia; subsequently, the autopsy also showed PiD (Wechsler et al., 1982).

Another variety of Pick complex pathology is characterized by ballooned neurons (Pick cells), subcortical neuronal inclusions (atypical Pick bodies) and tau positive glial pathology (astrocytic plaques, etc.), originally thought to be specific for CBD. A substantial number of PPA patients, however, have this pathology in our experience (Munoz, 1998). Many other pathological varieties of the Pick complex have features of CBD. The clinical overlap between CBD and PPA has already been reviewed.

The majority of cases of Pick complex do not have Pick bodies, but they are characterized by gliosis, neuronal loss, layers II and III spongiform changes with or without ballooned neurons, and have been labeled as "dementia lacking distinctive histology." More recently, histochemical investigation revealed that most, if not all, of these cases have ubiquitin positive, tau negative, synuclein negative inclusions that can also be seen in motor neuron disease. Although this kind of pathology may underlie PPA or FTD with motor neuron disease, it often occurs in cases where there is no clinical or pathological evidence of this. Therefore, the previous designation of this histological change as "FLD with motor neuron disease" is inappropriate.

Autosomal dominant inheritance of Pick complex or FTD have been observed and some of these families have shown linkage to chromosome-17 (Foster et al., 1997). In some of these a number of tau mutations have been demonstrated recently (Hutton et al., 1998). This provides further evidence for the biological cohesion of these clinical conditions, including PPA (Lendon et al., 1998). Although relatively little linguistic investigation has been done in these familial cases, many of them have progressive aphasia. The variations in the description of these cases reflect the variation in the anatomical involvement and the clinical data availability rather than fundamental biological differences.

REFERENCES

Alzheimer, A. (1907). On peculiar disease of the cerebral cortex. *Allgemeine Zeitschrift für Psychiatrie*, *64*, 146.
Appell, J., Kertesz, A., & Fisman, M. (1982). A study of language functioning in Alzheimer patients. *Brain and Language*, *17*, 73-91.
Benson, D. F. & Zaias, B. W. (1991). Progressive aphasia: A case with postmortem correlation. *Neuropsychiatry, Neuropsychology and Behavioral Neurology*, *4*, 215-223.
Caron, M. (1934). *Étude clinique de la maladie Pick*. Paris: Vigot.
Caselli, R. J., Jack, C. R., Petersen, R. C., Wahner, H. W., & Yanagihara, T. (1992). Asymmetric cortical degenerative syndromes. *Neurology*, *42*, 1462-1468.
Caselli, R. J., Windebank, A. J., Petersen, R. C., Komori, T., Parisi, J. E., Okazak, H., Kokmen, E. M., Iverson, R., Dinapoli, R. P., Graff-Radfor, N. R., & Stein, S. D. (1993). Rapidly progressive aphasic dementia and motor neuron disease. *Annals of Neurology*, *33*, 200-207.
Chawluk, J. B., Mesulam, M-M., Hurtig, H., Kushner, M., Weintraub, S., Saykin, A., Rubin, N., Alavi, A., & Reivich, M. (1986). Slowly progressive aphasia without generalized dementia: Studies with positron emission tomography. *Annals of Neurology*, *19*, 68-74.
Cohen, L., Benoit, N., Van Eeckhout, P., Ducarne, B., & Brunet, P. (1993). Pure progressive aphemia. *Journal of Neurology,Neurosurgery and Psychiatry*, *56*, 923-924.
Croisile, B. & Trillet, M. (1990). Cerebral blood flow and transient global amnesia. *Journal of Neurology, Neurosurgery, and Psychiatry*, *53*, 361.
Foster, N. L., Wilhelmsen, K., Sima, A. F. A., Jones, M. Z., D'Amato, C. J., Gilman, S., & conference participants. (1997). Frontotemporal dementia and Parkinsonism linked to chromosome 17: A consensus conference. *Annals of Neurology*, *41*, 706-715.
Gibb, W. R. G., Luthert, P. J., & Marsden, C. D. (1989). Corticobasal degeneration. *Brain*, *112*, 1171-1192.
Graff-Radford, N. R., Damasio, A. R., Hyman, B. T., Hart, M. N., Tranel, D., Damasio, H., Vanhoesen, G. W., & Rezai, K. (1990). Progressive aphasia in a patient with Pick's disease. *Neurology*, *40*, 620-626.
Gustafson, L., Brun, A., & Risberg, J. (1990). Frontal lobe dementia of non-Alzheimer type. In R. J. Wurtman, S. Corkin, J. Growdon, & E. Ritter-Walker (Eds.), *Alzheimer's disease* (pp. 65-71). New York: Raven Press.
Harasty, J. A., Halliday, G. M., Code, C., & Brooks, W. S. (1996). Quantification of cortical atrophy in a case of progressive fluent aphasia. *Brain*, *119*, 181-190.
Holland, A. L., McBurney, D. H., Moossy, J., & Reinmuth, O. M. (1985). The dissolution of language in Pick's disease with neurofibrillary tangles: A case study. *Brain and Language*, *24*, 36-58.
Hutton, M., Lendon, C. L., Rizzu, P., Baker, M., Froelich, S., Houlden, H., et al. (1998). Association of missense and 5'-splice-site mutations in tau with the inherited dementia FTDP-17. *Nature*, *393*, 702-705.
Karbe, H., Kertesz, A., & Polk, M. (1993). Profiles of language impairment in primary progressive aphasia. *Archives of Neurology*, *50*, 193-201.
Kertesz, A. (1998). Frontotemporal degeneration: Primary progressive aphasia, frontal lobe dementia and the Pick complex. In F. Fazekas, R. Schmidt, & A. Alavi (Eds.), *Neuroimaging of normal aging and uncommon causes of dementia* (pp. 111-127). Dordrecht, The Netherlands: ICG Publications.
Kertesz, A., Davidson, W., & McCabe, P. (1998). Primary progressive semantic aphasia: A case study. *Journal of the International Neuropsychological Society*, *4*, 388-398.
Kertesz, A. & Fisman, M. (1986). The dissolution of language in Alzheimer's disease. *Canadian Journal of Neurological Sciences*, *13*, 415-418.
Kertesz, A., Hudson, L., Mackenzie, I. R. A., & Munoz, D. G. (1994). The pathology and nosology of primary progressive aphasia. *Neurology*, *44*, 2065-2072.
Kertesz, A. & Munoz, D. (1998). Clinical and pathological overlap in Pick complex. In A. Kertesz & D. Munoz (Eds.), *Pick's disease and Pick complex* (pp. 281-286). New York: Wiley & Sons, Inc.
Kirshner, H. S., Tanridag, O., Thurman, L., & Whetsell, W. O., Jr. (1987). Progressive aphasia without dementia: Two cases with focal spongiform degeneration. *Annals of Neurology*, *22*, 527-532.
Kosaka, K. (1976). On aphasia of Pick's disease: A review of our own 3 cases and 49 autopsy cases in Japan (In Japanese). *Seishin Igaku*, *18*, 1181-1189, as quoted by Ohashi (1983).
Lang, A. E., Bergeron, C., Pollanen, M. S., & Ashby, P. (1992). Parietal Pick's disease mimicking cortical-basal degeneration. *Neurology*, *44*, 1436-1440.

Lendon, C. L., Lynch, T., Norton, J., McKeel, D. W., Busfield, F., Craddock, N., Chakraverty, S., Gopalakrishnan, G., Shears, S. D., Grimmett, W., Wilhelmsen, K. C., Hansen, L., Morris, J. C., & Goate, A. M. (1998). Hereditary dysphasic disinhibition dementia - A frontotemporal dementia linked to 17q21-22. *Neurology, 50*, 1546-1555.

Lüers, T. (1947). Über den Verfall der Sprache bei der Pickschen Krankheiten (umschriebene Atrophie der Grosshirnrinde). *Zeitschrift für die gesamte Neurologie und Psychiatrie, 179*, 94-131.

Malamud, N. (1940). Pick's disease with atrophy of the temporal lobes. *Archives of Neurology and Psychiatry, 43*, 210-222.

McDaniel, K. D., Wagner, M. T., & Greenspan, B. S. (1991). The role of brain single photon emission computed tomography in the diagnosis of primary progressive aphasia. *Archives of Neurology, 48*, 1257-1260.

Mesulam, M.-M. (1982). Slowly progressive aphasia without generalized dementia. *Annals of Neurology, 11*, 592-598.

Mesulam, M.-M. (1987). Primary progressive aphasia - differentiation from Alzheimer's disease *Annals of Neurology, 22*, 533-534.

Mesulam, M. M. & Weintraub, S. (1992). Primary progressive aphasia: Sharpening the focus on a clinical syndrome. In F. Boller, F. Forette, Z. Khachaturian, M. Poncet, & Y. Christen (Eds.), *Heterogeneity of Alzheimer's disease* (pp. 43-66). Berlin: Springer-Verlag.

Mesulam, M. M. & Weintraub, S. (1992). Spectrum of primary progressive aphasia. In B. Tindall (Ed.), *Baillière's clinical neurology* (pp. 583-609). Berlin: Springer-Verlag.

Munoz, D. G. (1998). The pathology of Pick complex. In A. Kertesz & D. G. Munoz (Eds.), *Pick's disease and Pick complex* (pp. 211-241). New York: Wiley & Sons, Inc.

Neary, D., Snowden, J. S., Northen, B., & Goulding, P. (1988). Dementia of frontal lobe type. *Journal of Neurology, Neurosurgery, and Psychiatry, 51*, 353-361.

Obler, L. K. & Albert, M. L. (1980). *Language and communication in the elderly*. Norwood, MA: D. C. Heath and Company.

Ohashi, H. (1983). An aphasiologic approach to Pick's disease. In A. Hirano & K. Miyoshi (Eds.), *Neuropsychiatric disorders in the elderly* (pp. 132-135). Tokyo: Igaku-Shoin.

Parkin, A. J. (1993). Progressive aphasia without dementia - A clinical cognitive neuropsychological analsysis. *Brain and Language, 44*, 201-220.

Pick, A. (1892). Über die Beziehungen der senilen Hirnatrophie zur Aphasie. *Prager Medizinische Wochenschrift, 17*, 165-167.

Pogacar, S. & Williams, R. G. (1984). Alzheimer's disease presenting as slowly progressive aphasia. *RI Medical Journal, 67*, 181-185.

Rebeiz, J.J., Kolodny, E.H., & Richardson, E.P., Jr. (1968). Corticodentatonigram degeneration with neuronal achromasia. *Archives of Neurology, 18*, 20-33.

Rosenfeld, M. (1909). Die partielle Grosshirnatrophie. *Journal of Psychology and Neurology, 14*, 115-130.

Sakurai, Y., Hashida, H., Uesugi, H., Arima, K., Murayama, S., Bando, M., Iwata, M. Momose, T., & Sakuta, M. (1996). A clinical profile of corticobasal degeneration presenting as primary progressive aphasia. *European Neurology, 36*, 134-137.

Snowden, J.S., Goulding, P.J., & Neary, D. (1989). Semantic dementia: a form of circumscribed cerebral atrophy. *Behavioral Neurology, 2*, 167-182.

Snowden, J. S., Neary, D., & Mann, D. M. A. (1996). *Fronto-temporal lobar degeneration: Frontotemporal dementia, progressive aphasia, semantic dementia*. London: Churchill Livingstone.

Snowden, J. S., Neary, D., Mann, D. M. A., Goulding, P. J., & Testa, H. J. (1992). Progressive language disorder due to lobar atrophy. *Annals of Neurology, 31*, 174-183.

Thompson, P. D. & Marsden, C. D. (1992). Corticobasal degeneration. In T. Baillière (Ed.), *Baillière's clinical neurology* (pp. 677-686). London: Baillière-Tindall.

Turner, R. S., Kenyon, L. C., Trojanowski, J. Q., Gonatas, N., & Grossman, M. (1996). Clinical, neuroimaging, and pathologic features of progressive nonfluent aphasia. *Annals of Neurology, 39*, 166-173.

Tyrell, P. J., Warrington, E. K., Frackowiak, R. S. J., & Rossor, M. N. (1990). Progressive degeneration of the right temporal lobe studied with positron emission tomography. *Journal of Neurology, Neurosurgery and Psychiatry, 54*, 1046-1050.

Wechsler, A. F. (1977). Presenile dementia presenting as aphasia. *Journal of Neurology, Neurosurgery, and Psychiatry, 40*, 303-305.

Wechsler, A. F., Verity, A., Rosenstein, L. D., Fried, I., & Scheibel, A. B. (1982). Pick's disease: A clinical, computed tomographic, and histologic study with Golgi impregnation observations. *Archives of Neurology, 39,* 287-290.

Weintraub, S., Rubin, N. P., & Mesulam, M.-M. (1990). Primary progressive aphasia: Longitudinal course, neuropsychological profile, and language features. *Archives of Neurology, 47,* 1329-1335.

Yamamoto, H., Tanabe, H., Kashiwagi, A., Ikejiri, Y., Fukuyama, H., Okuda, J., Shiraishi, J., & Nishimura, T. (1990). A case of slowly progressive aphasia without generalized dementia in a Japanese patient. *Acta Neurologica Scandinavica, 82,* 102-105.

PHARMACOTHERAPY OF APHASIA

Yutaka Tanaka and David L. Bachman

INTRODUCTION

Although the neurological and neurolinguistic literature has focused on the relation between cerebral anatomical localization and language, relatively little emphasis has been placed on the relation between neurotransmitter function and language. In 1988, Albert and colleagues (Albert, Bachman, Morgan, & Helm-Estabrooks, 1988) reported a case in which speech fluency in an aphasic patient was partially restored by administration of a dopamine agonist, bromocriptine. Since that initial report, other investigators have also explored the efficacy of dopamine agonists in treating aphasia. More recently, acetylcholinergic systems have also been implicated in the symptom complex of aphasia. These early efforts to understand the relation between specific pharmacological therapies and particular aphasic symptoms may offer insight into the contribution of neurotransmitter systems to language function. In particular, we wish to offer two hypotheses: (1) dopaminergic systems may be important for activation and initiation of speech output, and (2) acetylcholinergic systems may play a role in semantic memory. In this chapter, we will elaborate on these hypotheses and present clinical and anatomical data that support them.

DOPAMINERGIC SYSTEM

Anatomical Data

Before discussing the relation between the dopaminergic system and language, we will provide an anatomical overview. At least three of these systems – striatonigral, mesocortical, and mesolimbic – may have some relevance for language function. The dopamine cell bodies for these three systems are located within the anterior midbrain, situated primarily within the substantia nigra and ventral tegmental area. From the midbrain, dopaminergic projections ascend to innervate the caudate and putamen (basal ganglia), the cortex (especially the dorsal frontal cortex, including the supplementary motor area), and various limbic structures.

A number of studies have implicated the dorsal frontal regions, particularly the supplementary motor cortex, in the initiation of language. Based on electroencephalographic (EEG) findings, Penfield and Jasper (1954) hypothesized that the supplementary motor and lower motor cortices have specific roles to play in the actual motor production of speech, although the supplementary motor area also plays a more specifically linguistic role. Luders et al. (1991) surgically implanted subdural cortical electrodes that permitted stimulation and recording for days or weeks prior to anticipated epilepsy surgery. The most common language abnormality elicited was speech arrest, which resulted from stimulation of five areas: the primary motor areas for facial/buccal/lingual movement, a motor area adjacent to the primary motor area that included the supplementary motor area, Broca's area, Wernicke's area, and the infero-basal temporal regions. In addition, they reported that differences in stimulation intensities produced different results: at lower stimulation intensities, speech was slowed, anomia was present, and subjects had difficulty carrying out complex linguistic tasks; at high stimulation intensities, speech arrest was accompanied by a global aphasia. Wise et al. (1991) attributed the frontal activation, particularly in the dorsolateral posterior frontal cortex (DLPFC), to the process of retrieving verbal information from posterior language areas, particularly Wernicke's area. When subjects had to internally generate words, the primary activation site was the DLPFC.

Because of the mesocortical dopaminergic distribution in dorsofrontal regions, one could anticipate that speech output, which seems to depend especially on left frontal regions, may be linked to dopamine. In addition, it has been demonstrated from CT-scan correlation studies that the subcallosal fasciculus, a pathway connecting supplementary motor area and anterior cingulate with striatal sites, must be lesioned in order for there to be a persistent nonfluent aphasia (Naeser et al., 1989).

The striatonigral system also may play a role in speech initiation and maintenance. The striatonigral and mesolimbic systems may be important for species-specific motivational behavior (Bachman & Albert, 1984). It has long been known that lesions of the striatum and thalamus, placed to treat Parkinson's disease, may result in transient or persistent abnormalities of speech and language. It is highly likely, therefore, that dopamine may work via two separate neural pathways, and possibly, two separate mechanisms, to influence speech and language initiation. The mesocortical projection may be important in cortical mechanisms responsible for language formulation, whereas striatonigral and mesolimbic pathways may play a more general role in behavioral/motor initiation, including speech initiation.

Clinical Data

The idea of language-targeted dopaminergic therapy can be traced to ancient times. Bachman and Albert (1990) have extensively reviewed the history of the pharmacotherapy of aphasia. One of the earliest known treatments for aphasia is the cashew nut (*Anacardium*). Cashews were used to treat a variety of psychiatric and neurological symptoms, especially disorders of language. Although it is easy to dismiss as naive claims of their therapeutic efficacy, nevertheless, cashews are relatively rich in certain amino acids which may serve as precursors to neurotransmitters critical to cerebral function.

Other treatments of historical interest include hypnotherapy, amytal, and a variety of other drugs including caffeine, dibazol, phenamine, and glutamic acid, as well as curare-like muscle relaxants (see Table 1). Gheorghita et al. (1977) and Voinescu and Gheorghita (1978) investigated a multitude of pharmacological

Table 1. Previous reports of dopaminergic agents for language impairment

Reporter	Drug	Subjects	Language
Linn	sodium amytal	BI	vocabulary, word of choice
		S	fluency, attention
Bergman	sodium amytal	S etc.	fluency*
Solomonovici	imipramine	A	language
Kryshova	caffein	A	language
Gheoghita	pyrithioxine lucidril acetylsalicilic acid caffein ephedrine	A	repetition, naming reading, writing
Tanaka	L-dopa	A	naming, fluency
Albert	bromocriptine	A	initiation, naming fluency
Sabe	bromocriptine	A	fluency
Gupta	bromocriptine	A	fluency
Walker-Watoson	amphetamine	A	language
Liebson	L-dopa and bromocriptine	BI	dysarthria

A = aphasia
BI = brain injury
S = stroke
etc. = and so on
* many patients felt they were more fluent

agents in the treatment of aphasia, including pyrithioxine, lucidril, acetylsalicylic acid, ephedrine, and caffeine. These authors did not control for subtype of aphasia but did divide patients into groups according to general severity of aphasia. They examined the effect of the drugs on different components of aphasic symptoms, including repetition, naming, reading, writing, reception, and total score. There were different drug-effects on different components of language. Caffeine may be expected to have a general *activating* effect on all aspects of cognitive function, but it exhibited little long-term positive effect during testing. In contrast, pyrithioxine (encephabol) had a significant, and specific, effect on aphasic symptoms. Voinescu and Gheorghita hypothesized that the effect pyrithioxine exhibited was due to enhanced cortical metabolic activity. However, other studies suggest that pyrithioxine may exert its effect by increasing dopaminergic activity within the central nervous system (Stoica et al., 1972). In the United States, Benson (1970) utilized dexedrine in the treatment of a small number of aphasia patients. Samuels has routinely used L-dopa/carbidopa in the treatment of nonfluent aphasia.

The first modern reports of pharmacotherapy of aphasia were from Martin Albert's group at the Boston VA Hospital. In 1988, Albert et al. described a case which suggested that the dopamine agonist bromocriptine helped restore speech fluency in a patient with transcortical motor aphasia resulting from stroke. The patient was a 62 year-old man with residual moderate transcortical motor aphasia following left-frontal intracerebral hemorrhage. He was tested before treatment with bromocriptine, during treatment, and then after cessation of treatment. His major fluency problems, including impaired initiation and hesitancies (long response latencies) of speech, responded well to bromocriptine. Both the number and proportion of pauses between and within utterances diminished significantly during free conversation. His language returned to the baseline after cessation of the drug.

Bachman and Morgan (1988), from the same laboratory, reported two additional cases, one with stable mixed anterior aphasia and the other with severe Broca's aphasia. On bromocriptine, both subjects demonstrated increased use of novel words and reported increased likelihood of conversational initiation at home. However, other effects were not apparent on formal testing.

Other studies described beneficial effects of bromocriptine on fluency in aphasia. Gupta et al. (1992) reported two patients with left frontoparietal infarcts and non-fluent aphasia. These patients were treated with bromocriptine for three months and underwent comprehensive language testing before and during monthly treatment. Both patients improved markedly in speech fluency, but not in other aspects of language function. Sabe et al. (1992) reported a prospective open-label trial of bromocriptine in seven non-fluent aphasics with left frontal infarcts. They treated three patients with moderate nonfluent aphasia with 30 to 60 mg/day of bromocriptine. They reported statistically significant correlations between behavioral improvement and escalating doses, as well as between behavioral deterioration and declining doses of the drug.

Walker-Batson et al. (1991) reported a study of six aphasic patients who had ischemic stroke, all in the distribution of the left middle cerebral artery. All patients were evaluated by the PICA (Porch Index of Communicative Ability) (Porch, 1967). Each patient took d-amphetamine every four days, approximately one hour before a session of speech and language therapy, for a total of ten sessions. When evaluated after these periods, the patients scored more than 100 percent better than predicted by PICA norms.

In Japan in 1991, Tanaka et al. found that L-dopa enhanced word fluency in three of five patients with aphasia and improved productive communication of the aphasic person within the family, but had no effect on auditory comprehension. In addition, Tanaka et al. showed that L-dopa had a limited effect, not increasing above a certain threshold dose (Tanaka et al., 1993).

As described above, most drugs producing some increased catecholamine activity, including pyrithioxine, lucidril, ephedrine, caffeine, dexedrine, levodopa, L-dopa/carbidopa, and bromocriptine, resulted in improvement in initiation of speech. This finding suggests that dopmaninergic systems are likely important for language function, especially naming or initiation of speech.

However, it is important to note that several studies have failed to demonstrate such an effect (MacLennan et al., 1990; Gupta et al., 1995; Sabe et al., 1995). In 1994, Small carefully reviewed the topic of pharmacotherapy of aphasia. He correctly noted problems of methodology, pharmacological mechanism, or interpretation in all positive studies, observing that studies were uncontrolled, subjects samples were small, drug trials were unblinded, and no placebo phases were included. MacLennan et al. (1990) conducted a placebo-controlled study to verify the effect of bromocriptine on speech and language deficits. Although the number of words produced by their subjects increased during bromocriptine administration, the authors concluded that bromocriptine did not significantly affect any specific speech and language function, and they cautioned against uncritical acceptance of bromocriptine treatment for improving communication capabilities of aphasic patients. Despite the authors' critical comments, however, effects on language were similar to those seen in positive studies.

Gupta et al. (1995) reported that bromocriptine had no significant effect on aphasia and suggested that bromocriptine was not recommended as monotherapy for the treatment of chronic aphasia. Although this study employed a rigorous research protocol, it included a mixture of several different types of aphasia, and, more importantly, 8 of 20 subjects had aphasia for more than five years. Our data suggest that individuals with chronic aphasia may not show improvement of language function after administration of bromocriptine.

In Sabe et al.'s study (1995), the dose of bromocriptine was reported to be up to 60mg/day – an amount that may act as a dopamine antagonist. Among their subjects taking 3.5 mg of bromocriptine, scores of significant words, content units, pauses, and Boston Naming ability improved, but for those at doses above 3.75 mg, scores decreased compared to a placebo. These data suggest that bromocriptine, in particular, may be dose-dependent in its effect.

Except for one report (Tanaka et al., 1991), all patients who benefited from dopamine agonist treatment had nonfluent aphasia. It appears, however, that not all patients with nonfluent aphasia improve with drug administration. Results from cases reported thus far suggest that patients with transcortical motor aphasia respond more readily to dopamine agents than patients with other types of aphasia. This observation is consistent with the notion that transcortical motor aphasia may result from damage interrupting the mesocortical dopaminergic projection.

Dopamine and Language

Various neurological structures that connect with the frontal lobes are plausible targets of the dopamine system. The frontal lobes themselves play a key role in: (1) the integration of motor output, (2) interconnection of multimodal sensory association areas, and (3) integrating processes necessary for the initiation of volitional behavior. Almost all important language regions are linked directly to frontal lobe structures.

These considerations lead to the language-dopaminergic system network shown in Figure 1. These designated cerebral regions each receive dopamine innervation. Damage to any component or its connections will cause aphasia. Principal symptoms associated with lesions to these areas are impairments in word-finding and speech initiation. For example, damage to the supplementary motor area (SMA), to the prefrontal heteromodal cortex, or their interconnections may result in certain symptoms of nonfluent aphasia. The SMA, in particular, is thought to play a major role in the initiation and planning of speech output, and the prefrontal heteromodal cortex is thought to play a major role in the retrieval of

164 Neurobehavior of Language and Cognition

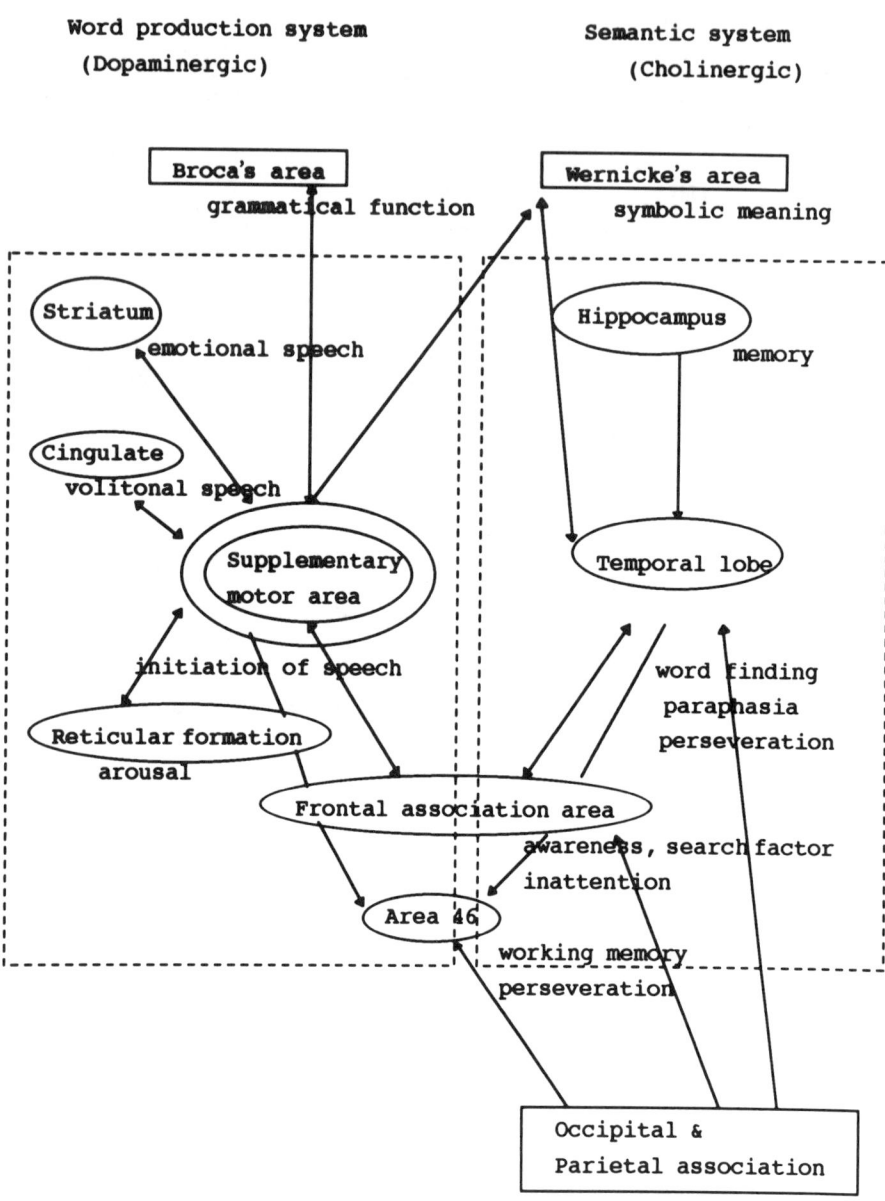

Figure 1. Testable model of dopaminergic system: direct related area and indirect related area.

words from superordinate categories. Other broad regions of the prefrontal lobes are thought to play roles in attention, awareness, and temporal integration with other associated language areas.

The SMA and other prefrontal regions are known to receive dopamine projections, especially from medial substantia nigra and the ventral tegmental region. Interruption of dopamine projections, as demonstrated in animal studies, has resulted in symptoms similar to direct lesions of the frontal lobes (Alexander, 1989). Therefore, if direct lesions of these cerebral areas result in specific language deficits, it is likely that interruption of dopaminergic projections to these areas may also result in similar language symptoms. Certain cerebral lesions, such as strokes to ascending mesocortical projections, may interrupt dopaminergic projections without directly involving the frontal lobes themselves. If this postulated mechanism is correct, some aphasic patients with specific language symptoms such as speech initiation difficulties due to appropriately placed lesions may be good candidates for treatment with bromocriptine or other dopaminergic agents.

A second mechanism by which dopamine agonists may alleviate aphasic symptoms involves dopaminergic innervation of the basal ganglia. The ventromedial component of the striatum is involved primarily with motor limbic function, and a dorsolateral component is involved primarily with volitional motor control (Nauta & Domesick, 1984). These specialized areas of the striatum receive topographically-organized dopamine projections from the midbrain. Iversen and Fray (1982) have hypothesized that the ventral striatal-dopamine system may be important for "species-specific motivational behavior." It has long been recognized by clinicians that emotionally charged words may be more easily produced by aphasic patients (Hughlings Jackson, 1878). If this ventral striatal-dopamine system is used by aphasic patients spontaneously to produce emotionally significant speech, perhaps a dopamine agonist is working by enhancing utilization of the alternative motor system for accessing language.

It is also possible that other mechanisms may exist for dopamine to enhance language function in aphasic patients. Dopamine agonists may simply have a nonspecific effect on the activation of cognition in a general way, rather than a specific effect on language function. There are insufficient data to support or refute this hypothesis at this time.

ACETYLCHOLINERGIC SYSTEM AND LANGUAGE

The cognitive operations that produce language have been divided into components including phonetics, syntax, and semantics. It has been postulated that Wernicke's area is located at the semantic-lexical pole of the neural-language network, and that Broca's area lies at the syntactic-articulatory pole (Mesulam, 1990). Although anomia or word-finding difficulty is described in most aphasic syndromes, it is quite likely that lesions of different neural systems, including different neurotransmitter systems, may underlie similar clinical aphasic features, including anomia. In particular, we hypothesize that the anomia that is characteristic of Wernicke's aphasia shares neural systems in common with certain memory systems and is likely to be dependent on intact acetylcholine system function.

Several lines of evidence support the above hypothesis. First, the activity of choline acetyltransferase, the rate-limiting enzyme necessary for the synthesis of acetylcholine, is reduced in Alzheimer's disease (AD) (Amaducci et al., 1981; Sorbi et al., 1984). Anomia is a common symptom of AD. Second, anomia and verbal memory deficits may both result from damage to the left temporal lobe (Albert, 1989; Milner, 1978). Third, the activity of choline acetyltransferase is higher in the left (language-dominant) than right temporal lobes (Amaducci et al., 1981; Sorbi et al., 1984). Fourth, when the anticholinergic agent scopolamine has been given to normal volunteers, not only have deficits in attention and memory been demonstrated but also impairments in reading, spelling, verbal fluency, and object naming (Aarsland et al., 1994). Fifth, physostigmine, an acetylcholin-esterase inhibitor, increases the brain concentration of acetylcholine when administered in clinical trials (Cohen & Wurtman, 1975). There is a case report of a patient with a basal forebrain lesion who demonstrated selectively enhanced left hippocampal blood flow after the administration of physostigmine (Chatterjee et al., 1993). In addition, physostigmine has been reported to increase regional cerebral blood flow in Alzheimer's disease in the left cerebral cortex, especially left frontal and higher frontal regions (Hunter et al., 1991). Clinical improvement after administration of physostigmine was especially pronounced on measures of word-finding, more so than on memory or other cognitive tasks. Physostigmine also appears to improve naming ability in patients with anomia (Jacobs et al., 1996).

Dopaminergic agents may improve naming ability by facilitating motor systems for speech initiation. Tanaka and Albert (1997) have hypothesized that the ability to name is dependent on features of semantic memory that, in turn, may be dependent on cholinergic system links to the temporal lobe. Speech initiation and word-finding, although mutually interdependent language processes, may depend on different neural systems and neurotransmitter systems.

Anatomical Data

Fedio and Van Buren (1974) found increased naming deficits (semantic retrieval) with stimulation of posterior temporo-parietal cortex, suggesting a common substrate for a generalized language-based retrieval system. Intra-operative stimulation trials demonstrated the highest proportion of naming sites within the left posterior, superior temporal gyrus. The largest proportion of memory sites were in the middle superior temporal and inferior parietal zones. Memory sites were also identified well into the anterior middle temporal lobe, although there was considerable inter-individual variability. Naming sites within the posterior temporo-parietal region appeared to be adjacent to memory sites.

Clinical Data

Little research has looked directly at the effect of cholinergic agents on speech and language functions. A summary can be seen in Table 2.

Luria et al. (1969) utilized galanthamine, a powerful cholinergic agent, to obtain a "deinhibitory" effect on complex gnostic, praxic, and speech functions in brain damage. Galanthamine was said to have improved a wide range of cognitive

Table 2. Previous reports of cholinergic agents for language impairment

Reporter	Drug	Subjects	Language
Luria	galantamine	A	articulation, araphasia fluency, aphonia
Scolyarova	piracetam	A	speech, language
Moscowitch	ameridin	A	naming, comprehension
Willmes	piracetam	A	language
Tanaka	bifemelane CDP-choline	A VD	naming naming, digit span fluency
Kabasawa	bifemelane	A	fluency, naming, comprehension
Farlow	tacrine	AD	naming, word finding, language
Jacob	physostigmine	M	naming*

A = aphasia
VD = vascular dementia
AD = Alzheimer's disease
* impairment

dysfunctions. They concluded that galanthamine was effective in sensory disorders of speech: the range of acoustic perception of the patients became wider, their understanding of the speech of others was improved, the phenomena of alienation of word meaning were diminished, phonemic discrimination was improved, and the time required for naming objects was shortened. EEG was used during treatment with galanthamine to obtain evidence of change in cortical neurodynamics. Activation of cortical function, as measured by EEG following administration of galanthamine, was found to take place only if anatomical connections between cortex and mesencephalon remained intact. These observations suggest that galanthamine acts through cholinergic structures in the reticular formation of the mesencephalon. The drug may have a general activating effect on cortical activity, rather than an effect specific to targeted cerebral centers.

Following Luria, Stolyarova et al. (1978) examined the effect of the nootropic agent piracetam on aphasic patients. Piracetam is a cyclic derivative of gamma-amino butyric acid (GABA). In addition to its central nervous system (CNS) effect of increasing adenosine triphosphate (ATP) synthesis, piracetam may also enhance acetylcholine release from presynaptic neurons. These investigators found that administration of piracetam resulted in improvement in speech and language of 20 of 35 aphasic patients. Moscowitch et al. (1991) reported that a cholinergic agent (ameridin) selectively improved language performance in semantic aphasia. Eight patients with semantic aphasia who were administered ameridin showed improvement in comprehension of grammatical structures and in naming after treatment, compared with 13 control patients (age- and severity-matched).

In Germany, Willmes et al. (1988) conducted a double-blind, placebo-controlled pilot study in which patients with aphasia treated with piracetam showed greater improvement than the control group in certain subtests of the Aachen Aphasia Test. In Japan, Tanaka et al. (1997) administered bifemelane, a cholinergic agonist, to aphasic patients and showed that it improved naming ability. Kabasawa et al. (1994) used bifemelane in a series of stroke patients. In case 1 there was improvement in comprehension, writing, and naming. Case 2 demonstrated improvement in fluency, naming, and repetition. Case 3 revealed improvement in comprehension and naming. All subtests of language improved in case 4, and case 5 showed improvement of comprehension, repetition, naming, writing, and reading. In addition to clinical improvement, all cases showed increased cerebral blood flow and metabolism in the left hemisphere after treatment (through pre- and post-treatment positron emission tomography).

In addition, as noted earlier, a number of studies have suggested that enhancement of acetylcholine function in AD may result in measurable improvement in word finding. Farlow et al. (1992) demonstrated that 80 mg of tacrine, an acetylcholinesterase inhibitor, improved language function in patients with AD. Although other cognitive functions may also respond to treatment, improvement in word-finding, when examined, appears to be a consistent finding.

Effects of Anticholinergic Agents on Language

Recently, there have been two reports of the effects of anticholinergic agents on language function. Aarsland et al. (1994) performed tests of reading, spelling, and oral language after administration of scopolamine in 22 healthy women to investigate the effect of cholinergic blockade on language. After scopolamine administration, there were dose-dependent impairments in reading, spelling, verbal fluency, and object naming. In 25 to 60 percent of subjects receiving 0.6 mg of scopolamine, there were clinically significant impairments on tests assessing lexical and phonological strategies. The authors suggest, based on the similarity of their findings with the pattern of deficits in reading and spelling observed in AD, that cholinergic blockade may be responsible for the type of language impairments found in AD.

Dubois et al. (1990) compared the neuropsychological performance of a group of 20 subjects treated with anticholinergic drugs to a control group. There was no significant difference between the two groups of patients for intellectual, visuospatial, instrumental, and memory function. In contrast, the group that received anticholinergic agents demonstrated the greatest impairment on verbal tests, digit span, and the Wisconsin Card Sorting Test. The authors speculated that the administration of anticholinergic agents may affect some aspects of learning/memory interpretation.

Cholinergic Hypothesis

In this chapter, we propose a testable model of the relation between acetylcholine systems to language function (depicted in Figure 2).

The studies outlined above suggest that the cholinergic system plays a prominent role in regulating left temporal lobe cortical function. This region may include portions of Wernicke's area, but is not coterminous with that area. The

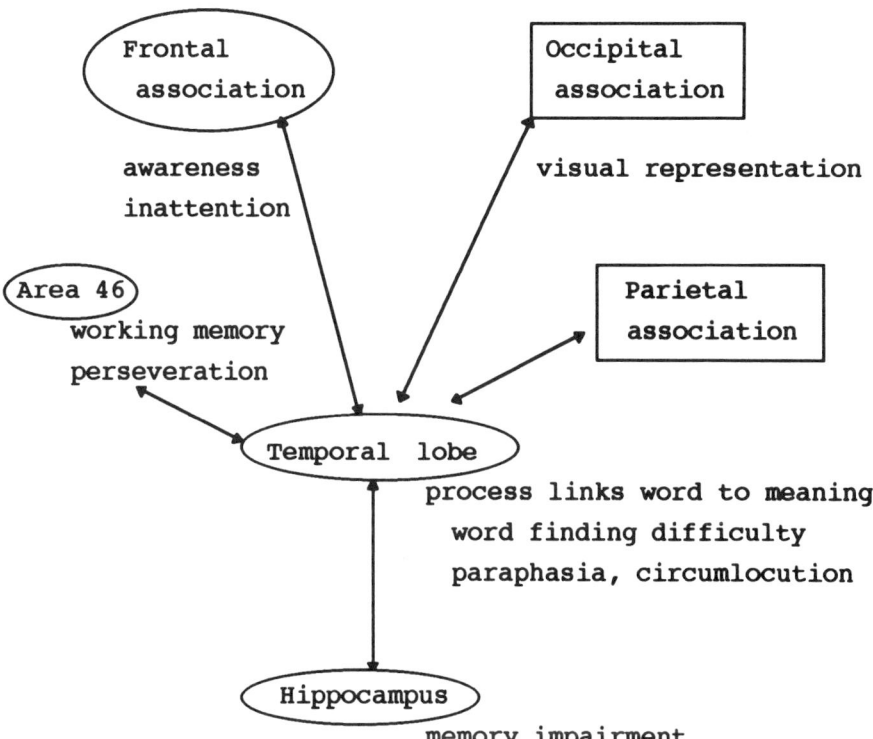

Figure 2. Testable model of cholinergic system: direct related area and indirect related area.

language function of the left temporal lobe almost certainly includes the process of linking phonemic word sounds to word meaning. When this region is lesioned, a variety of clinical symptoms may occur, including anomia. In addition, left temporal cortical structures are linked in a feed-forward and feed-back relation to frontal and parietal language areas. Consequently, lesions of the temporal lobe may also reasonably be expected to have an impact on language self-monitoring mechanisms, resulting in additional clinical symptoms such as paraphasias or perseveration.

Cholinergic agents may enhance word-finding via a number of possible mechanisms. First, by increasing cortical activation, cholinergic agents may increase the likelihood of a match between phonemic strings (or visual images) and semantic meaning. They may enhance the cortical interaction of temporal cortices with frontal and parietal language areas, allowing for greater feedback monitoring of semantic choices. This may reduce the likelihood of paraphasic or perseverative errors in naming.

Second, the hippocampal formations, located in the medial region of both temporal lobes, are critical structures for establishing new memories. Although a lesion to the left hippocampus may result in anterograde amnesia without language deficit, more often than not, some degree of anomia is present when the left basal temporal region is also involved – suggesting that a true memory impairment is responsible for some types of anomia. Cholinergic agents may enhance the cholinergic neurons' function within the hippocampus, resulting in improvement in memory. They may enhance verbal memory retrieval in a general way, thereby broadening mnemonic associations with phonemic strings or visual images, increasing the likelihood of successful word retrieval. Thus, one would expect an improvement in naming ability.

Third, lesions of left frontal language association area may disrupt language function in a number of ways. Temporal integration of language production (including initiation), attentional mechanisms (including aspects of search), self-monitoring, and so-called working memory are processes dependent on frontal function. As noted above, frontal function is sensitive to activity within the dopamine system. However, cholinergic systems may enhance frontal cortical function directly, perhaps producing a synergistic effect with dopamine activation. Improved frontal activity, via positive effects on attention and other functions, may increase the efficiency of temporal lobe word retrieval. Overall, cholinergic agents may enhance memory function and naming ability.

OTHER NEUROTRANSMITTERS

We have reviewed the relevance of two specific neurotransmitter systems, the dopamine and acetylcholine systems, in the production or alleviation of specific symptoms of aphasia. It is quite possible that, in the future, other neurotransmitter systems will also be found to play important roles. At this time, however, information on other systems is extremely scanty. Many neurochemical substances have been identified as neurotransmitters in the human brain. Some of these substances appear promising as "cognitive enhancers" that may secondarily and nonspecifically have beneficial effects on speech and language. Almost all neurotransmitter systems influence other neurotransmitter systems. For example, CDP-choline mainly plays a role in the regulation of the cholinergic system but also weakly activates the dopaminergic system. A GABA system, likewise, projects to the dopaminergic system.

There has been much less evidence in adrenergic and serotonergic systems of direct effects on specific language function than in dopaminergic and cholinergic systems. Even if other neurotransmitters do not influence language function directly, it is possible that improvement of memory or emotion could indirectly result in improved language function.

CONCLUSION

A Neurochemical Model of Language

In this chapter, we are proposing a model focused on relations between language function and neurotransmitter systems (see Figure 3). We hypothesize that language-related cortical and subcortical centers are influenced in characteristic ways by dopaminergic, cholinergic, or combined systems. The supplementary motor area (SMA) is a key target for dopamine innervation, regulating speech initiation, while the temporal lobe is the primary target for cholinergic innervation, playing a pivotal role in word retrieval. The relative balance between cerebral dopaminergic and cholinergic activity may itself be important in maintaining the integrity of language or in the manifestation of certain language symptoms in the face of brain injury.

The interaction between the SMA and Wernicke's area (and thus between dopamine and cholinergic function) may explain certain language symptoms seen in aphasia. For instance, if the left temporal lobe is damaged, cholinergic activity may be diminished, resulting in relative compensatory activation of the dopaminergic system. The effect of increased dopamine function on the SMA could result in increased speech initiation and, thus, pressured speech, typical of Wernicke's aphasia. In addition, the combination of increased speech initiation and diminished frontal monitoring may also contribute to jargon aphasia.

Frontal association areas are regulated by both systems. Interactions between the two neurotransmitters may affect local circuits and may be the basis for some spontaneous and treatment-induced language changes. For instance, lesions of either of these two neurotransmitter systems may disrupt distant cerebral function. Perhaps this is the reason that some unexpected lesions, particularly those in subcortical areas, produce classical aphasic syndromes in certain patients. Classic language areas may be affected indirectly by the disruption of ascending dopaminergic or cholinergic pathways. If dopaminergic pathways are interrupted, the aphasic syndrome may be biased towards a nonfluent aphasia with impaired speech initiation. If cholinergic pathways are predominantly interrupted, the aphasic syndrome may be biased towards a fluent aphasia with word finding difficulties, paraphasias, and perhaps pressured speech with jargon aphasia.

Despite clinical and theoretical evidence that neurotransmitter systems, especially the dopaminergic and cholinergic systems, may be involved in language regulation, the effects of pharmacological agents on aphasic symptoms remain

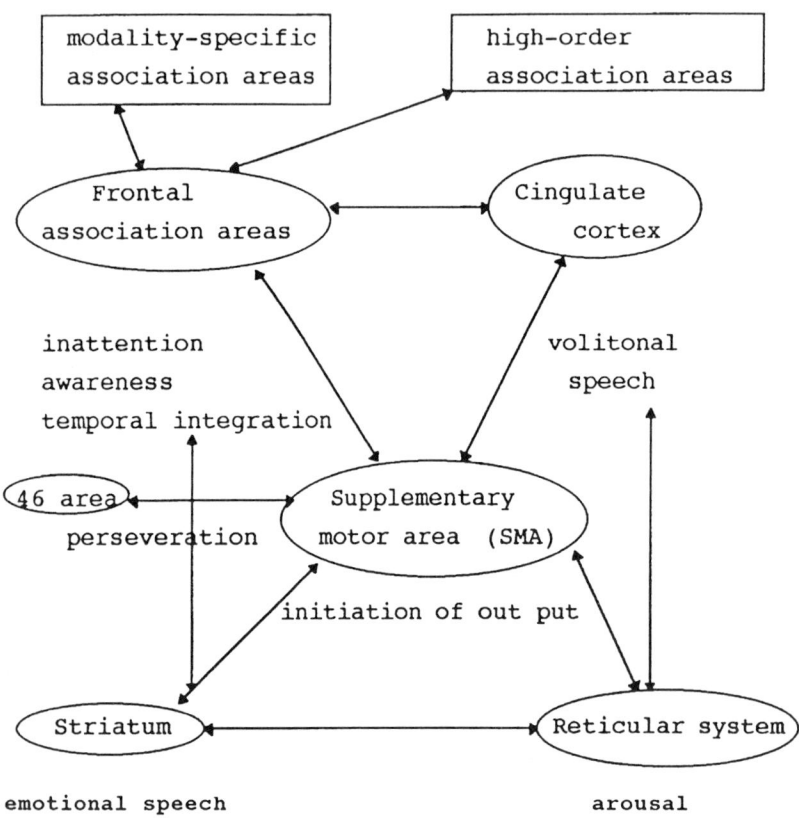

Figure 3. Testable model of neurotransmitter and language: direct related area and indirect related area.

unpredictable. One may reasonably ask why. There are a number of reasons why the clinical effects of dopaminergic- and cholinergic-enhancing agents may vary substantially from patient to patient: lesion size, lesion site, multiple lesions, associated disorders, and sensitivity of receptors or distribution of neurotransmitter systems.

Lesion Size

If lesion size extends to a sufficiently large area, the number of damaged neurons or post-synaptic receptors is, clearly, greater. There may be, therefore, too few target receptors in appropriate language regions for the drug to act upon.

Lesion Site

If lesion site is sufficiently large and centered primarily on language cortex, the absolute loss of critical language cortex may outweigh the relative contribution of the neurotransmitter pathways.

Multiple Lesions

Multiple cerebral lesions may result in a cumulative effect that mimics either of the above-stated effects.

Associated Disorders

If patients with aphasia also have another associated neurobehavioral syndrome with diffuse pathology, such as Alzheimer's disease, then the relative impact of the specific neurotransmitter system on language function may be masked by other cognitive and behavioral symptoms.

Sensitivity of Receptors or Distribution of Neurotransmitter Systems

It is possible that there is individual variability of receptor sensitivity among patients that would explain some inter-patient differences in treatment response. Dosages of bromocriptine sufficient to produce receptor activation in some patients may result in inhibition in other patients. In addition, the relative asymmetry of neurotransmitter systems for the right and left cerebral hemispheres may differ from individual to individual. In three sets of studies Albert (1987) demonstrated that the right cerebral hemisphere is involved in certain aspects of language. Other investigators have postulated a role for the right cerebral hemisphere for language recovery. It is unknown at this time whether cerebral asymmetry of dopaminergic and cholinergic activity plays a role in recovery of aphasia or the persistence of aphasic symptoms. It is not impossible that the neurochemical role in recovery or persistence of aphasia may vary from patient to patient depending on lesion site, number, and extent.

In summary, the mechanisms of language recovery after brain damage remain controversial. It is possible that neurotransmitter systems may be activated to compensate for certain language symptoms. This speculation gives us the opportunity not only to create new models of language function but to anticipate new drug treatments for specific aphasic symptoms.

REFERENCES

Aarsland, D., Larsen, J. P., Reinvang, I., & Aasland, A. M. (1994). Effects of cholinergic blockade on language in healthy young women: Implications for the cholinergic hypothesis in dementia of the Alzheimer type. *Brain, 117,* 1377-1384.

Albert, M. L. (1988). Neurological aspects of aphasia therapy. *Aphasiology, 2,* 215-218.

Albert, M. L., Bachman, D. L., Morgan, A., & Helm-Estabrooks, N. (1988). Pharmacotherapy for aphasia. *Neurology, 38,* 877-879.

Albert, M. L. (1987). New thoughts on functions of the right hemisphere. *Japanese Journal of Neuropsychology, 3,* 4-10.

Albert, M. L. (1989). The role of perseveration in language disorders. *Journal of Neurolinguistics, 4,* 471-478.

Alexander, M. P. (1989). Frontal lobes and language. *Brain and Language, 37,* 656-691.

Amaducci, L., Sorbi, S., Albanese, A., & Gainotti, G. (1981). Choline acetyltransferase (ChAT) activity differs in right and left human temporal lobes. *Neurology, 31,* 799-805.

Bachman, D. L. & Morgan, A. (1988). The role of pharmacotherapy in the treatment of aphasia: Preliminary results. *Aphasiology, 2,* 225-228.

Bachman, D. L. & Albert, M. L. (1990). The pharmacotherapy of aphasia: Historical perspective and directions for future research. *Aphasiology, 4,* 407-413.

Bachman, D. L. & Albert, M. L. (1991). The cerebral organization of language. In A. Peters & E. G. Jones (Eds.), *Cerebral Cortex: Normal altered states of function* (Vol. 9, pp. 213-262). New York: Plenum Press.

Bachman, D. L. & Albert, M. L. (1984). The dopaminergic syndromes of dementia. In G. Pilleri & F. Teagliliavini (Eds.), *Cerebral aging and degenerative dementia* (Vol. 1, pp. 91-113). Bern, Switzerland: Brain Anatomy Institute.

Benson, D. F. (1970). Presentation 10. In A. L. Benton (Ed.), *Behavioral changes in cerebrovascular disease* (pp. 77). New York: Harper & Row.

Bergman, P. S. & Green, M. (1949). Aphasia: Effect of intravenous sodium amytal. *Neurology, 1,* 471-475.

Billow, B. W. (1949). Observation on the use of sodium amytal in the treatment of aphasia. *Medical Records, 162,* 12-13.

Chatterjee, A., Morris, M. K., Bowers, D., Williamson, D. J., Doty, L., & Heilman, K. M. (1993). Cholinergic treatment of an amnestic man with a basal forebrain lesion: Theoretical implications. *Journal of Neurology, Neurosurgery and Psychiatry, 56,* 1282-1289.

Cohen, E. L. & Wurtman, R. J. (1975). Brain acetylcholine: Increase after systemic choline administration. *Life Sciences, 16,* 1095-1102.

Dubois, B., Pilon, B., L'hermitte, F., & Agid, Y. (1990). Cholinergic deficiency and frontal dysfunction in Parkinson's disease. *Annals of Neurology, 28,* 117-121.

Farlow, M., Gracon, S. I., Hershey, L. A., Lewis, K. W., Sadowsky, C. H., & Dolan-Ureno, J. (1992). A controlled trial of tacrine in Alzheimer's disease. *Journal of the American Medical Association, 268,* 2523-2529.

Fedio, P. & Van Buren, J. M. (1974). Memory deficits during electrical stimulation of the speech cortex in conscious man. *Brain and Language, 1,* 29-42.

Gheorghita, N. (1977). Immediate effects of neurodynamic substances on verbal performance in the treatment of aphasia. *Revue Roumaine de Neurologie et de Psychiatrie, 15,* 95-101.

Gupta, S. R. & Mlcoch, A. G. (1992). Bromocriptine treatment of nonfluent aphasia. *Archives of Physical Medicine and Rehabilitation, 73,* 373-376.

Gupta, S. R., Mlcoch, A. G., Scolaro, C., & Moritz, T. (1995). Bromocriptine treatment of nonfluent aphasia. *Neurology, 45,* 2170-2173.

Hughlings Jackson, J. (1878). On the affections of speech from disease of the brain. *Brain, 1,* 304-330.

Hunter, R., Wyper, D. J., Patterson, J., Hansen, M. T., & Goodwin, G. M. (1991). Cerebral pharmacodynamics of physostigmine in Alzheimer's disease investigated using single-photon computerised tomography. *British Journal of Psychiatry, 158,* 351-357.

Iversen, S. D. & Fray, P. J. (1982). Brain catecholamines in relation to affect. In A. Beckman (Ed.), The neural basis of behavior. New York: Spectrum.
Jacobs, D. H., Shuren, J., Gold, M., Adair, J. C., Bowers, D., Williamson, D. J. G., & Heilman, K. M. (1996). Physostigmine pharmacotherapy for anomia. *Neurocase*, *2*, 83-91.
Kabasawa, H., Matsubara, M., Kamimoto, K., Hibino, H., Banno, T., & Nagai, H. (1992). Effects of bifemelane on cerebral circulation and metabolism in patients with aphasia. *Clinical Therapeutics*, *16*, 471-482.
Liebson, E., Walsh, M. J., Jankowiak, J., & Albert, M. L. (1994). Pharmacotherapy for post-traumatic dysarthria. *Neuropsychiatry, Neuropsychology, and Behavioral Neurology*, *7*, 122-124.
Linn, L. & Stein, M. H. (1946). Sodium amytal in treatment of aphasia. Preliminary report. *Bulletin of the US Army Medical Department*, *5*, 705-708.
Luders, H., Lesser, R. P., Hahn, J., Dinner, D. S., Morris, H. H., Wyllie, E. & Godoy, J. (1991). Basal temporal language area. *Brain*, *114*, 743-754.
Luria, A. R., Naydin, V. L., Tsvetkova, L. S., Vinarskaya E.N. (1969). Restoration of higher cortical function following local brain damage. In P. J. Vinken & G. W. Bruyn (Eds.), *Handbook of clinical neurology: Disorders of higher nervous activity* (Vol. 3, pp. 368-433). Amsterdam: North Holland Publishing.
MacLennan, D. L., Nicholas, L. E., Morley, G. K., & Brookshire, R. H. (1990). The effects of bromocriptine on speech and language function in a man with transcortical motor aphasia. In T. E. Prescott (Ed.), *Clinical aphasiology, 20* (pp. 145-155). Boston: College Hill
Mesulam, M. M. (1990). Large-scale neurocognitive networks and distributed processing for attention, language, and memory. *Annals of Neurology*, *28*, 597-613.
Milner, B. (1978). Clues to the cerebral organization of memory. In P. A. Bruser & A. Rougeul-Bruser (Eds.), *Cerebral correlates of conscious experiences* (pp. 139-153). Amsterdam: Elsevier.
Mimura, M., Albert, M. L., & McNamara, P. (1995). Towards a pharmacotherapy for aphasia. In H. S. Kirshner (Ed.), *Handbook of neurological speech and language disorders* (pp. 465-482). New York: Marcel Dekker.
Moscowitch, L., McNamara, P., & Albert, M. L. (1991). Neurochemical correlates of aphasia. *Neurology*, *41* (1), 410.
Naeser, M. A., Palumbo, C. L., Helm-Estabrooks, N., Stiassny-Eder, D., & Albert, M. L. (1989). Severe non-fluency in aphasia: Role of the medial subcallosal fasciculus plus other white matter pathways in recovery of spontaneous speech. *Brain*, *112*, 1-38.
Nauta, W. J. H. & Domesic, V. B. (1984). Afferent and efferent relationships of the basal ganglia. In D. Evered, M. O'Connor (Eds.), *Functions of the basal ganglia*. Ciba Foundation Symposium (Pitman, London).
Penfield, W. & Jasper, H. (1954). *Epilepsy and the functional anatomy of the human brain*. Boston, Little Brown.
Porch, B. E. (1967). *Porch Index of Communicative Ability, I: Theory and development*. Palo Alto, CA, Consulting Psychologists Press.
Sabe, L., Leiguarda, R., & Starkstein, S. E. (1992). An open-label trial of bromocriptine in nonfluent aphasia. *Neurology*, *42*, 1637-1638.
Sabe, L., Salvarezza, F., Garcia Cuerva, A., Leiguarda, R., & Starkstein, S. (1995). A randomized, double-blind, placebo-controlled study of bromocriptine in nonfluent aphasia. *Neurology*, *45*, 2272-2274.
Sitaram, N., Weingartner, H., & Gillin, J. C. (1978). Human serial learning: Enhancement with arecoline and choline and impairment with scopolamine. *Science*, *201*, 274-276.
Small, S. L. (1994). Pharmacotherapy of aphasia: A critical review. *Stroke*, *25*, 1282-1289.
Solomonovici, A., Fradis, A., Mihallescu, L., Sevastopol, M. (1972). Tratamental cu imipramina in afrazille de origine vasculara. *Studii si Cercetari de Neurologie*, *7*, 257-263.
Sorbi, S., Bracco, L., Piacentini, S., Morandi, A., & Amaducci, L. (1984). Chemical lateralization in human temporal cortex. *Monographs in Neural Sciences*, *11*, 157-162.
Stoica, E., Stefanescu, E., & Gheoghiu, M. (1972). The restoration of the reactivity of higher autonomic centers by pyrithioxine administration in cerebral infarct patients. *European Neurology*, *7*, 348-363.
Stolyarova, L., Kadykov, A., Kistenev, B., et al. (May, 1978). The role of piracetam in complex rehabilitation therapy of patients with residual manifestations of a cerebral stroke. In E. A. Babayan, N. V. Lebedeva, G. M. Rudenko et al (Eds.). Nootropil in Neurological and Psychiatric Practice: Materials of a Symposium. Moscow.

Tanaka, Y., Minematsu, K., Hirano, T., Hayashida, K., & Yamaguchi, T. (1994). Effects of CDP-choline on dynamic changes in LCBF and cognitive function in demented subjects - An H215O-PET study. *Rinsho Shinkeigaku [Clinical Neurology], 34,* 877-881 (In Japanese with English abstract).

Tanaka, Y., Miyashita, T., Miyazaki, M., Kuroda, Y., Kuzuhara, S. (1993). The relationship between the prognosis of aphasia and chronological changes of HVA levels in CSF during L-dopa therapy. *Neurologia Medico-Chirurgica, 38,* 42-46 (in Japanese with English abstract).

Tanaka, Y., Tsuda, M., Miyazaki, M., Kuroda, Y., Kuzuhara, S. (1991). L-dopa therapy for aphasia. *Neurologia Medico-Chirurgica, 34,* 532-534. (in Japanese).

Tanaka, Y., Bachman, D. L., & Miyazaki, M. (1993). Pharmacotherapy for akinesia following anterior communicating artery aneurysm hemorrhage. *Japanese Journal of Medicine, 32,* 641-643.

Tanaka, Y., Miyazaki, M., & Albert, M. L. (1997). Effects of increased cholinergic activity on naming in aphasia. *Lancet, 350,* 116-117.

Voinescu, I. & Gheorghita, N. (1973). Tratamentul afraziel cu imipramina. *Neurologia, Psihiatria, Neurochirurgia, 18,* 423-430.

Voinescu, I. & Gheorghita, N. (1978). Adjuvant drug therapy with psychologopedic rehabilitation of aphasic patients. *Revue Roumaine de Neurologie et de Psychiatrie, 16,* 155-161.

Walker-Batson, D., Devous, M., Curtis, S., Unwin, D.H., Greenlee, R.G. (1991). Response to amphetamine to facilitate recovery from aphasia subsequent to stroke. *Clinical Aphasiology, 21,* 137-143.

Willmes, K., Huber, W., Poeck, K., et al. (1988). Die Wirkung von Piracetam bei der logopadischen Intensivtherapie von chronish aphasischen Patienten. In Von Helmchen (Ed.), Sonderd ruck ans Wirlumgen und Wirksamkeit von Nootropika (pp. 177-187). Berlin, Springer-Verlag.

Wise, R., Chollet, F., Hadar, U., Friston, K., Hoffner, E., & Frackowiak, R. (1991). Distribution of cortical neural networks involved in word comprehension and word retrieval. *Brain, 115,* 1803-1817.

UNDERSTANDING COGNITIVE FUNCTIONING THROUGH BRAIN DAMAGE

THE NEURAL BASIS OF WORKING MEMORY: EVIDENCE FROM NEUROPSYCHOLOGICAL, PHARMACOLOGICAL AND NEUROIMAGING STUDIES

Mark D'Esposito

INTRODUCTION

The frontal lobes in man represent a portion of the cerebral cortex whose function still stands as quite a mystery. The famous patient Phineas Gage, who was described over 100 years ago, is an example of the consequences of damage to this brain region. Prior to his accident, he was a religious, family-loving, honest, and hard working man who was described after his frontal injury as being

> fitful, irreverent, indulging at times in the grossest profanity... impatient of restraint or advice when it conflicts with his desires... obstinate... devising many plans of operation, which are no sooner arranged than they are abandoned in turn for others appearing more feasible (Harlow, 1868).

Adding to the mystery of the consequences of his brain injury was the observation that his intelligence seemed relatively intact, as well as his motor and sensory functions. In recent years, the field of cognitive neuroscience has exploded, and new neuroscientific methods have been developed to study brain function of both human and non-human primates providing clues to the function of the largest, yet least well-understood area of the cerebral cortex.

As researchers strive to characterize the cognitive processes subserved by the frontal lobes or, specifically, the prefrontal cortex (PFC), the term *executive function* has emerged and gained prominence in the taxonomy of cognition used in psychology and neuroscience. The clinical neuropsychological literature, for example, includes, under the rubric of executive function, a wide range of cognitive processes such as focused and sustained attention, fluency and flexibility of thought in the generation of solutions to novel problems, and planning and regulating adaptive and goal directed behavior (Hécaen & Albert, 1978; Lezak, 1995; Luria, 1966). As is evident by the wide scope of these processes, executive function has been used to capture the highest order of cognitive abilities. Such abilities are not only difficult to define but are also difficult to measure, and the elusive nature of the cognitive functions that are governed by the PFC has hampered the investigation of their physiological bases. Part of the problem has been the common error of using the term *executive function* synonymously with *frontal lobe function* and the treatment of the frontal lobes as an undifferentiated cortical mass. It is likely that not all measures thought to tap executive function are subserved by the PFC, that the PFC is not the only brain region contributing to executive function, and that particular portions of the PFC are specialized to contribute to specific aspects of executive function and other higher cognitive processes.

THE CONCEPT OF EXECUTIVE FUNCTION

Several theoretical models of executive function exist. For example, Baddeley (1986; 1992) has proposed the existence of *a central executive system* (CES). Based on behavioral studies of normal subjects, he proposes that this system actively regulates the distribution of limited attentional resources and coordinates information within limited capacity verbal and spatial memory storage buffers. The CES and the analogous *supervisory attentional system* (SAS) proposed by Norman and Shallice (1986) are proposed to take control over cognitive processing when novel tasks are engaged and/or when existing behavioral routines have to be overridden. Because the CES is thought to have a limited capacity, each additional cognitive process that a subject performs places increasing demands on this system. The dual-task paradigm has been used as an effective tool for probing this system. Sequential performance of two tasks or parallel performance of two unrelated tasks that engage separate processing mechanisms are thought to make minimal demands on a system such as the CES. However, two tasks performed concurrently that require similar processing structures will make greater demands on the CES and will lead to a decrement in performance.

Both Baddeley and Shallice have argued that an *executive controller* is a distinct cognitive module that is supported by neuronal networks in the PFC and that failure of this module, or system, accurately describes the behavior of patients with frontal lobe damage. We have tested the idea that the PFC is an important neural substrate of the CES in two ways. First, using functional MRI (fMRI), we investigated whether activation of the PFC would be observed while normal human subjects performed a dual-task experiment (D'Esposito et al., 1995). During scanning, subjects concurrently performed a spatial task and a verbal task, cognitive challenges that were selected because they have been reported to activate predominantly posterior brain regions (i.e., not frontal). We reasoned that any activation in frontal regions would be due to the dual-task nature of the experiment and not to the performance of either of the individual tasks per se. Our study did in fact demonstrate lateral PFC activation only during the dual-task condition (see Figure 1).

Because the dual-task condition was more difficult than either task condition performed alone, it was necessary to eliminate the possibility that PFC activation was simply due to a non-specific increase in mental effort required to perform the dual-task. We addressed this issue by having subjects perform the spatial task alone, but at different levels of difficulty. Even during the more difficult condition,

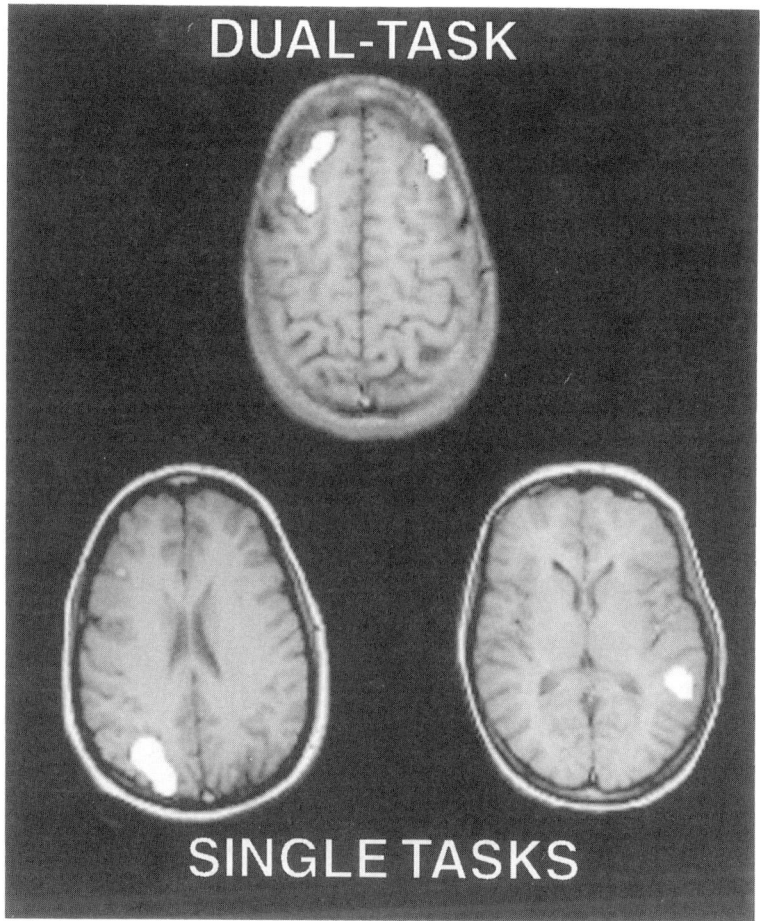

FIGURE 1. The top brain slice reveals prefrontal cortical activation during the dual-task whereas the bottom-two brain slices reveal posterior (temporal/parietal) brain activation during the single tasks. The two tasks were verbal tasks which required subjects to identify exemplars of a target category (e.g., *vegetable*) in a series of aurally presented words whereas the spatial task required subjects to indicate which of two squares had a dot in the same location, relative to a double line, as a spatially rotated target square.

when performance was worse than that seen for the spatial task performed during the dual-task condition, we did not observe any PFC activation. This finding suggested that the PFC activation observed during the dual-task experiment was related specifically to the executive control process required to organize and execute two tasks simultaneously.

Because neuroimaging methods such as fMRI cannot determine whether a brain region is *necessary* for a specific cognitive process, but only whether it is engaged in association with a certain type of behavior (Sarter, Bernston, & Cacioppo, 1996), we sought next to determine if patients with prefrontal damage would be impaired on dual-task paradigms. In a study of a group of traumatic brain injury patients, we demonstrated that, indeed, despite performing comparably to healthy control subjects under single task conditions, performance of the patients was significantly inferior to control subject performance under dual-task conditions (McDowell, Whyte, & D'Esposito, 1997). We have also found a similar deficit in patients with Parkinson's disease (D'Esposito & Postle, in press), who have been described clinically as exhibiting a similar neurobehavioral picture to patients with frontal lobe damage (Taylor, Saint-Cyr, & Lang, 1986).

Taken together, our imaging and behavioral studies with patients provide converging evidence for an association between executive control and prefrontal cortical function. However, both the Baddeley and Shallice models propose that there is a system or controller module that is doing the controlling of behavior. And, even though empirical evidence that we have accumulated supports a link between normal PFC function and the ability to perform tasks that require executive control, an important question to consider is whether one needs to propose that a unitary controller exists in the brain to mediate executive function.

IS THERE AN EXECUTIVE CONTROLLER IN THE BRAIN?

Evidence from studies of patients with brain damage suggests that if there is a controller there is not likely to be only one (e.g., a central executive). For example, patients with frontal-lobe damage are typically not impaired on all clinical measures of executive function. Baddeley and colleagues (Baddeley, Della Sala, Papagano, & Spinnler, 1997) have reported that patients with frontal lobe lesions who showed a behaviorally assessed *dysexecutive* syndrome had a greater dual-task impairment as compared to frontal lobe patients who were behaviorally normal (non-dysexecutive). However, these two groups of patients did not differ significantly from each other on other measures of executive function such as the Wisconsin Card Sorting Task or verbal fluency. Thus, to adequately explain these empirical data, one would need to propose that each of these tasks represent different types of executive processes that are each subserved by different parts of the PFC.

Other investigators have attempted to provide a parsimonious account of the computations underlying the diverse processes considered to be executive in nature. Such an account of prefrontal function had been proposed by Kimberg and Farah (1993). Their model proposes that executive dysfunction is due to a weakening of associations among working memory representations, including mental representations of internal goals, stimuli in the environment, and stored declarative knowledge. In this model, the representations themselves remain intact. Evidence for this hypothesis has come from a computational model that accounted for performance on four very different measures of executive function (motor sequencing, the Stroop task, the Wisconsin Card Sorting Task, and a context memory task) by weakening the associations among the goal, stimuli, and knowledge elements constituting working memory. Rather than requiring an explanation for performance on each task, these investigators were able to explain performance on these seemingly disparate measures of executive function based on one disruption: the weakening of associations among working memory representations. In this model, there is no controller module. This interesting approach represents another way to consider prefrontal function. However, the importance this model places on working memory requires a much better understanding of this concept.

THE CONCEPT OF WORKING MEMORY

Working memory is an evolving concept that refers to the short-term storage of information that is not accessible in the environment and the set of processes that keep this information active for later use in behavior (Fuster, 1997; Goldman-Rakic, 1987). It is critically important in cognition and seems necessary in the course of performing many other cognitive functions such as reasoning, language comprehension, planning, and spatial processing. Evidence for the neuroanatomical basis of working memory has been derived in part from monkey studies of delayed-response tasks. In these tasks, the monkey must keep *in mind* a stimulus over a short delay. There is abundant evidence from such experiments to support the claim that the lateral PFC plays a critical role during tasks that involve working memory. For example, neurons within the PFC are found to be persistently activated during the delay period of a delayed-response task when the monkey is maintaining information in memory prior to making a motor response (Funahashi, Bruce, & Goldman-Rakic, 1989; Fuster & Alexander, 1971). The necessity of this region for working memory has been demonstrated in monkey studies that have shown that lesions of the lateral PFC impair performance on these tasks (Bauer & Fuster, 1976; Funahashi, Bruce, & Goldman-Rakic, 1993). Thus, it is proposed that the PFC allows the integration of events that are separated in time and utilizes stored representational knowledge to guide an appropriate motor response.

Human studies have provided converging evidence to support the hypothesis that working memory is subserved in part by the PFC. For example, working memory impairments have been demonstrated in humans following restricted PFC damage (Pierrot-Deseilligny, Rivaud, Gaymard, & Agid, 1991; Ptito, Crane, Leonard, Amsel, & Caramanos, 1995; Verin et al., 1993). Also, functional neuroimaging studies of working memory in healthy young adults have provided empirical evidence for the link between working memory and the PFC (Cohen et al., 1997; Courtney, Ungerleider, Keil, & Haxby, 1997). In fact, there now seems to be a critical mass of studies that have used functional imaging to show that the PFC is engaged during the working memory tasks (D'Esposito, Aguirre, Zarahn, & Ballard, 1998). For example, Jonides and colleagues performed the first study that showed that the PFC was activated during performance of a spatial working memory task that was analogous to the one used in the monkey studies. In this study, PFC activation was present when a block of trials with a delay period were compared to a block of trials without a delay period (Jonides et al., 1993).

A potential problem in interpretation of an imaging study such as that of Jonides is that it relies on the assumptions of the method of *cognitive subtraction*. Cognitive subtraction attempts to correlate brain activity with specific processes by pairing two tasks that are assumed to be matched perfectly for every sensory, motor, and cognitive process except the process of interest (Posner, Petersen, Fox, & Raichle, 1988). For example, in the Jonides study it was assumed that the only difference between the two experimental conditions was the delay period and, therefore, the process of memory storage. Although the application of cognitive subtraction to imaging was a major innovation when originally introduced (Petersen, Fox, Posner, Mintun, & Raichle, 1988), it has become clear that it is a potentially flawed methodology that may lead to erroneous interpretation of imaging data.

DEVELOPMENT OF A NEW IMAGING METHOD TO STUDY PREFRONTAL FUNCTION

The assumptions that must be relied upon for cognitive subtraction methodology can be faulty for at least two reasons. First, it involves the assumption of *additivity* (or *pure insertion*), the idea that a cognitive process can be added to a pre-existing set of cognitive processes without affecting them (Sternberg, 1969). For example, the delayed-response paradigm, typically used to study working memory, is comprised of a memory-requiring delay period between a *perceptual* process (the presentation of the item(s) to be stored) and a *choice* process (a required decision based upon the item that was stored). The neural substrates of the memory process are proposed to be revealed by a subtraction of the integrated (i.e., averaged, summed, or totaled) functional hemodynamic signal during a no-delay condition (e.g., a block of trials without a delay period) from that during a delay condition (e.g., a block of trials with a delay period). In this example, failure to meet the assumptions of cognitive subtraction will occur if the insertion of a delay period between the perceptual and choice processes interacts with these other behavioral processes in the task. For example, these non-memory processes may be different in delay trials as compared to no-delay trials.

In neuroimaging, an additional requirement must be met in order for cognitive subtractive methodology to yield non-artifactual results: the transform between the neural signal and the neuroimaging signal must be linear. In two studies thus far, some non-linearities have been observed in this system (Boynton, Engel, Glover, & Heeger, 1996; Vazquez & Noll, 1998). In our example of a delayed-response paradigm, failure will occur if the sum of the transform of neural activity to hemodynamic signal for the perceptual and choice processes differs when a delay is inserted as compared to when it is not present. In this example, artifacts of cognitive subtraction might lead to the inference that a region displayed delay-correlated increases in neural activity when in actuality it did not. To overcome these potential problems, we have developed an *event-related* fMRI design that does not rely on cognitive subtraction (Zarahn, Aguirre, & D'Esposito, 1997). With this method we have found that the PFC is activated during the delay. But more importantly, we have found empirical evidence of a cognitive subtraction failure (Zarahn, Aguirre, & D'Esposito, 1999).

As mentioned, spatial delayed-response tasks, designed to probe spatial working memory, typically have a stimulus presentation period, an ensuing delay (of a few seconds), and a choice period. Changes in single unit neural activity have been observed during each of these task components in electrophysiological studies of non-human primates. For example, Fuster and colleagues, using a visual delayed-response task, observed that responses of single prefrontal cortical neurons to the initial stimulus presentation ended within a few hundred milliseconds of stimulus offset (Fuster, Bauer, & Jervey, 1982). They also observed changes in firing rate in single neurons in the lateral PFC during the delay period that were sustained for several seconds. If these results also characterize human PFC function, it should be possible with fMRI to resolve temporally functional changes correlated with the delay period from those correlated with the stimulus presentation/early delay period in a population of neurons.

The logic of our new fMRI design is as follows: A single behavioral trial may be hypothesized to be associated with one brief neural event, or several brief neural events, that are subcomponent processes that are engaged within a trial. A neural event will cause a brief fMRI signal change, which we will call an impulse response function (IRF). If we wish to model the evoked fMRI response caused by a single neural event, the IRF would seem an appropriate *a priori* candidate. Similarly, the fMRI signal evoked by a series of shifted neural events (e.g., sequential events in time such as the presentation of a cue or a motor response) would be modeled appropriately by a set of IRFs shifted to the appropriate time period where the event occurs. Most importantly, a combination of IRFs could theoretically model any neural event, even if the event is sustained, such as delay period activity. An illustration of this method is presented in Figure 2.

DOES THE PFC IN HUMANS SUBSERVE WORKING MEMORY?

Analyzed in the manner described above, during the performance of a spatial delayed-response task, we observed that several brain regions, including the PFC, consistently displayed activity that correlated with the delay period across subjects (Zarahn, Aguirre, & D'Esposito, 1998). This finding suggests that these regions may be involved in temporary maintenance of spatial representations in humans. With this event-related fMRI design we could be confident that activity observed was not due to differences in other components of the task (i.e., presentation of the cue or motor response) during the behavioral trials. Most importantly, these results do not rely on the assumptions of cognitive subtraction.

An example of the time series of the fMRI signal averaged across trials for a PFC region displaying delay-correlated activity is shown in Figure 3. In this study, we also found direct evidence for the failure of cognitive subtraction. We found a region in the PFC that did not display sustained activity during the delay (in a single trial analysis) yet showed greater activity in the delay trials as compared to the trials without a delay (in a blocked trial analysis). In a blocked neuroimaging study, which compared delay versus no-delay trial with subtraction, such a region would be detected and likely assumed to be a memory region. Thus, this result provides

186 Neurobehavior of Language and Cognition

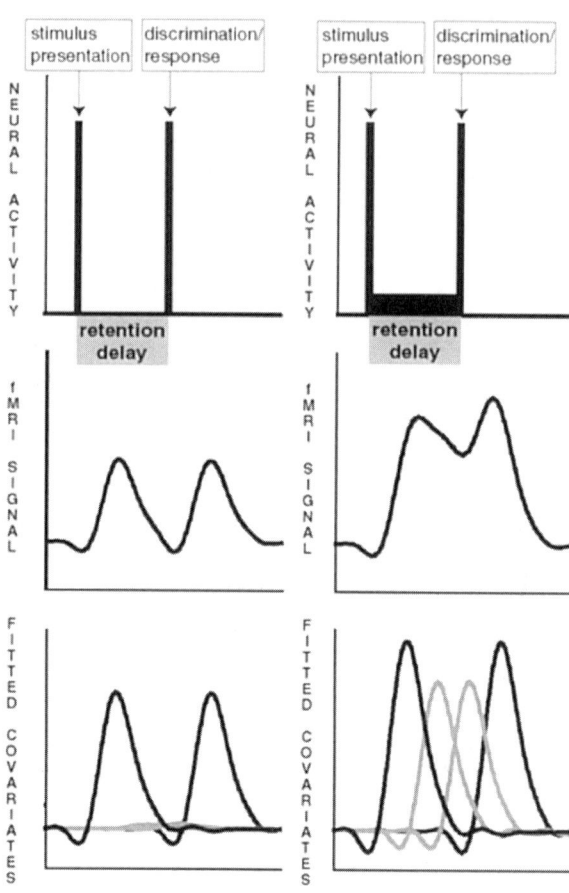

FIGURE 2. In the left panel, neural activity is evoked only during the presentation of the stimulus and during the motor response. In this scenario, there is no activity modeled by impulse response functions that are placed in the appropriate time period to capture delay period activity (grey lines). Alternatively, in the right panel, neural activity is present during the delay period (as well as during the cue and response). In this example, appropriately placed IRFs capture delay period activity (grey lines).

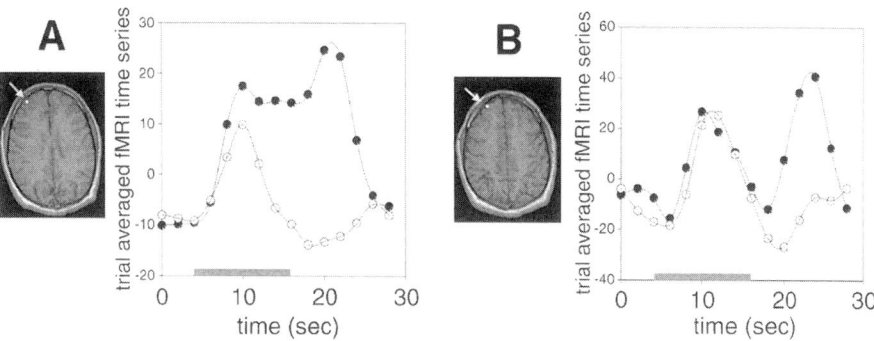

FIGURE 3. (A) An example of the time series of the fMRI signal averaged across trials for a PFC region that displayed delay-correlated activity is shown; filled black circles represent activity for delay trials and open circles are trials without a delay. (B) An example of a time series where the integrated activity for the presentation of the cue and response during the delay trials (filled black circles) is greater than that observed during the combined presentation of the cue and response in the no-delay trials (open circles).

grounds for being somewhat wary of the inferences drawn from imaging studies that have relied on cognitive subtraction.

DOES HUMAN PFC HAVE FUNCTIONAL SUBDIVISIONS?

While the evidence presented above suggests that the PFC appears to be critical for the processing of temporarily stored information, it is unclear whether there are functional subdivisions within the PFC that are specialized for particular aspects of working memory. We believe there are at least four ways to think about how PFC operations might be organized neuroanatomically (illustrated in Figure 4).

First, there may be a single PFC region involved in all working memory processes (e.g., simple maintenance operations such as rehearsal and more complex operations such as retrieval, reordering, performing spatial transformations, etc.) that can be directed at distributed representations in posterior brain regions (Model 1). Second, there may be different PFC regions for different types of representations (e.g., spatial, object) regardless of operation (Model 2). Third, there may be different PFC regions required for different operations (e.g., maintenance, manipulation) regardless of the type of representation (Model 3). Finally, there may be different PFC regions for combinations of operation and type of representation (Model 4).

Goldman-Rakic and colleagues have proposed that the different regions of the PFC are critical for the temporary maintenance of different types of stimuli. Specifically, they have provided evidence that the monkey PFC is segregated into one region that retains information about an object's color and shape (inferior or ventral PFC) and a second region that retains the object's location in space (superior or dorsal PFC) (Wilson, Scalaidhe, & Goldman-Rakic, 1993). This was demonstrated by recording from neurons within a more ventral region, the inferior prefrontal convexity, while monkeys performed spatial-delayed or pattern-delayed response tasks and finding that a greater number of neurons in this region responded during the delay period selectively to pattern rather than location information. Also, lesions comprising the dorsal PFC have been shown to impair spatial working memory (Funahashi, Bruce, & Goldman-Rakic, 1993; Gross, 1963) whereas other studies reveal impaired non-spatial working memory following more ventral lesions (Mishkin & Manning, 1978; Passingham, 1975).

These findings have led to the hypothesis that the lateral PFC is organized in a dorsal/ventral fashion subserving the temporary storage of *what* and *where* information. This hypothesis has the appeal of parsimony, as a similar organization has been identified in the visual system (Ungerleider & Haxby, 1994). Also, anatomical studies in monkeys have demonstrated that the parietal cortex (i.e., spatial vision regions) predominantly projects to a dorsal region of the lateral PFC (Cavada & Goldman-Rakic, 1989; Petrides & Pandya, 1984), whereas the temporal cortex (i.e., object vision regions) projects more ventrally within the lateral PFC (Barbas, 1988).

Functional MRI may be able to address this question in humans by determining the pattern of PFC activity during spatial and non-spatial working memory tasks. Several studies of this kind have been conducted previously, and we have critically examined this literature for evidence for or against the *what* versus

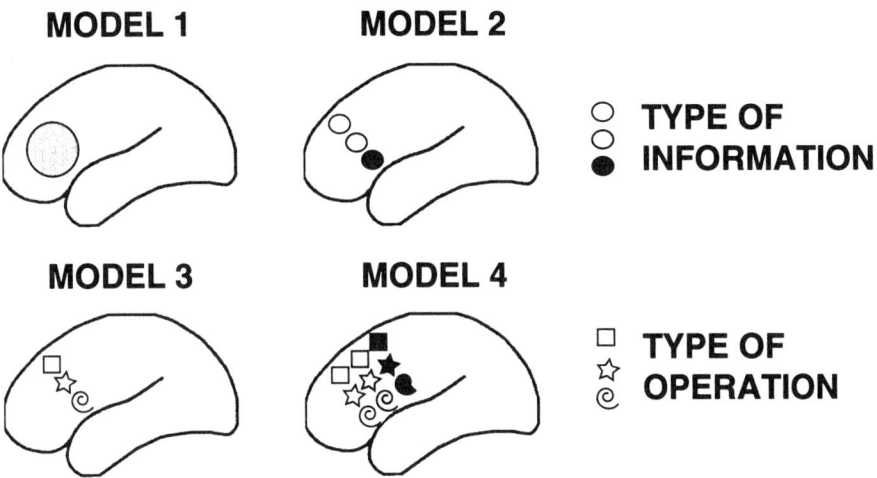

FIGURE 4. Models of prefrontal cortical organization.

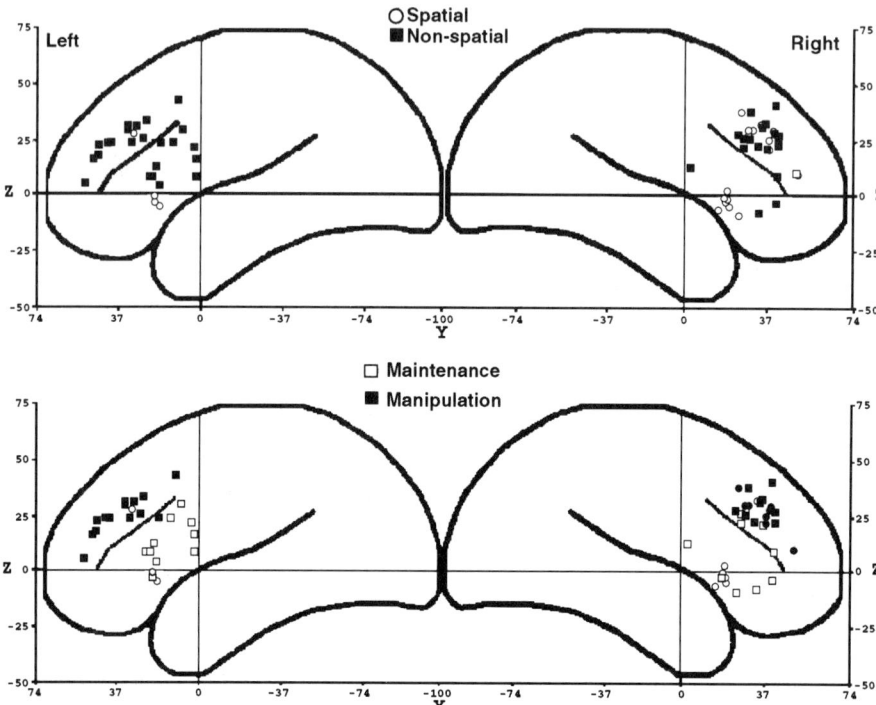

FIGURE 5. Meta-analysis of published functional neuroimaging studies of working memory. Each symbol represents a significant activation reported in a standardized atlas (Talairach & Tournoux, 1988). Top panel shows activations from either *spatial* or *non-spatial* studies whereas bottom panel reports activations from the same studies reclassified as requiring *maintenance* or *manipulation*. Studies classified as *manipulation*, which observed ventral PFC activation, in addition to dorsal PFC activation, are represented by gray symbols. The black line indicates the boundary between the middle and inferior frontal gyrus (inferior frontal sulcus) representing dorsal (areas 9 and 46) and ventral regions (areas 44, 45, and 47) of lateral PFC, respectively.

where model of prefrontal organization as well as performed our own empirical studies (D'Esposito et al., 1998). In our meta-analysis, we plotted the locations of activation from all reported functional-neuroimaging studies of spatial and non-spatial working memory on a standardized brain. Based on the animal literature, it is proposed that the human homologue of the principal sulcal region of the lateral PFC, the middle frontal gyrus (Brodmann's area 46), would subserve spatial working memory whereas non-spatial working memory would be subserved by a more ventral region such as the inferior frontal gyrus (Brodmann's areas 47, 44, and 45). We found no evidence for this dorsal/ventral dissociation in this analysis as illustrated in Figure 5.

In an empirical study, we have tested subjects during two different working memory tasks with different sets of stimuli during fMRI. In the memory condition, subjects attended to serially-presented stimuli and determined if a letter or location of a square was the same as that presented two stimuli back. In the control condition, subjects were asked to identify a single predetermined letter or location. Group and individual subject analyses revealed activation in the right middle frontal gyrus that did not differ between spatial and non-spatial working memory conditions. Again, we did not find evidence for dorsal/ventral organization of the PFC based on the type of information held in working memory. Several other investigators using virtually identical tasks have found similar results (Cohen et al., 1998; Postle, Stern, Rosen, & Corkin, 1997). Recently, we have performed a follow-up to this study using event-related fMRI. Even when we modeled only the delay period and did not rely on cognitive subtraction, identical regions of the PFC were activated when subjects remembered spatial or object information. Reliable spatial/object differences in the delay period activity were observed, in contrast, in posterior cortical regions (Postle & D'Esposito, in press).

As it turns out, several investigators studying non-human primates have questioned whether a dorsal/ventral what/where functional subdivision in monkeys actually exists. For example, several other single-unit recording studies of dorsal and ventral regions within the lateral PFC during delayed response tasks have found a mixed population of neurons in both regions that are not clearly segregated by the type of information (e.g., spatial versus nonspatial) that is being stored (Fuster, Bauer, & Jervey, 1982; Quintana, Yajeya, & Fuster, 1988; Rao, Rainer, & Miller, 1997; Rosenkilde, Bauer, & Fuster, 1981). Also, cooling of a dorsal region of the lateral PFC has been demonstrated to cause impairments on both spatial and non-spatial tasks (Bauer & Fuster, 1976; Fuster & Bauer, 1974; Quintana & Fuster, 1993). Finally, lesions of a dorsal region of the lateral PFC have been demonstrated to cause impairments on nonspatial working memory tasks (Mishkin, Vest, Waxler, & Rosvold, 1969; Petrides, 1995), and more ventral lesions in the lateral PFC have caused spatial impairments (Butters, Butter, Rosen, & Stein, 1973; Iversen & Mishkin, 1970; Mishkin et al., 1969). Moreover, a recent paper has found that the ventral PFC lesions in monkeys did not cause delay-dependent defects on a visual pattern association task and color matching task (Rushworth, Nixon, Eacott, & Passingham, 1997).

Another possible axis along which the human lateral PFC may be organized is according to the processing performed upon information being stored in working memory rather than the type of information being temporarily stored. Petrides has proposed a two-stage model in which there are two processing systems, one dorsal and the other ventral, within the lateral PFC (Petrides, 1994). It is proposed that ventral PFC (Brodmann's areas 45/47) is the site where information is initially received from posterior association areas and where active comparisons of information held in working memory are made. In contrast, the dorsal PFC (areas 9/46) is recruited only when monitoring and manipulation within working memory are required.

To test this alternative hypothesis of prefrontal organization, we again analyzed the data derived from previously reported working memory functional neuroimaging studies. We divided all working memory tasks according to the conditions under which information is being temporarily maintained rather than the type of information being maintained. For example, delayed-response tasks require a subject to maintain information across a non-distracted delay period. To achieve accurate performance on this type of task no additional processing of the stored information is necessary except for its maintenance across a delay period that has no distracting stimuli. Alternatively, all other working memory paradigms reported in the literature either require (1) reshuffling of the information being temporarily maintained and/or (2) processing of intervening stimuli during the maintenance of stored information. For example, in self-ordered tasks, subjects must update, in working memory, each stimulus that they choose in order to correctly pick a new stimulus. The continuous nature of the *n-back* tasks requires constant reshuffling of the contents held in working memory since different stimuli are simultaneously being stored, inhibited, and dropped from memory. Finally, other tasks, such as one in which subjects must compare the first and last notes of an eight-note melody, simply require the maintenance of information across a distracted delay. Thus, we made an operational distinction between two general types of working memory tasks used in neuroimaging studies: *maintenance* and *manipulation*.

When all locations of the lateral PFC activation reported in the literature are plotted onto a standardized brain according to the classification of tasks into either maintenance or manipulation, a dorsal/ventral dissociation becomes evident (see bottom panel of Figure 5). A challenge for the further development of the hypothesis that the human lateral PFC is organized by processing requirements is determining the psychological constructs that differ between tasks that activate the dorsal versus ventral PFC. Certainly, there are many possible component processes that may be necessary in tasks that activate the dorsal PFC. The component processes that we have labeled *manipulation* will need to be determined. Also, if the lateral PFC is functionally subdivided, it will be important to determine if it is organized hierarchically with information passing from the ventral to dorsal PFC. If a hierarchical organization does exist, it is expected that those tasks that we classified as manipulation tasks would activate the ventral as well as dorsal PFC.

We have begun to test this process-specific organization of PFC using our event-related FMRI method (D'Esposito, Postle, Ballard, & Lease, in press). In our study, subjects were presented two types of trials in random order in which they were required to either (1) maintain a sequence of letters across a delay period or (2) manipulate (alphabetize) this sequence during the delay in order to respond correctly to a probe. Similar to the spatial working memory study described above, we identified brain activity related to the three periods of our task: stimulus presentation, delay, and response. In each subject, activity during the delay period was found in both the dorsal and ventral PFC in both types of trials PFC. However, the dorsal PFC activity was greater in trials during which information held in working memory was manipulated. These findings suggest that the dorsal PFC may exhibit greater recruitment during conditions where additional processing of information held in working memory is required and support a process-specific organization of the PFC.

THE SPECIFICITY OF THE PFC FOR WORKING MEMORY

Single unit recording studies in monkeys during delayed-response tasks have also observed the PFC neurons that are active during periods in addition to the delay period. For example, the PFC neurons have been shown to respond during any combination of cue, delay and response periods (Funahashi, Bruce, & Goldman-Rakic, 1989; Fuster, Bauer, & Jervey, 1982). Although delay-specific neurons are most common, other types are identified frequently. Thus, the PFC appears to be involved in non-mnemonic processes that may include stimulus encoding, sustained attention to stimuli, preparation for a motor response, and the motor response itself. Most human functional imaging studies of working memory using cognitive subtraction methodology have not emphasized the role of the PFC in non-mnemonic cognitive processes and sometimes suggest that the PFC is specific for working memory. Moreover, the interpretation of some functional imaging studies of other cognitive domains (e.g., language, visuoperception) have relied upon post-hoc interpretations of observed PFC activation by their task as being due to the engagement of working memory processes. Such an interpretation tacitly assumes that the PFC is specific for working memory. The demonstration that the same PFC region activated during tasks that engage working memory is also recruited during non-memory processes would dispute this assumption. In light of the results of electrophysiological studies cited above, we predicted that this pattern of the PFC activation would be observed. In fact, we have several lines of evidence to support this claim (D'Esposito, Ballard, Aguirre, & Zarahn, 1998; Zarahn, Aguirre, & D'Esposito, 1999). In one example, if we revisit the spatial working memory experiment described above, it can be seen in Figure 3 (left panel showing fMRI signal) that there is significant activity above the baseline in a region of the PFC that displayed activity above the baseline even during trials without a delay period. This result does not support models that posit neural substrates subserving memory-specific processing, but rather is supportive of models which posit that memory is a property of neural networks which also mediate perceptuomotor processes.

IS WORKING MEMORY SUBSERVED BY A SPECIFIC NEUROTRANSMITTER SYSTEM?

Human cognitive neuroscience research has given much more emphasis to identifying the neuroanatomical correlates of specific cognitive processes and much less emphasis to their neurochemical basis. The brain is certainly comprised of numerous networks of interconnected regions that support cognitive function.

These regions, however, communicate via chemical messengers, and it is becoming increasingly clear that neurotransmitter systems in the brain are highly organized and, in many cases, highly specific. For example, there is a significant anterior/posterior concentration gradient for the neurotransmitter dopamine in the brain. Thus, the concentration of dopamine in the PFC is among the highest of all cortical areas in primates (Brown, Crane, & Goldman, 1979). As might be expected from this unique cortical distribution of dopamine, abundant evidence exists from monkeys that dopamine plays a critical role in working memory. For example, depletion of dopamine in the PFC or pharmacological blockade of dopamine receptors induces impairment in the spatial delayed-response task (Sawaguchi & Goldman-Rakic, 1991). Furthermore, dopaminergic agonists administered to those same monkeys can reverse their delayed-response impairments (Arnsten, Cai, Murphy, & Goldman-Rakic, 1994; Brown, Crane, & Goldman, 1979). These findings provide evidence that impairments in working memory function can be caused by dopamine deficiency, and replacement of dopamine can lead to improvement.

One method of assessing dopamine's influence on cognitive function in humans is by testing Parkinson's disease (PD) patients on and off their dopaminergic replacement medication. This is possible because the half-life of levodopa is quite short, and the CNS levels of dopamine can be monitored by observing deterioration in the patient's motor status. Several studies have been reported using this method and have tested patients on measures that are thought to be sensitive to frontal lobe dysfunction. In each of these studies, patients were impaired on frontal lobe measures (e.g., the Tower of London, a spatial working memory task, a test of attentional set-shifting) when they were off dopaminergic medications (Bowen, Kamienny, Burns, & Yahr, 1975; Cooper et al., 1992; Lange, Paul, Naumann, & Gsell, 1995; Lange et al., 1992). Recently, we have looked directly at the process of executive control during relative dopamine depletion or supplementation. Similar to other studies, PD patients were tested in the on and off state during the performance of dual-task paradigms. PD patients' reaction time for responding to visual stimuli presented randomly on a computer display was measured as a baseline and during the concurrent performance of two secondary tasks with different processing demands. Preliminary analyses suggest that dual-task performance of PD patients during the on state was better than during the off state. On a control task that measured overall attention and arousal there was no difference in performance during the on and off state, ruling out the possibility that dopamine acts as a nonspecific CNS stimulant (D'Esposito, unpublished observation). Taken together, these studies provide further evidence for a link between dopamine and prefrontal function.

Administration of dopamine receptor agonists, which stimulate dopamine receptors in the same way dopamine does, also provides a viable methodology for examining the role of dopaminergic systems in higher cognitive functions in humans. Most dopamine receptor agonists are relatively selective for a particular receptor subtype, the two most common being D-1 and D-2. The selectivity of these drugs for cognitive functions is poorly understood. Two such drugs approved for human use are bromocriptine, which is relatively selective for the D-2 receptor subtype, and pergolide, which affects D-1 and D-2 subtypes. Because both drugs are relatively safe to administer to normal human populations and have well-understood agonist properties, they offer a useful probe for investigating the relationship between dopamine and prefrontal function.

As mentioned above, dopamine receptors are found in great concentrations in the PFC. D-2 dopamine receptors are present in much lower concentrations in the cortex than D-1 receptors and are mostly within the striatum (Camps, Cortés, Gueye, Probst, & Palacios, 1989). However, D-2 receptors are at their highest concentrations in layer V of the PFC (Goldman-Rakic, Lidow, & Gallager, 1990), which makes them especially well positioned to have a strong impact on behavior. And while D-1 receptors have been implicated in mnemonic functions in monkeys (Arnsten et al., 1994), there is evidence from animal studies that some prefrontal functions may depend on a synergistic interaction between these two dopamine receptor types (Sawaguchi & Goldman-Rakic, 1991).

Two studies have reported the effects of bromocriptine on human working memory. Luciana and colleagues (Luciana, Depue, Arbisi, & Leon, 1992) found that normal subjects were significantly better at a spatial working memory task after having taken bromocriptine than after having taken a placebo. In this task (similar to that used in animal studies), subjects had to remember the location on a computer monitor of a briefly presented dot. Subjects were required to report the location of the dot either immediately after its presentation or after an eight-second delay. In the immediate condition, subjects performed similarly both on and off the drug. In the delay condition, subjects were significantly more accurate when on bromocriptine than after having taken a placebo. Müller and colleagues (Müller, Pollmann, & von Cramon, 1997) tested the effects of bromocriptine, pergolide, and a placebo on a visuospatial delayed matching task with various delay periods. It was found that pergolide, and not bromocriptine, reduced the error rates in the longest delay period. They performed a reaction-time analysis that determined that the error reduction was not due to a speed-accuracy tradeoff. No effect of either drug was found on two basic attentional tasks. These authors pointed out that their task had minimal motor demands unlike the task by Luciana and colleagues that required a pointing response. Thus, they postulated that D-2 receptors might be more important for preparation and release of motor programs rather than working memory per se. Although preliminary, these results again suggest a link between dopamine and specific cognitive processes and a possible difference in the role of different dopamine receptors.

No human studies have examined the effects of dopaminergic agonists on complex human behavior. Because of the importance of dopamine in prefrontal function demonstrated in monkeys and the presumed role of the PFC in more complex cognitive behavior, we carried out a more elaborate bromocriptine study with 30 normal subjects. We found that the effects of bromocriptine were not the same for all subjects, but that bromocriptine interacted with the subject's working memory capacity (Kimberg, D'Esposito, & Farah, 1997). Subjects with low capacity tended to demonstrate cognitive improvement on the drug while high-capacity subjects worsened. This interaction is especially interesting in light of the recent study from Goldman-Rakic's laboratory in which they describe dose-dependent effects of a dopamine receptor antagonist in monkeys (Williams & Goldman-Rakic, 1995). They reported that low doses of the drug enhanced delay-period activity of mnemonic neurons, while higher doses inhibited firing for all units, including those showing delay-period activity. Findings in monkeys and humans suggest that there is an optimal level of dopamine for working memory and the cognitive processes that depend on it and that at higher levels of dopamine and/or working memory capacity additional dopamine impairs rather than facilitates performance.

Traumatic brain injury (TBI) patients often suffer prefrontal damage, and we have shown that they have deficits in high-level executive and integrative functions. Based on our results with normal young and elderly subjects, we tested the hypothesis that a dopaminergic medication would improve performance on prefrontal measures in traumatic brain injury patients. Again, we administered the same battery of cognitive tasks given to young and older normal subjects to 24 TBI patients twice (on and off bromocriptine) in a double-blind procedure (McDowell, Whyte, & D'Esposito, 1998). We found that there was a significant main effect of bromocriptine across subjects on all measures requiring executive control. However, on other measures that depended on active maintenance of information but not executive control, improvement on bromocriptine was not noted. Also, performances on the control task, as well as the baseline conditions of the other executive measures that assess basic attentional and sensorimotor processes, were not improved on bromocriptine. These findings demonstrate a selective effect of bromocriptine, a dopamine agonist, on tasks that probe cognitive processes thought to depend on prefrontal function. Moreover, the functional subdivisions of the PFC, as supported by anatomical and behavioral studies, may also be differentially dependent on dopamine.

THE UTILITY OF CONVERGING EVIDENCE FROM MULTIPLE METHODS

In the research described above, we have frequently collected empirical data from experiments utilizing multiple methods including behavioral studies of brain damaged patients, neuroimaging experiments of healthy subjects, and pharmacological studies of healthy and brain damaged subjects. We propose that, because of the inferential limitations of any one empirical method in isolation, it is preferable to obtain converging evidence from many methods. The inferential power of imaging studies can be limited because the behaviors under study are enormously complicated. We have also argued that any attempt to isolate them by subtraction is questionable. New methods such as event-related fMRI (D'Esposito, Zarahn, & Aguirre, 1999) have allowed us to increase our inferential power. A second shortcoming of neuroimaging is that the evidence that derives from such studies cannot support a claim that a specific neuroanatomical region is necessary for a given cognitive process, only that the region is computationally involved in that process. However, analysis of loss of a specific behavior after damage to a brain region provides stronger evidence for such a claim. Of course, mechanisms such as diaschisis and retrograde trans-synaptic degeneration can somewhat limit inferences of lesions studies as well. Therefore, the strongest level of inference comes from combining lesion, pharmacological, and neuroimaging studies. For example, we have provided evidence for combinations such as (*i*) lesions to a cortical area impaired a cognitive process and (*ii*) that cognitive process, when engaged by intact subjects, evokes neural activity in the same cortical area. Thus, in a complementary way, each type of study provides inferential support that the other lacks. Pharmacological probe studies, such as the ones we outlined above, have been rarely used in cognitive neuroscience, but provide an additional important method that certainly complements both imaging and lesion studies.

CONCLUSION

Studies with multiple methods, including behavioral, neuroimaging and pharmacological studies of healthy and brain damaged patients, have been used to provide converging evidence for the role of the PFC in cognition. One process thought to be subserved by the PFC, executive function, remains difficult to characterize, but progress is being made. The physiological basis of this process as well as other processes thought to be subserved by the PFC (such as working memory) are beginning to be mapped out, both on a neuroanatomical and neurochemical level. An improved understanding of the PFC function will make an important contribution to our goal of understanding the normal human brain. It will also have an important impact on our goal of using this knowledge to improve care of patients with damage to this region. Although many individuals with frontal lobe pathology perform well on standard neuropsychological tests, they often exhibit significant functional difficulties (Eslinger & Damasio, 1985; Shallice & Burgess, 1991). These practical difficulties, which seem to be caused by cognitive deficits in organization, planning, and goal integration, are likely due to impairments in the processes being investigated in our studies. Because incomplete recovery of prefrontal function prevents full re-integration into society, development of more effective treatment approaches for these patients, such as pharmacological intervention, will be an extremely important component of their care. Thus, our findings provide a foundation for potential therapies that may not only improve cognitive function in patients with prefrontal damage, but also may decrease the disability associated with those cognitive impairments.

ACKNOWLEDGMENTS

Supported by the American Federation for Aging Research, the Charles A. Dana Foundation and NIH grants NS 01762 and AG 09399.

REFERENCES

Arnsten, K. T., Cai, J. X., Murphy, B. L., & Goldman-Rakic, P. S. (1994). Dopamine D1 receptor mechanisms in the cognitive performance of young adult and aged monkeys. *Psychopharmacology*, *116*, 143-151.
Baddeley, A. (1986). *Working memory*. New York: Oxford University Press.
Baddeley, A. (1992). Working memory. *Science*, *255*, 556-559.
Baddeley, A., Della Sala, S., Papagano, C., & Spinnler, H. (1997). Dual-task performance in dysexecutive and nondysexecutive patients with a frontal lesion. *Neuropsychology*, *11*, 187-194.
Barbas, H. (1988). Anatomic organization of basoventral and mediodorsal visual recipient prefrontal regions in the rhesus monkey. *The Journal of Comparative Neurology*, *276*, 313-342.

Bauer, R. H. & Fuster, J. M. (1976). Delayed-matching and delayed-response deficit from cooling dorsolateral prefrontal cortex in monkeys. *Journal of Comparative and Physiological Psychology, 90,* 293-302.

Bowen, F. P., Kamienny, R. S., Burns, M. M., & Yahr, M. D. (1975). Parkinsonism: Effects of levodopa treatment on concept formation. *Neurology, 25,* 701-704.

Boynton, G. M., Engel, S. A., Glover, G. H., & Heeger, D. J. (1996). Linear systems analysis of functional magnetic resonance imaging in human V1. *The Journal of Neuroscience, 16,* 4207-4221.

Brown, R. M., Crane, A. M., & Goldman, P. S. (1979). Regional distribution of monoamines in the cerebral cortex and subcortical structures of the rhesus monkey: concentrations and in vitro synthesis rates. *Brain Research, 168,* 133-150.

Butters, N., Butter, C., Rosen, J., & Stein, D. (1973). Behavioral effects of sequential and one-stage ablations of orbital prefrontal cortex in monkey. *Experimental Neurology, 39,* 204-214.

Camps, M., Cortés, R., Gueye, B., Probst, A., & Palacios, J. M. (1989). Dopamine receptors in human brain: Autoradiographic distribution of D1 sites. *Neuroscience, 28,* 275-290.

Cavada, C. & Goldman-Rakic, P. S. (1989). Posterior parietal cortex in rhesus monkey: II. Evidence for segregated corticocortical networks linking sensory and limbic areas with frontal lobe. *The Journal of Comparative Neurology, 287,* 422-445.

Cohen, J. D., Nystrom, L. E., Braver, T. S., Sabb, F. W., Delgado, M. R., & Noll, D. C. (1998). fMRI studies of the topographic organization of working memory representations in prefrontal cortex. *Cognitive Neuroscience Society Abstracts, 5,* 87.

Cohen, J. D., Perlstein, W. M., Braver, T. S., Nystrom, L. E., Noll, D. C., Jonides, J., & Smith, E. E. (1997). Temporal dynamics of brain activation during a working memory task. *Nature, 386,* 604-607.

Cooper, J. A., Sagar, H. J., Doherty, M., Jordan, N., Tidswell, P., & Sullivan, E. V. (1992). Different effects of dopaminergic and anticholinergic therapies on cognitive and motor function in Parkinson's disease. *Brain, 115,* 1701-1725.

Courtney, S. M., Ungerleider, L. G., Keil, K., & Haxby, J. V. (1997). Transient and sustained activity in a distributed neural system for human working memory. *Nature, 386,* 608-611.

D'Esposito, M., Aguirre, G. K., Zarahn, E., & Ballard, D. (1998). Functional MRI studies of spatial and non-spatial working memory. *Cognitive Brain Research, 7,* 1-13.

D'Esposito, M., Detre, J. A., Alsop, D. C., Shin, R. K., Atlas, S., & Grossman, M. (1995). The neural basis of the central executive system of working memory. *Nature, 378,* 279-281.

D'Esposito, M. & Postle, B. R. (in press). Neural correlates of component processes of working memory: Evidence from neuropsychological and pharmacological studies. In S. Monsell & J. Driver (Eds.), *Attention and performance XVIII: Control of cognitive processes.* Cambridge, MA: MIT Press.

D'Esposito, M., Zarahn, E., & Aguirre, G. K. (1999). Event-related fMRI: Implications for cognitive psychology. *Psychological Bulletin, 125,* 155-164.

D'Esposito, M., Ballard, D., Aguirre, G., & Zarahn, E. (1998). Human prefrontal cortex is not specific for working memory. *NeuroImage, 8,* 274-282.

D'Esposito, M., Postle, B. R., Ballard, D., & Lease, J. (in press). Maintenance and manipulation of information held in working memory: An event-related fMRI study. *Brain & Cognition.*

Eslinger, P. J. & Damasio, A. R. (1985). Severe disturbance of higher cognition following bilateral frontal lobe ablation: Patient EVR. *Neurology, 35,* 1731-1741.

Funahashi, S., Bruce, C. J., & Goldman-Rakic, P. S. (1989). Mnemonic coding of visual space in the monkey's dorsolateral prefrontal cortex. *Journal of Neurophysiology, 61,* 331-349.

Funahashi, S., Bruce, C. J., & Goldman-Rakic, P. S. (1993). Dorsolateral prefrontal lesions and oculomotor delayed-response performance: Evidence for mnemonic "scotomas". *The Journal of Neuroscience, 13,* 1479-1497.

Fuster, J. (1997). *The prefrontal cortex: Anatomy, physiology, and neuropsychology of the frontal lobes* (3rd ed.). New York: Raven Press.

Fuster, J. M. & Alexander, G. E. (1971). Neuron activity related to short-term memory. *Science, 173,* 652-654.

Fuster, J. M. & Bauer, R. H. (1974). Visual short-term memory deficit from hypothermia of frontal cortex. *Brain Research, 81,* 393-400.

Fuster, J. M., Bauer, R. H., & Jervey, J. P. (1982). Cellular discharge in the dorsolateral prefrontal cortex of the monkey in cognitive tasks. *Experimental Neurology, 77,* 679-694.

Goldman-Rakic, P. S. (1987). Circuitry of the prefrontal cortex and the regulation of behavior by representational memory. In F. Plum & V. Mountcastle (Eds.), *Handbook of physiology. Sec 1. The nervous system.* (Vol. 5, pp. 373-417). Bethesda, MD: American Physiological Society.

Goldman-Rakic, P. S., Lidow, M. S., & Gallager, D. W. (1990). Overlap of dopaminergic, adrenergic, and serotoninergic receptors and complementarity of their subtypes in primate prefrontal cortex. *The Journal of Neuroscience, 10,* 2125-2138.

Gross, C. G. (1963). A comparison of the effects of partial and total lateral frontal lesions on test performance by monkeys. *Journal of Comparative and Physiological Psychology, 56,* 41-47.

Harlow, J. (1868). Recovery from the passage of an iron bar through the head. *Proceedings of the Massachusetts Medical Society, 2,* 725-728.

Hécaen, H. & Albert, M. L. (1978). *Human neuropsychology.* New York: John Wiley & Sons.

Iversen, S. D. & Mishkin, M. (1970). Perseverative interference in monkeys following selective lesions of the inferior prefrontal convexity. *Experimental Brain Research, 11,* 376-386.

Jonides, J., Smith, E. E., Koeppe, R. A., Awh, E., Minoshima, S., & Mintun, M. A. (1993). Spatial working memory in humans as revealed by PET. *Nature, 363,* 623-625.

Kimberg, D., D'Esposito, M., & Farah, M. (1997). Effects of bromocriptine on human subjects depend on working memory capacity. *NeuroReport, 8,* 3581-3585.

Kimberg, D. & Farah, M. (1993). A unified account of cognitive impairments following frontal damage: The role of working memory in complex, organized behavior. *Journal of Experimental Psychology: Learning, Memory & Cognition, 122,* 411-428.

Lange, K. W., Paul, G. M., Naumann, M., & Gsell, W. (1995). Dopaminergic effects of cognitive performance in patients with Parkinson's disease. *Journal of Neural Transmission Supplement, 46,* 423-432.

Lange, K. W., Robbins, T. W., Marsden, C. D., James, M., Owen, A. M., & Paul, G. M. (1992). L-Dopa withdrawal in Parkinson's disease selectively impairs cognitive performance in tests sensitive to frontal lobe dysfunction. *Psychopharmacology, 107,* 394-404.

Lezak, M. (1995). *Neuropsychological assessment* (3rd ed.). New York: Oxford University Press.

Luciana, M., Depue, R. A., Arbisi, P., & Leon, A. (1992). Facilitation of working memory in humans by a D2 dopamine receptor agonist. *Journal of Cognitive Neuroscience, 4,* 58-68.

Luria, A. (1966). *Higher cortical functions in man.* New York: Basic Books.

McDowell, S., Whyte, J., & D'Esposito, M. (1997). Working memory impairments in traumatic brain injury: Evidence from a dual-task paradigm. *Neuropsychologia, 35,* 1341-1353.

McDowell, S., Whyte, J., & D'Esposito, M. (1998). Differential effect of a dopaminergic agonist on prefrontal function in traumatic brain injury patients. *Brain, 121,* 1155-1164.

Mishkin, M. & Manning, F. J. (1978). Non-spatial memory after selective prefrontal lesions in monkeys. *Brain Research, 143,* 313-323.

Mishkin, M., Vest, B., Waxler, M., & Rosvold, H. E. (1969). A re-examination of the effects of frontal lesions on object alternation. *Neuropsychologia, 7,* 357-363.

Müller, U., Pollmann, S., & von Cramon, D. Y. (in press). D1 versus D2-receptor stimulation of visuo-spatial short-term memory. *Journal of Neuroscience.*

Norman, D. A. & Shallice, T. (1986). Attention to action: Willed and automatic control of behavior. In R. J. Davidson, G. E. Schwartz, & D. Shapiro (Eds.), *Consciousness and self-regulation* (pp. 1-18). New York: Plenum Press.

Passingham, R. (1975). Delayed matching after selective prefrontal lesions in monkeys. *Brain Research, 92,* 89-102.

Petersen, S. E., Fox, P. T., Posner, M. I., Mintun, M., & Raichle, M. E. (1988). Positron emission tomographic studies of the cortical anatomy of single word processing. *Nature, 331,* 585-589.

Petrides, M. (1994). Frontal lobes and working memory: Evidence from investigations of the effects of cortical excisions in nonhuman primates. In F. Boller & J. Grafman (Eds.), *Handbook of neuropsychology.* Amsterdam: Elsevier Science B.V.

Petrides, M. (1995). Impairments on nonspatial self-ordered and externally ordered working memory tasks after lesions of the mid-dorsal lateral part of the lateral frontal cortex of monkey. *The Journal of Neuroscience, 15,* 359-375.

Petrides, M. & Pandya, D. N. (1984). Projections to the frontal cortex from the posterior parietal region in the rhesus monkey. *The Journal of Comparative Neurology, 228,* 105-116.

Pierrot-Deseilligny, C., Rivaud, S., Gaymard, B., & Agid, Y. (1991). Cortical control of memory-guided saccades in man. *Experimental Brain Research, 83,* 607-617.

Posner, M. I., Petersen, S. E., Fox, P. T., & Raichle, M. E. (1988). Localization of cognitive operations in the human brain. *Science, 240*, 1627-1631.

Postle, B. R. & D'Esposito, M. (in press). "What" - then- "Where" in visual working memory; an event-related fMRI study. *Journal of Cognitive Neuroscience.*

Postle, B. R., Stern, C. E., Rosen, B. R., & Corkin, S. (1997). fMRI of spatial and nonspatial visual working memory reveals differences in posterior, but not prefrontal, cortex. *Society for Neuroscience Abstracts, 23*, 1679.

Ptito, A., Crane, J., Leonard, G., Amsel, R., & Caramanos, Z. (1995). Visual-spatial localization by patients with frontal-lobe lesions invading or sparing area 46. *NeuroReport, 6*, 1781-1784.

Quintana, J. & Fuster, J. M. (1993). Spatial and temporal factors in the role of prefrontal and parietal cortex in visuomotor integration. *Cerebral Cortex, 3*, 122-132.

Quintana, J., Yajeya, J., & Fuster, J. (1988). Prefrontal representation of stimulus attributes during delay tasks. I. Unit activity in cross-temporal integration of motor and sensory-motor information. *Brain Research, 474*, 211-221.

Rao, S. C., Rainer, G., & Miller, E. K. (1997). Integration of "what" and "where" in the primate prefrontal cortex. *Science, 276*, 821-824.

Rosenkilde, C. E., Bauer, R. H., & Fuster, J. M. (1981). Single cell activity in ventral prefrontal cortex of behaving monkeys. *Brain Research, 209*, 375-394.

Rushworth, M. F. S., Nixon, P. D., Eacott, M. J., & Passingham, R. E. (1997). Ventral prefrontal cortex is not essential for working memory. *The Journal of Neuroscience, 17*, 4829-4838.

Sarter, M., Bernston, G., & Cacioppo, J. (1996). Brain imaging and cognitive neuroscience: toward strong inference in attributing function to structure. *American Psychologist, 51*, 13-21.

Sawaguchi, T. & Goldman-Rakic, P. S. (1991). D1 dopamine receptors in prefrontal cortex: Involvement in working memory. *Science, 251*, 947-950.

Shallice, T. & Burgess, P. W. (1991). Deficits in strategy application following frontal lobe damage in man. *Brain, 114*, 727-741.

Sternberg, S. (1969). The discovery of processing stages: Extensions of Donders' method. *Acta Psychologica, 30*, 276-315.

Talairach, J. & Tournoux, P. (1988). *Co-planar stereotaxic atlas of the human brain.* New York: Thieme.

Taylor, A. E., Saint-Cyr, J. S., & Lang, A. E. (1986). Frontal lobe dysfunction in Parkinson's disease: The cortical focus of neostriatal outflow. *Brain, 109*, 279-292.

Ungerleider, L. G. & Haxby, J. V. (1994). "What" and "where" in the human brain. *Current Opinion in Neurobiology, 4*, 157-165.

Vazquez, A. L. & Noll, D. C. (1998). Nonlinear aspects of the BOLD response in functional MRI. *NeuroImage, 7*, 108-118.

Verin, M., Partiot, A., Pillon, B., Malapani, C., Agid, Y., & Dubois, B. (1993). Delayed response tasks and prefrontal lesions in man: Evidence for self generated patterns of behavior with poor environmental modulation. *Neuropsychologia, 31*, 1379-1396.

Williams, G. V. & Goldman-Rakic, P. S. (1995). Modulation of memory fields by dopamine D1 receptors in prefrontal cortex. *Nature, 376*, 572-575.

Wilson, F. A., Scalaidhe, S. P., & Goldman-Rakic, P. S. (1993). Dissociation of object and spatial processing domains in prefrontal cortex. *Science, 260*, 1955-1958.

Zarahn, E., Aguirre, G. K., & D'Esposito, M. (1997). A trial-based experimental design for functional MRI. *NeuroImage, 6*, 122-138.

Zarahn, E., Aguirre, G. K., & D'Esposito, M. (1999). Temporal isolation of the neural correlates of spatial mnemonic processing with fMRI. *Cognitive Brain Research, 7*, 255-268.

LANGUAGE FUNCTIONS IN PARKINSON'S DISEASE: EVIDENCE FOR A NEUROCHEMISTRY OF LANGUAGE

Patrick McNamara and Raymon Durso

INTRODUCTION

In this chapter, we evaluate the claim that dopamine plays a crucial role in certain aspects of language processing by reviewing language processing deficits in Parkinson's Disease (PD) and other more circumstantial clinical evidence. PD is a progressive neurodegenerative disorder characterized by tremor, rigidity, gait disorder, bradykinesia, and dopaminergic deficit (Hoehn & Yahr, 1967). PD-associated speech and language dysfunction will be reviewed below. The claim that speech and language functions are influenced by dopaminergic activity is supported by the PD data, a small body of circumstantial clinical evidence, and by the chemical neuroanatomy of dopamine itself.

PD PATHOLOGY

Although several other neurotransmitter systems are implicated in PD (Dubois & Pillon, 1992), the primary pathology involves loss of dopaminergic cells in the substantia nigra (SN) and in the ventral tegmental area (VTA) (Agid, Javoy-Agid, & Ruberg, 1987). These two subcortical dopaminergic sites give rise to two projection systems important for motor and cognitive (as well as other) functioning. The nigrostriatal system originates in the pars compacta of the SN and terminates in the striatum. The mesocortical system originates in the VTA and terminates in the ventral striatum, amygdala, frontal lobes, and some other basal forebrain areas. In the mid-late stages of the disease, dopamine levels in the ventral striatum, frontal lobes, and hippocampus are approximately 40% of normal levels (Agid, Javoy-Agid, & Ruberg, 1987; Javoy-Agid & Agid, 1980; Scatton, Javoy-Agid, Rouquier, Dubois, & Agid, 1982; Shinotoh & Calne, 1995). The degree of VTA-mesocortical dopaminergic impairment correlates positively with the degree of intellectual impairment (German, Manaye, Smith, Woodward, & Saper, 1989; Rinne, Rummukainen, Paljari, & Rinne, 1989) in affected individuals.

Approximately 80% of PD patients develop significant cognitive impairment as the disease progresses (Cooper, Sagar, Jordan, Harvey, & Sullivan, 1991;

Heitanen & Teräväinen, 1986; 1988; Lees & Smith, 1983). While 60% of these patients exhibit a variable *mix* of specific deficits that are similar to those found in patients who have suffered prefrontal lesions (Brown & Marsden 1990; Dubois, Bollen, Pillon, & Agiol, 1991; Dubois, Pillon, Malapani, Deweer, Vérin, Partiaud, Fontaines, Sirigu, Texeira, & Agid, 1995; Gotham, Brown, & Marsden, 1988; Levin, Eisenberg, & Benton, 1991; Wolters & Scheltens, 1995; Taylor & Saint-Cyr, 1991; 1995, Taylor, Saint-Cyr, & Lang, 1986), the remaining 20% develop a global intellectual deterioration severe enough to be considered dementia. We focus here on non-demented PD patients who exhibit language-related cognitive deficits.

SPEECH AND LANGUAGE FUNCTIONS

With regard to speech and language production, PD patients often exhibit fluency and motor speech disorders (Critchley, 1981; Darkins, Frankin, & Benson, 1988; Illes, 1989; Illes, Metter, Hanson, & Iritani, 1988), word-finding difficulties (Auriacombe, Grossman, Carvell, Gollomp, Stern, & Hurtig, 1993; Cooper, Sagar, Jordan, Harvey, & Sullivan, 1991; Matison, Meyeux, Rosen, & Fahn, 1981), and grammatical difficulties. They tend, for example, to use simplified sentence structures with an increase in the ratio of open-class items (nouns, verbs, and adjectives) to closed-class items (determiners, auxiliaries, prepositions, etc.) as well as an increase in the frequency and duration of hesitations and pauses (Cummings, Derkins, Mendez, Mill, & Benson, 1988; Illes, Metter, Hanson, & Iritani, 1988; Illes, 1989; McNamara, Obler, Au, Durso, & Albert, 1992) at critical sites in a sentence.

With regard to language comprehension, these patients often exhibit what appears to be a mild to moderate syntactic comprehension deficit (Geyer & Grossman, 1995; Grossman, Carvell, Gollomp, Stern, Vernon, & Hurtig, 1991; Grossman, Crino, Stern, Reivich, & Hurtig, 1992; Grossman, Carvell, Stern, Gollomp, & Hurtig, 1992; Grossman et al., 1993; Grossman, Carvell, & Peltzer, 1993; Grossman, Stern, Gollomp, Vernon, & Hurtig, 1994; Grossman, in press; Kemmerer, in press; Lieberman, Friedman, & Feldman, 1990; Lieberman, Kako, Friedman, Tajchman, Feldman, & Jiminez, 1992; McNamara, Krueger, O'Quinn, Clark, & Durso, 1996; Natsopoulos, Katsarou, Bostantzopoulos, Grouios, Metenopoulos, & Logothetis, 1991; Seidl, Onishi, White, D'Esposito, & Grossman, 1995). While the exact nature and source of this comprehension deficit is controversial, there is now no doubt that it is reproducible with standard testing materials.

SYNTACTIC COMPREHENSION DEFICITS IN PD

Lieberman et al. (1990, 1992) administered the Rhode Island Test of Linguistic Structure (RITLS) to two groups of PD patients. This test includes 100 sentences representing 20 different types of constructions. Eleven of the constructions included a single verb (called *simple*) and the remaining nine constructions involved two verbs (called *complex*). In both experiments, roughly half of the PD patients exhibited syntactic comprehension difficulties especially with the complex constructions. Natsopoulos et al. (1991) tested the ability of 20 nondemented Greek-speaking PD patients in their understanding of four different types of relative clause constructions. They found substantial impairment for some patients on some sentence types and claimed that patients' errors were consistently based on certain kinds of heuristic strategies. Grossman, Carvell, et al. (1992) tested a group of 20 nondemented PD patients on a syntactic comprehension battery that included active, passive, and relative clause constructions. They found that slightly more than half of the patients performed significantly worse than the control subjects and that patient performance steadily declined as grammatical complexity increased. Center embedded relative clauses were more difficult for patients than active or passive sentences. McNamara et al. (1996) tested 15 non-demented patients on a grammaticality judgment task and then a comprehension test involving the same constructions used in the grammaticality test. These were systematically varied dative constructions. On the comprehension test, patients were required to listen to a long sentence and then answer in sequence five different probe questions about the meaning of the sentence. PD patients were significantly impaired on the comprehension task relative to control subjects but less impaired relative to a group of five Broca's aphasics. Grammaticality judgments were largely intact in all three groups. Kemmerer (in press) tested 15 non-demented PD patients on a variety of carefully constructed sentences designed to test competing hypotheses short term memory deficit, a parsing deficit, and attentional deficit on the source of the PD language deficit. A pattern of performance dissociations on canonical versus noncanonical subject-to-subject raising, canonical versus non-canonical object-to-subject raising, subject-subject versus subject-object relatives, object-subject versus object-object relatives, and subject clefts versus object clefts supported the attentional hypothesis, according to Kemmerer.

It should be noted here that all of these syntactic comprehension studies used materials or tasks that required patients to respond from memory, that is to make their decisions based on post-interpretative processing of the stimulus materials. Thus, none of these studies speak to the issue of whether these patients exhibit primary syntactic or parsing difficulties. Only on-line studies can dissect the abilities of patients to rapidly and appropriately assign syntactic structure. Nevertheless, these initial *off-line* studies are suggestive and point to the need for more sophisticated investigation of linguistic processing in these patients.

ATTENTIONAL DYSFUNCTION

Grossman, Carvell, et al. (1992) were the first to suggest attentional dysfunction as the source of the PD sentence comprehension deficit. These investigators claimed that PD patients evidence their greatest difficulties when required to process non-canonically ordered sentence types under conditions of attentional interference (Seidl, Onishi, White, D'Esposito, & Grossman, 1995). For example, in sentences with center embedded subject relative clauses (*The truck that hit the car was green*) the Noun Phrases involved in the relative clause have a canonical order such that the Noun Phrase playing the role of actor precedes the verb and the Noun Phrase playing the role of object follows the verb. However, in sentences with center embedded object relative clauses (*The truck that the car hit was green*) the Noun Phrases have a non-canonical order around the verb –

specifically object-subject-action. For constructions like this with *unexpected* or non-canonical ordering, executive attention is needed to suppress the canonical template and promote the noncanonical interpretation. Although the passive construction *(The car was hit by the truck)* involves noncanonical ordering of thematic roles, PD patients performed normally on these in virtually every sentence comprehension study cited above. Geyer and Grossman (1995) argue that PD patients perform normally on these because of the passive morphology or surface cues associated with the sentence type (e.g., the preposition *by*, the auxiliary verb, and so on).

ON/OFF STUDIES IN PD PATIENTS

Language-related Cognitive Functions

When patients with PD are withdrawn from their dopaminergic medications, various higher cognitive functions (particularly those dependent on prefrontal sites) are affected (Jahanshahi, Brown, & Marsden, 1992; Taylor, Saint-Cyr, & Lang, 1987; Wolters & Scheltens, 1995). Gotham et al. (1988), for example, assessed the performance of PD patients on four tests that are known to be sensitive to prefrontal cortical dysfunction: (1) the Wisconsin Card Sort Test, (2) two measures of verbal fluency, one with a single category as cue and another with alternation between two categories, (3) a self-ordered pointing task where the patient was presented with a card depicting 12 figures and then required to point to a different figure on each trial, and (4) a task that involved learning to match abstract figures with particular colors. The patients were tested with these materials under two conditions: first while on levodopa medication, and then while off the medication. Performance on the verbal fluency test varied with the patient's dopaminergic levels. Verbal fluency was within normal limits while on levodopa but declined significantly (at least with the alternation task) while off levodopa. Wisconsin Card Sort Test performance was impaired both on and off levodopa. Patients showed largely normal performance on self-ordered pointing and the matching task while off levodopa, but they were significantly impaired while on levodopa. Lange et al. (1992) tested ten PD patients on a battery of tests sensitive to prefrontal functioning. These tests included a Tower of Hanoi task, set shifting (internally vs. externally driven), working memory, and spatial attention span. Patients were dramatically impaired on these *frontal* tests (but not non-frontal tests) only when withdrawn from levodopa medication.

Bradyphrenia when Off Levodopa

The issue of cognitive slowing or bradyphrenia is relevant for language processing functions in PD (Rogers, Lee, Smith, Trimble, & Stern, 1987). Bradyphrenia is frequently associated with early-stage PD. Speed of cognitive processing is thought to be modifiable by administration of dopaminergic agents, and some language-related functions depend on rapid automatized processing of constituent structures into messages or sentences, etc. While there has been a substantial body of work produced on cognitive slowing and aging (Cerella,

Rybash, Hoyer, & Commons, 1993), very little has been published on cognitive slowing and language processing in PD. Pillon and colleagues (1989) administered a test they call the *15 Objects Test* to 70 PD patients. This timed, visual discrimination test requires patients to identify 15 superimposed images of everyday objects (e.g., a lamp). These authors found that PD patients' performance on this test did not correlate with the patients' akinesia scores when withdrawn from dopaminergic medications, but did correlate with the parkinsonian disability score which is a measure of residual axial motor function not usually affected by dopaminergic treatment. Although the time needed to identify 12 of the 15 objects increased by 58% in 70 patients while off levodopa, and almost half of the 32 patients improved their performance while on levodopa, the authors nevertheless concluded that non-dopaminergic transmitter systems were responsible for cognitive slowing in PD.

Language Comprehension

We are aware of only two studies that assessed PD language comprehension functions both on and off dopaminergic medications (Grossman, in press; McNamara, Krueger, O'Quin, Clark, & Durso, 1996). In the Grossman studies, sentence comprehension was assessed in 20 Stage-1 PD patients when on their dopamine medication and then when off for 12 hours. The patients were assessed on two occasions separated by about four weeks with the order of assessment randomized. The comprehension tasks involved sentence picture matching and oral responses to comprehension queries under conditions of dual task performance. Ten (50%) of the 20 patients demonstrated a pattern of poorer performance on center-embedded than on terminal subordinate constructions under the off condition relative to performance under the on condition. When these ten patients were compared with the other ten better-performing PD patients, no performance differences were found when on medications. By contrast, when off medication, performance differences emerged for the more complex center-embedded but not the terminal subordinate sentences. Correlational analysis revealed that greater difficulty with sentence comprehension during the off condition was associated with worse performance on the dual task measure during the off condition. In the McNamara et al. (1996) study, eight mild to severe patients were tested both on and off dopaminergic medicines using queries to test for comprehension of orally presented target sentences. McNamara et al. found that comprehension declined relative to the on state for all sentence types probed except *direct object sentences*. Taken together, these studies provide weak but suggestive evidence concerning a selective dependence of comprehension abilities on mesocortical dopaminergic activity.

In summary, PD patients exhibit significant syntactic comprehension deficits for constructions involving non-canonical ordering and increased attentional resources. This processing deficit is sensitive to dopaminergic activity. What is the basis of PD language-related impairments?

PREFRONTAL DYSFUNCTION

One possibility is that mesocortical dopaminergic activity supports rapid attentional switching or deployment of prefrontal cortical working memory processing resources. Grossman's work on the attentional hypothesis has been mentioned above. With regard to working memory, Fuster (1980), Goldman-Rakic (1987; 1995a; 1995b), and others utilizing a variety of experimental approaches, including delayed response paradigms, have found cells in the dorsolateral prefrontal cortex of the rhesus monkey that remain active during a brief delay period between presentation of a stimulus and execution of the response. Pharmacological blocking of these cell groups and the dopamine receptors in this cortical area (Brozoski, Brown, Rosvold, & Goldman, 1979) abolishes the monkey's ability to carry out the delayed response (Diamond & Goldman-Rakic, 1989). Dopamine replacement therapy, in turn, restores delayed-response function (Brozoski, Brown, Rosvold, & Goldman, 1979). Thus, dopaminergic activity apparently supports some aspects of prefrontal working memory capacity.

Prefrontally-based executive or attentional control functions appear to be impaired in PD (Brown & Marsden, 1988a; 1988b; Caltagirone, Carlesimo, Nocentini, & Vicari, 1989; Hietanen & Teräväinen, 1986; Lees & Smith, 1983; Reitan & Boll, 1971; Taylor, Saint-Cyr, & Lang, 1986) despite intact functioning in those components of working memory (Baddeley, 1986; 1992) that tap the so-called articulatory loop (Hietanen & Teräväinen 1988; Cooper, Sagar, Jordan, Harvey, & Sullivan, 1991) and the visual-spatial scratch pad (Morris, Downes, Sahakian, Evenden, Heald, & Robbins, 1988; Sullivan & Sagar, 1989). There is a well-established PD attentional switching deficit on certain verbal fluency paradigms, namely *category alternation paradigms*, where the patients are required to generate names in one category for about a minute and then switch to another category. It is not clear whether the difficulty for patients on this task is due to set-shifting problems or to naming problems or to some other more general response initiation problems (Brown & Marsden, 1988a; 1988b; Cools, Van der Berken, Horstink, Van Spaendonck, & Berger, 1984; Cools, Berger, Buytenhuijs, Horstink, & Van Spaendonck, 1995; Downes, Sharp, Costall, Sagar, & Howe, 1993; Lees & Smith 1983; Pillon, Dubois, Bonnet, Esteguy, Guimaraes, Vigouret, L'hermitte, & Agid, 1989; Taylor, Saint-Cry, & Lang, 1986). These category fluency tasks, however, point to the larger verbal fluency problem mentioned above that most PD patients must cope with as the disease progresses.

DOPAMINE AND VERBAL FLUENCY

As reviewed above, verbal fluency performance in PD appears to vary slightly with medication status. Performance declines when patients are withdrawn from dopaminergic medications. In addition, Blonder, Gur, Gur, Saykin, and Hurtig (1984) found that PD patients with predominantly right sided symptoms had greater verbal fluency deficits in controlled word association, animal naming, confrontation naming, and fluency than PD patients with left-sided symptoms. Similarly, some aspects of verbal fluency and language deficits in aphasia may be amenable to pharmacologic treatment with dopaminergic medications. Albert and colleagues

(Mimura, Albert, & McNamara, 1995) were the first to investigate the use of bromocriptine (a D2 dopamine receptor agonist) for treatment of non-fluent aphasia. While initial results based on case studies were promising, no controlled clinical studies of the effects of dopaminergic agonists on aphasic symptoms have yet been published (but see reviews on pharmacologic treatment of aphasia in the Tanaka and Bachman chapter in this volume). Bromocriptine appears to work best for patients with transcortical motor aphasia.

There is some evidence that dopaminergic activity needs to be optimal or balanced (rather than *high*) in order to facilitate fluency. Speech dysfluencies in the stutterer can be reduced or eliminated with haloperiodol, an antidopaminergic agent (Andrews & Dozsa, 1977; Rosenberger, 1980; Wingate, 1988). Several authors have suggested that stuttering may be linked to a central excess in dopaminergic activity (Yeudall, 1985; Rastatter & Harr, 1988). These suggestions regarding stuttering are similar to those made to explain the linguistic disturbances associated with schizophrenia, another dopamine-related disorder.

CHEMICAL NEUROANATOMY

Dopaminergic projections to the frontal lobes are more numerous dorsally than laterally and mesially (Williams & Goldman-Rakic, 1993) and more dense in the left- than the right-hemisphere (Glick, Ross, & Hough, 1982; Tucker & Williamson, 1984). Oke, Keller, Mefford, and Adams (1978) and Glick, Ross, and Hough (1982) found greater cathecholaminergic activity in left forebrain sites than in right sided sites in the post mortem human brain.

In the monkey and the rat, biochemical and histochemical analyses have revealed that the density of DA innervation decreases in a rostrocaudal gradient such that only trace amounts of DA are found in caudal occipital areas, while primary motor cortex exhibits very dense DA innervation (Foote & Morrison, 1987). Area 7 of the inferior parietal lobe is densely innervated as is the prefrontal cortex. Sensory regions and layer IV neurons are sparsely innervated (Foote & Morrison, 1987). Physiologically, DA appears to boost signal-to-noise ratios in the striatum, thus serving as a reinforcement signal that guides both the learning and the maintenance of adaptive behaviors (Wickens & Kötter, 1995). Dopaminergic activity dampens excitatory corticostriatal and thalamostriatal activity (Schultz, Romo, Ljungberg, Mirenowicz, Hollerman, & Dickinson, 1995) with the ultimate effect of enabling only the strongest, most task-relevant inputs to pass through to the impulse-generating mechanism at the cell body; the weakest, most task-irrelevant inputs are filtered out (Robbins & Brown, 1990; Schultz, Romo, Ljungberg, Mirenowicz, Hollerman, & Dickinson, 1995; Saint-Cyr, Taylor, & Nicholson, 1995).

ROLE OF THE ANTERIOR CINGULATE CORTEX

Grossman, Carvell, Gollomp, et al. (1993) found that the ability of PD patients to understand center embedded object relative clauses and to detect errors in various sentence constructions correlated with glucose metabolism levels in the anterior cingulate cortex, a site known to be implicated in attentional processing (Cabeza &

Nyberg, 1997; Posner, 1994; Posner & Dehaene, 1994). Grossman, Crino, et al. (1992) measured regional cerebral blood flow in PD patients and control subjects as they processed sentences that varied in grammatical complexity. For the control subjects, blood flow increased in the anterior cingulate cortex when performing sentence tasks. For PD patients, no such increased blood flow was demonstrated.

A number of neuroimaging studies have found activation of the anterior cingulate cortex when attentional switching is required (Corbetta, Miezin, Dobmeyer, Shulman, & Peterson, 1991; Devinsky, Morrell, & Vogt, 1995; Frith, Friston, Liddle, & Frackowiak, 1991). Destruction of the anterior cingulate gyrus or the supplementary motor area may cause mutism. Electrical stimulation of the periaqueductal gray substance in the midbrain and upper pons elicits species-specific vocalizations in mammals and in humans. The anterior cingulate gyrus sends efferents directly onto the central gray and appears to control the initiation and voluntary control of vocalization. The anterior cingulate gyrus in turn receives efferents from the supplementary motor area in the cortex. The fiber tracts connecting the supplementary motor area (SMA) in the cortex and the anterior cingulate gyrus are believed to be dopaminergic. Patients with bilateral lesions within the cingulate area undergo a period of mutism followed by slow recovery where speech is aprosodic and initiations are rare. Electrical stimulation within the SMA elicits vocalizations in both humans and monkeys. Regional cerebral blood flow studies have demonstrated activation of SMA associated with both silent speech and automatic speech production. Left-sided SMA lesions are associated with transcortical motor aphasia as well as transient mutism.

SUMMARY

PD patients exhibit mild to moderate difficulty both in production and in comprehension of language. Both the fluency and the comprehension impairments are sensitive to dopaminergic levels. Because PD patients also exhibit selective dysfunction in working memory and attentional systems, the language impairment may be related to functioning in these other cognitive systems. The dopaminergic prefrontal and anterior cingulate systems are particularly affected in those PD patients evidencing language-related disorder. The available evidence suggests that language functions depend in part on these dopaminergic neural networks.

ACKNOWLEDGMENTS

The authors would like to thank David Kemmerer, Ph.D. for detailed comments on earlier drafts of this chapter.

REFERENCES

Agid, Y., Javoy-Agid, F., & Ruberg, M. (1987). Biochemistry of neurotransmitters in Parkinson's disease. *Movement Disorders*, 2,166-230.
Andrews, G. & Dozsa, M. (1977). Haloperiodol and the treatment of stuttering. *Journal of Fluency Disorders*, 2, 217-224.
Auriacombe, S., Grossman, M., Carvell, S., Gollomp, S., Stern, M., & Hurtig, H. (1993). Verbal fluency deficits in Parkinson's disease. *Neuropsychologia*, 7, 182-192.

Baddeley, A. (1986). *Working memory*. Oxford: Oxford University Press.
Baddeley, A. (1992). Working memory. *Science, 255*, 556-559.
Blonder, L. X., Gur, R. E., Gur, R. C., Saykin, A. J., & Hurtig, H. I. (1989). Neuropsychological functioning in hemiparkinsonism. *Brain and Cognition, 9*, 244-257.
Brown, R. & Marsden, C. (1988). An investigation of the phenomenon of "set" in Parkinson's disease. *Movement Disorders, 3*, 152-161.
Brown, R. & Marsden, C. (1988). Internal vs. external cues and the control of attention in Parkinson's disease. *Brain, 11*, 323-345.
Brown, R. & Marsden, C. (1990). Cognitive function in Parkinson's disease: From description to theory. *Trends in Neurosciences, 13*, 21-29.
Brozoski, T., Brown R., Rosvold H., & Goldman P. (1979). Cognitive deficit caused by regional depletion of dopamine in prefrontal cortex of rhesus monkey. *Science, 205*, 929-931.
Cabeza, R. & Nyberg, L. (1997). Imaging cognition: An empirical review of PET studies with normal subjects. *Journal of Cognitive Neuroscience, 9*, 1-26.
Caltagirone, C., Carlesimo, A., Nocentini, U., & Vicari, S. (1989). Defective concept formation in Parkinson's disease is independent from mental deterioration. *Journal of Neurology, Neurosurgery, and Psychiatry, 52*, 334-337.
Cerella, J., Rybash, J., Hoyer, W., & Commons, M. L. (Eds.). (1993). *Adult information processing: Limits on loss*. New York: Academic Press.
Cools, A., Berger, H., Buytenhuijs, E., Horstink, M., & Van Spaendonck, K. (1995). Manifestations of switching disorders in animals and man with dopamine deficits in A^{10} and/or A^9 circuitries. In E. Wolters & P. Scheltens (Eds.), *Mental dysfunction in Parkinson's disease* (pp. 49-68). The Netherlands: ICG.
Cools, A., Van Der Berken, J., Horstink, M., Van Spaendonck, K., & Berger, H. (1984). Cognitive and motor shifting aptitude disorder in Parkinson's disease. *Journal of Neurology, Neurosurgery, and Psychiatry, 47*, 443-453.
Cooper, J. H., Sagar, N., Jordan, N., Harvey, N., & Sullivan, E. (1991). Cognitive impairment in early, untreated Parkinson's disease and its relationship to motor disability. *Brain, 114*, 2095-2122.
Corbetta, M., Miezin, S., Dobmeyer, S., Shulman, G., & Petersen, S. (1991). Selected and divided attention during visual discriminations of shape, color and speed: Functional anatomy by positron emission tomography. *Journal of Neuroscience, 11*, 2383-2402.
Critchley, E. (1981). Speech disorders of Parkinsonism: A review. *Journal of Neurology, Neurosurgery, and Psychiatry, 44*, 751-758.
Cummings, J., Darkins, A., Mendez, M., Hill, M., & Benson, D. (1988). Alzheimer's disease and Parkinson's disease: Comparison of speech and language alterations. *Neurology, 38*, 680-684.
Darkins, A., Fromkin, V., & Benson, D. (1988). A characterization of the prosodic loss in Parkinson's disease. *Brain and Language, 34*, 315-327.
Devinsky, O., Morrell, M., & Vogt, B. (1995). Contributions of anterior cingulate cortex to behavior. *Brain, 118*, 279-306.
Diamond, A. & Goldman-Rakic, P. (1989). Comparison of human infants and rhesus monkeys on Piaget's "A not B" task: Evidence for dependence on dorsolateral prefrontal cortex. *Experimental Brain Research, 74*, 24-40.
Downes, J., Sharp, H., Costall, B., Sagar, H., & Howe, J. (1993). Alternating fluency in Parkinson's disease: An evaluation of the attentional control theory of cognitive impairment. *Brain, 116*, 887-902.
Dubois, B., Boller, F., Pillon, B., & Agid, Y. (1991). Cognitive deficits in Parkinson's disease. In F. Boller & J. Grafman (Eds.), *Handbook of neuropsychology* (pp. 195-240). New York: Elsevier.
Dubois, B. & Pillon, B. (1992). Biochemical correlates of cognitive changes and dementia in Parkinson's disease. In S. Huber & J. Cummings (Eds.), *Parkinson's disease: Neurobehavioral aspects* (pp. 178-198). Oxford: Oxford University Press.
Dubois, B., Pillon, B., Malapani, C., Deweer, B., Vérin, M., Partiaud, A., Fontaines, B., Sirigu, A., Texeira, C., & Agid, Y. (1995). Subcortical dementia and Parkinson's disease: What are the cognitive functions of the basal ganglia? In E. Wolters & P. Scheltens (Eds.), *Mental dysfunction in Parkinson's disease* (pp. 195-210). The Netherlands: ICG.
Foote, S. & Morrison, J. (1987). Extrathalamic modulation of cortical function. *Annual Review of Neuroscience, 10*, 67-95.
Frith, C., Friston, K., Liddle, P., & Frackowiak, R. (1991). Willed action and the prefrontal cortex in man: A study with PET. *Proceedings of the Royal Society of London, Series B, 244*, 241-246.

Fuster, J. (1980). *The prefrontal cortex*. New York: Raven Press.
German, D., Manaye, K., Smith, W., Woodward, D., & Saper, C. (1989). Midbrain dopaminergic cell loss in Parkinson's disease: Computer visualization. *Annals of Neurology, 26*, 507-514.
Geyer, H. & Grossman, M. (1995). Investigating the basis for the sentence comprehension deficit in Parkinson's disease. *Journal of Neurolinguistics, 8*, 191-205.
Glick, S., Ross, D., & Hough, L. (1982). Lateral asymmetry of neurotransmitters in human brain. *Brain Research, 234*, 53-63.
Goldman-Rakic, P. (1987). Circuitry of primate prefrontal cortex and regulation of behavior by representational memory. In V. Mountcastle & F. Plum (Eds.), *Handbook of physiology: Higher cortical function* (pp. 373-413). American Physiological Society.
Goldman-Rakic, P. (1995a). Toward a circuit model of working memory and the guidance of voluntary motor action. In J. Houk, J. Davis, & D. Beiser (Eds.), *Models of information processing in the basal ganglia* (pp. 131-148). Cambridge, MA: The MIT Press.
Goldman-Rakic, P. (1995b). Architecture of the prefrontal cortex and the central executive. *Annals of the New York Academy of Sciences, 769*, 71-83.
Gotham, A., Brown, R., & Marsden, C. (1988). "Frontal" cognitive functions in patients with Parkinson's disease "on" and "off" levodopa. *Brain, 111*, 299-321.
Grossman, M. (in press). Sentence comprehension in Parkinson's disease: A review.
Grossman, M., Carvell, S., Gollomp, S., Stern, M., Vernon, G., & Hurtig, H. (1991). Sentence comprehension and praxis deficits in Parkinson's disease. *Neurology, 41*, 1620-1626.
Grossman, M., Crino, P., Stern, M., Reivich, M., & Hurtig, H. (1992). Attention and sentence processing deficits in Parkinson's disease: The role of anterior cingulate cortex. *Cerebral Cortex, 2*, 513-525.
Grossman, M., Carvell, S., Stern, B., Gollomp, S., & Hurtig, H. (1992). Sentence comprehension in Parkinson's disease: The role of attention and memory. *Brain and Language, 42*, 347-384.
Grossman, M., Carvell, S., Gollomp, S., Stern, M., Reivich, M., Morrison, D., Alavi, A., & Hurtig, H. (1993). Cognitive and physiological substrates of impaired sentence processing in Parkinson's disease. *Journal of Cognitive Neuroscience, 5*, 480-498.
Grossman, M., Carvell, S., & Peltzer, L. (1993). The sum and substance of it: The appreciation of mass/count information in Parkinson's disease. *Brain and Language, 44*, 351-384.
Grossman, M., Stern, M., Gollomp, S., Vernon, G., & Hurtig, H. (1994). Verb learning in Parkinson's disease. *Neuropsychology, 8*, 413-423.
Hietanen, M. & Terävainen, H. (1986). Cognitive performance in early Parkinson's disease. *Acta Neurologica Scandinavia, 73*, 151-159.
Hietanen, M. & Terävainen, H. (1988). The effect of age of disease onset on neuropsychological performance in Parkinson's disease. *Journal of Neurology, Neurosurgery, and Psychiatry, 51*, 244-249.
Hoehn, M. & Yahr, M. (1967). Parkinsonism: Onset, progression, and mortality. *Neurology, 17*, 427-442.
Illes, J. (1989). Neurolinguistic features of spontaneous language production dissociate three forms of neurodegenerative disease: Alzheimer's, Huntington's, and Parkinson's. *Brain and Language, 37*, 628-642.
Illes, J., Metter, E., Hanson, W., & Iritani, S. (1988). Language production in Parkinson's disease: Acoustic and linguistic considerations. *Brain and Language, 33*, 146-160.
Jahanshahi, M., Brown, R., & Marsden, C. (1992). The effect of withdrawal of dopaminergic medication on simple and choice reaction time and the use of advance information in Parkinson's disease. *Journal of Neurology, Neurosurgery, and Psychiatry, 58*, 1168-1176.
Javoy-Agid, F. & Agid, Y. (1980). Is the mesocortical dopaminergic system involved in Parkinson's disease? *Neurology, 30*, 1326-1330.
Kemmerer, D. (in press). Syntactic comprehension deficits in Parkinson's disease.
Lange, K. W., Robbins, T. W., Marsden, C. D., James, M., Owen, A. M., & Paul, G. M. (1992). L-dopa withdrawal in Parkinson's Disease selectively impairs cognitive performance in tests sensitive to frontal lobe dysfunction. *Psychopharmacology, 107*, 394-404.
Lees, A. & Smith, E. (1983). Cognitive deficits in the early stages of Parkinson's disease. *Brain, 106*, 257-270.
Levin, H., Eisenberg, H., & Benton, A. (Eds.). (1991). *Frontal lobe function and dysfunction*. Oxford: Oxford University Press.
Lieberman, P., Friedman, J., & Feldman, L. (1990). Syntax comprehension in Parkinson's disease. *Journal of Nervous and Mental Disease, 178*, 360-366.

Lieberman, P., Kako, E., Friedman, J., Tajchman, G., Feldman, L., & Jiminez, E. (1992). Speech production, syntax comprehension, and cognitive deficits in Parkinson's disease. *Brain and Language, 43*, 169-189.

Matison, R., Mayeux, R., Rosen, J., & Fahn, S. (1982). "Tip of the tongue" phenomenon in Parkinson's disease. *Neurology, 32*, 567-570.

McNamara, P., Obler, L. K., Au, R., Durso, R., & Albert, M. (1992). Speech monitoring skills in Alzheimer's Disease, Parkinson's Disease and normal aging. *Brain and Language, 42*, 38-51.

McNamara, P., Krueger, M., O'Quin, K., Clark, J., & Durso, R. (1996). Grammaticality judgments and sentence comprehension in Parkinson's Disease: A comparison with Broca's aphasia. *International Journal of Neuroscience, 86*, 151-166.

Mimura, M., Albert, M., & McNamara, P. (1995). Toward a pharmacotherapy for aphasia. In H. Kirshner (Ed.), *Handbook of neurological speech and language disorders* (pp. 465-482). New York: Marcel Dekker.

Morris, R., Downes, J., Sahakian, B., Evenden, J., Heald, A., & Robbins, T. (1988). Planning and spatial working memory in Parkinson's disease. *Journal of Neurology, Neurosurgery, and Psychiatry, 51*, 757-766.

Natsopoulos, D., Katsarou, Z., Bostantzopoulos, S., Grouios, G., Mentenopoulos, G., & Logothetis J. (1991). Strategies in comprehension of relative clauses in Parkinsonian patients. *Cortex, 27*, 255-268.

Oke, A., Keller, R., Mefford, I., & Adams, R. (1978). Lateralization of norepinephrine in human thalamus. *Science, 200*, 1411-1413.

Pillon, B., Dubois, F., Bonnet, A., Esteguy, M., Guimaraes, J., Vigouret, J., L'hermitte, F., & Agid, Y. (1989). Cognitive "slowing" in Parkinson's disease fails to respond to levodopa treatment: The 15 objects test. *Neurology, 39*, 762-768.

Posner, M. (1994). Attention: The mechanisms of consciousness. *Proceedings of the National Academy of Science, USA, 91*, 7398-7403.

Posner, M. & Dehaene, S. (1994). Attentional networks. *Trends in Neurosciences, 17*, 75-79.

Rastatter, M. P. & Harr, R. (1988). Measurement of plasma levels of adrenergic neurotransmitters and primary amino acids in five stuttering subjects: A preliminary report (Biochemical aspects of stuttering). *Journal of Fluency Disorders, 13*, 127-139.

Reitan, R. & Boll, T. (1971). Intellectual and cognitive functions in Parkinson's Disease. *Journal of Consulting and Clinical Psychology, 37*, 364-369.

Rinne, J., Rummukainen, J., Paljarvi, L., & Rinne, U. (1989). Dementia in Parkinson's disease is related to neuronal loss in the medial substantia nigra. *Annals of Neurology, 26*, 47-50.

Robbins, T. & Brown, V. (1990). The role of the striatum in the mental chronometry of action: A theoretical review. *Reviews in the Neurosciences, 2*, 181-213.

Rogers, D., Lees, A., Smith, E., Trimble, M., & Stern, G. (1987). Bradyphrenia in Parkinson's disease and psychomotor retardation in depressive illness: An experimental study. *Brain, 110*, 761-776.

Rosenberger, P. B. (1980). Dopaminergic systems and speech fluency. *Journal of Fluency Disorders, 5*, 255-267.

Saint-Cyr, J., Taylor, A., & Nicholson, K. (1995). Behavior and the basal ganglia. In W. Weiner & A. Lang (Eds.), *Behavioral neurology and movement disorders, advances in neurology* (pp. 1-28). New York: Raven Press.

Scatton, B., Javoy-Agid, F., Rouquier, L., Dubois, B., & Agid, Y. (1982). Reduction of cortical dopamine, noradrenaline, serotonin, and their metabolites in Parkinson's disease. *Brain Research, 275*, 321-328.

Schultz, W., Romo, R., Ljungberg, T., Mirenowicz, J., Hollerman, J., & Dickinson, A. (1995). Reward-related signals carried by dopamine neurons. In J. Houk, J. Davis, & D. Beiser (Eds.), *Models of information processing in the basal ganglia* (pp. 233-248). Cambridge, MA: MIT Press.

Seidl, A., Onishi, K., White, H., D'Esposito, M., & Grossman, M. (1995). Resource limitations and grammatical complexity in the sentence comprehension of patients with Parkinson's disease [Abstract]. *Brain and Language, 51*, 106-108.

Shinotoh, H. & Calne, D. (1995). The use of PET in Parkinson's disease. *Brain and Cognition, 28*, 297-310.

Sullivan, E. & Sagar, H. (1989). Nonverbal recognition and recency discrimination deficits in Parkinson's disease and Alzheimer's disease. *Brain, 112*, 1503-1517.

Taylor, A. & Saint-Cyr, J. (1991). Executive function. In S. Huber & J. Cummings (Eds.), *Parkinson's disease: A neurobiological perspective* (pp. 74-85). Oxford: Oxford University Press.

Taylor, A. & Saint-Cyr, J. (1995). The neuropsychology of Parkinson's disease. *Brain and Cognition, 28*, 281-296.

Taylor, A., Saint-Cyr, J., & Lang, A. (1986). Frontal lobe dysfunction in Parkinson's disease. *Brain, 110*, 35-51.

Taylor, A., Saint-Cyr, J., & Lang, A. (1987). Parkinson's disease: Cognitive changes in relation to treatment response. *Brain, 110*, 35-51.

Tucker, D. M. & Williamson, P. A. (1984). Asymmetric neural control systems in human self-regulation. *Psychological Review, 9* (2), 185-218.

Wickens, J. & Kotter, R. (1995). Cellular models of reinforcement. In J. Houk, J. Davis, & D. Beiser (Eds.), *Models of information processing in the basal ganglia* (pp. 187-214). Cambridge, MA: MIT Press.

Williams, S. & Goldman-Rakic, P. (1993). Characterization of the dopaminergic innervation of the primate frontal cortex using a dopamine-specific antibody. *Cerebral Cortex, 3*, 199-222.

Wingate, M. E. (1988). *The structure of stuttering. A psycholinguistic analysis*. New York-Berlin: Springer-Verlag.

Wolters, E. & Scheltens, P. (Eds.). (1995). *Mental dysfunction in Parkinson's disease*. The Netherlands: ICG.

Yeudall, L. T. (1985). A neuropsychological theory of stuttering. *Seminars in Speech and Language, 6* (3), 197-222.

ASYMMETRIES OF BRAIN FUNCTION IN ALCOHOLISM: RELATIONSHIP TO AGING

Marlene Oscar-Berman and Haline E. Schendan

INTRODUCTION

Alcohol-related brain impairment has been associated with a variety of behavioral changes, indicating deficits in perceptual, emotional, and other cognitive functions. The present report reviews recent accomplishments in cognitive neuroscientific research on asymmetries of cerebral functioning that may be altered as a residual consequence of long-term chronic alcoholism. Residual effects – in contrast to acute effects – can be studied only in people who have abused alcohol for a lengthy period of time but who have been sober for at least four weeks prior to testing. In addition, they must be free of other comorbid medical complications that can affect brain functioning. Comorbid conditions (e.g., head injury, history of abuse of other drugs, concurrent psychiatric diagnoses, liver disease, HIV infection, etc.) are exclusionary criteria because cormorbidities may contribute to artifactual results that complicate interpretation.

Not all alcoholics are equally at risk for brain changes and neuropsychological deficits. The locus and extent of brain damage, as well as the type and degree of impairment, differ across individuals. These differences suggest that (a) certain subgroups of people (e.g., the elderly and women) are especially vulnerable to the neurotoxic sequelae of alcoholism, (b) that the susceptibility of particular brain regions (e.g., cerebral cortex and limbic and diencephalic structures) to alcoholism-related damage varies among individuals (e.g., with age and gender). To account for the diversity of findings, researchers have proposed different models. For context, Table 1 lists common current theoretical frameworks proposed to explain the residual neuropsychological impairments in abstinent long-term alcoholics. The models tend to focus on the vulnerability of particular participant populations, brain regions, or cognitive functions, but these factors are related. In this chapter, our discussion focuses upon the influence of alcoholism on the functioning of the cerebral hemispheres, particularly in relation to increased vulnerability associated with aging. Toward this end, our review covers primarily recent research on alcoholism and aging, as well as relevant cognitive neuroscience findings with nonalcoholic populations.

RIGHT-HEMISPHERE FUNCTIONS AND ALCOHOLISM

Clinical reports and experimental studies have provided evidence that each hemisphere of the human brain is important for mediating different functions. The left hemisphere of the brain has a dominant role in communication and in understanding the spoken and written word, while the right hemisphere plays a dominant role in coordinating interactions with the three dimensional world around us (e.g., spatial cognition). Processing modes of the two hemispheres also complement each other, depending upon context and task demands (Banich & Heller, 1998). The left hemisphere plays a special role in processing piecemeal information analytically and sequentially, and the right hemisphere plays a special role in integrating information holistically. Differences between the two cerebral hemispheres can be seen easily in cases of unilateral brain damage, and standard clinical neuropsychological tests are helpful for educing this dichotomy (e.g., see Lezak, 1995). Patients with left-hemispheric damage often have problems with language, and patients with right-hemispheric damage often have difficulty with maps, designs, music, and other nonlinguistic materials. Of interest to the present discussion is the fact that alcoholic and aging individuals have difficulty on tasks that resemble those on which patients with damage to the right hemisphere also encounter problems. In particular, patients with right-hemisphere lesions, as well as alcoholic and elderly individuals, are disproportionately impaired on nonverbal visuospatial tasks, as assessed by Performance IQ subtests (compared with Verbal IQ subtests) of the Wechsler Adult Intelligence Scale (WAIS) (Wechsler, 1981).

These observations led, independently, to the *right-hemisphere hypothesis* in both the alcoholism literature and the aging literature (Parsons, 1987). The right-hemisphere hypothesis states simply that the right half of the brain is more vulnerable to the effects of alcoholism (or the effects of aging) than the left half of the brain. In other words, a disproportionate decline in visuospatial and other nonlinguistic functions has been attributed to a greater sensitivity of the right hemisphere to the neurobiological consequences of alcoholism or aging. Later research on right-hemisphere contributions to cognitive (e.g., spatial and attentional) functions in alcoholism and aging has provided only equivocal support for the hypothesis that alcoholism and aging – alone or together – differentially affect the functioning of the two cerebral hemispheres (Bates & Convit, in press; Ellis & Oscar-Berman, 1989; Oscar-Berman, 1992; Parsons & Nixon, 1993; Rourke & Løberg, 1996).

ALCOHOLISM AND AGING

Neuropathological analyses provided some of the earliest insights into the relationship between alcoholism and aging. In *post mortem* specimens of alcoholic brains, cerebral atrophy was noted to resemble the brain shrinkage that occurs with normal chronological aging (Courville, 1966). The atrophy was most prominent in the frontal lobes, and it extended backwards to the parietal lobes. This finding was replicated by others who reported abnormal ventricular enlargement and widening of the cerebral sulci of alcoholics in relation to increasing age (Pfefferbaum et al., 1993). From the observed similarities among the brains of alcoholic and aging individuals came a search for parallels in functional decline associated with alcoholism and aging.

MODELS EMPHASIZING VULNERABILITY IN TERMS OF SUBJECT VARIABLES
Premature Aging Premature Aging Hypotheses posit that alcoholism accelerates aging. Brains of alcoholics resemble brains of chronologically older nonalcoholics.
Gender Alcoholism affects women more than men.
Vitamin Deficiency Thiamine deficiency contributes to brain lesions, especially in patients with Wernicke-Korsakoff's syndrome.
MODELS EMPHASIZING VULNERABILITY OF BRAIN REGIONS/SYSTEMS OR FUNCTIONAL PROCESSES
Diffuse Cortical Atrophy Cerebral atrophy occurs throughout the brain.
Right-hemispheric Functions Are more vulnerable to the effects of alcoholism than are left-hemispheric functions. (The same hypothesis has been applied to normal chronological aging, hence, more fuel for the premature aging hypothesis.)
Frontal Lobe Systems Are more vulnerable to the effects of alcoholism than other cortical systems.
Limbic and Diencephalic Brain Regions Are vulnerable to the effects of alcoholism in Korsakoff's syndrome.
Neurotransmitter Systems Emphasis is placed on the disruption of neurotransmitter systems, such as acetylcholine, dopamine, GABA, glutamate, and serotonin systems.
Reduction in Efficiency of Mental Operations Emphasis is placed on impairments of underlying cognitive processes.

<u>Table 1</u>. **Models proposed to explain the neuropsychological consequences of alcohol-related brain damage.** The hypotheses are not mutually exclusive; some are interrelated. There are supporting data for these hypotheses from neurobehavioral studies, brain scans, electrophysiological studies, and *post mortem* neuropathology.

The *premature aging hypothesis* has been put forth in two versions (reviewed by Ellis & Oscar-Berman, 1989). According to the first version, the *accelerated aging* (or *cumulative effects*) model, alcoholism is accompanied by the precocious onset of neurobiological and behavioral changes typically associated with advancing age. Cognitively, or neuropsychologically, alcoholics become old before their time. This version proposes that alcoholics at all ages are impaired compared to age-matched nonalcoholics.

The second version places the timing of the changes somewhat differently. In this view, which has been labeled the *increased vulnerability* model, the aging brain is more vulnerable to the deleterious influences of toxic substances, including ethanol, than is the brain of a younger person. Therefore, the cognitive decline associated with normal chronological aging (beginning at around age 50) receives added momentum when combined with alcoholism. This version proposes that older alcoholics are impaired compared to age-matched nonalcoholics; however, this would not be the case for younger alcoholics.

EMPIRICAL INVESTIGATIONS

Neuropathology, Neuroimaging, and Neurobehavior

Taken together, most of the evidence from neuropathological and neuroradiological investigations indicates that there is a link between alcoholism and premature aging (Oscar-Berman, 1998; Sullivan, Rosenbloom, & Pfefferbaum, 1998). Furthermore, studies favoring the increased vulnerability model are more common than those supporting the accelerated aging model (Oscar-Berman, 1998), although results of one recent study favor the latter. Belzunegui, Insausi, Ibanez, and Gonzalo (1995) examined the neuronal nuclear size and the neuronal population of the mammillary bodies and anterior thalamic complex in alcoholics and controls of ages 30 to 75. These subcortical structures are of particular interest because lesions to them are thought to be critical for establishing the memory impairment in alcoholic Korsakoff's amnesia (for review see Kopelman, 1995). Belzunegui et al. (1995) found significant reductions in neuronal size and number in the alcoholics, but the youngest alcoholics showed the greatest differences.

Most data, however, support the idea that older alcoholics are especially susceptible to the effects of alcoholism. Elderly alcoholics have an increased risk of accidents, side effects, and toxicity resulting from alcohol intake. This is because older people have a decreased ability to metabolize alcohol, and they may have concomitant medical problems (NIAAA, 1997). As predicted by the increased vulnerability model, certain brain structures show greater reduction in size in older alcoholics than in younger alcoholics. These are the cerebral cortex (Nicolás et al., 1997; Pfefferbaum, Sullivan, Mathalon, & Lim, 1997), the hippocampus (but see Harding, Wong, Svoboda, Kril, & Halliday, 1997; Sullivan, Marsh, Mathalon, Lim, & Pfefferbaum, 1995), and the cerebellum (Sullivan et al., 1996; for review see Sullivan et al., 1998). Alcoholics also have shown a stronger association between ventricular dilation and age compared with nonalcoholic controls (Di Sclafani et al., 1995).

More important for the issue of neurobehavioral hemispheric asymmetries in alcoholism and aging, the callosal area is notably reduced with age in alcoholics (Pfefferbaum, Lim, Desmond, & Sullivan, 1996); the corpus callosum enables communication between the cerebral hemispheres. Abnormalities in the structure of the corpus callosum can occur as a consequence of diffuse cortical damage and subsequent degeneration of cortical axons. Diffuse cortical damage, in turn, would be interpreted in conventional neuropsychological testing as a selective right-hemisphere functional deficit either because right-hemisphere functions have less cortical representation than left-hemisphere functions or because nonverbal tasks tend to be more difficult or less familiar than verbal tasks (Ellis & Oscar-Berman, 1989). Alternatively, diffuse cortical and/or callosal atrophy could interfere with cross-callosal transfer of information, causing some of the cognitive deficits observed in alcoholics and aging individuals (Hutner & Oscar Berman, 1996; Rourke & Løberg, 1996). For example, if the left hemisphere's contribution to nonverbal tasks normally is greater than the right hemisphere's contribution to verbal tasks, an interhemispheric transfer dysfunction would affect visuospatial functions more than verbal functions. Because the characteristics of hemispheric dominance are specific to each functional brain area, the altered patterns of hemispheric dominance from alcoholism and aging may be idiosyncratic to those brain areas and behavioral functions. It is, therefore, important to appreciate which brain regions are affected by chronic alcoholism and aging.

Cortical changes have been reported throughout the brain, but there is evidence that some cortical regions, especially the frontal and parietal lobes, are more consistently vulnerable to the effects of chronic alcoholism, as well as aging (Adams et al., 1998; Davila, Shear, Lane, Sullivan, & Pfefferbaum, 1994; Estruch et al., 1997; Kril, Halliday, Svoboda, & Cartwright, 1997; Pfefferbaum & Rosenbloom, 1993; Shear, Sullivan, Lane, & Pfefferbaum, 1996; Sullivan et al., 1995; Wang et al., 1993). Frontal, cingulate, parietal, parieto-occipital, and mesial temporal cortices in alcoholics show reduced metabolic activity with positron emission tomography (PET) (e.g., Adams et al., 1993; Gilman et al., 1996; Volkow et al., 1995; Volkow et al., 1997) and significantly smaller gray and/or white matter volume with structural magnetic resonance imaging (MRI) (e.g., Jernigan et al., 1991; Sullivan, Mathalon, Lim, Marsh, & Pfefferbaum, 1998). Selective neuronal loss in the frontal lobes has also been observed at a microscopic level (e.g., Kril et al., 1997). Additionally, Pfefferbaum, Sullivan, Mathalon, and Lim (1997) conducted a regional MRI analyses of cortical integrity and found evidence that cortical volume loss in alcoholism and aging is selective. The frontal lobes were especially vulnerable to chronic alcoholism at any age, but the effects were exacerbated in elderly people; temporal-parietal loss occurred mainly in aged alcoholics. These results favor the increased vulnerability model of premature aging in alcoholism. Another recent study by Sullivan et al. (1998) showed fewer regional abnormalities, but the investigators did note a relative sparing of gray matter (but loss of white matter) in the posterior superior temporal region that was also noted in the Pfefferbaum et al. (1997) study.

Neurobehavioral findings also tend to support the view that aging increases one's vulnerability to alcohol-related decline, but controversy prevails (see review by Evert & Oscar-Berman, 1995). With behavioral measures, the association between alcoholism and aging is less reliable than with imaging techniques. More importantly, when neurobiological and behavioral changes are examined together in the same study, concomitant brain damage with performance impairments are not always found.

Some studies of frontal lobe function with older alcoholics have confirmed reports of a correlation between impaired neuropsychological performance on tests of frontal functioning (e.g., executive control skills) and decreased frontal lobe perfusion or metabolism (Adams et al., 1998; 1993). However, in another study, Nicolás, Catafau, Estruch, Lomeña, Salamero, Herranz, Monforte, Cardenal, and Urbano-Marquez (1993) obtained cerebral blood flow measures and computerized tomography (CT) scans in a sample of 40 chronic alcoholic patients and related the neuroradiological findings to the results of neuropsychological testing. The researchers found evidence of significant brain hypoperfusion in the alcoholics. In 26 of the 40, the reduced blood flow was mainly in the frontal lobes, but only about 25% of them (11 of the 40) had CT evidence of frontal atrophy. Furthermore, the alcoholics exhibited significant impairments on tests of frontal-lobe functioning and visuospatial skills. Despite finding brain and behavioral changes, there was an independent relationship between frontal-lobe test performance and both frontal atrophy and frontal hypoperfusion. Age was not a relevant variable in this study.

In a study of other neural structures, Sullivan and her colleagues (1995) reported clear evidence of brain abnormalities but no differences on explicit memory tests in alcoholics relative to nonalcoholic controls aged 21 to 70 years. Explicit memory refers to the ability to consciously remember facts and events. It is assessed by recognition and recall tests and is impaired in alcoholic Korsakoff and other amnesic patients (for recent reviews see Kopelman, 1995; Mayes, 1995). The hippocampus and adjacent cortical areas have been strongly implicated in explicit memory by a host of neuropsychological, brain imaging, and nonhuman animal studies (for recent review see Eichenbaum, 1997). Sullivan et al. (1995) evaluated whether there were correlations between MRI measures of hippocampal volume and behavioral measures of verbal and nonverbal delayed recall, as defined by the Wechsler Memory Scale (WMS) (Wechsler & Stone, 1945). Anterior portions of the hippocampus were found to be smaller in the alcoholics than in the controls, and this difference was even greater in older than in younger alcoholics. While the MRI findings support the increased vulnerability model, the behavioral significance of the neuroanatomical reduction (i.e., increased hippocampal vulnerability in aging and alcoholism) was unclear because the explicit memory scores did not correlate with hippocampal volumes. Indeed, the alcoholics were not impaired on the memory tests. Furthermore, contrary to the right-hemisphere hypothesis, hippocampal reductions were bilateral, and verbal and nonverbal explicit memory performance did not differ. Sullivan et al. (1995) did, nonetheless, observe the oft-reported visuospatial impairments on the WAIS-R Digit Symbol subtest. While this subtest has a memory component, there were also no correlations between Digit Symbol performance and hippocampal volume.

Another study found no evidence of cortical atrophy but did show aging-related cognitive deficits. Di Sclafani et al. (1995) scanned older alcoholics and controls using MRI and gave them numerous neuropsychological tests in order to compare brain measures with cognitive abilities. The alcoholics displayed clear impairments on visuospatial and memory tasks, especially visuospatial memory. Despite the behavioral deficits, there were no group differences in global cerebral atrophy (although two alcoholics had significant atrophy). One reason for cognitive dysfunction in the absence of changes in gross brain morphology is that there can be synaptic neuronal changes that alter processing but are undetectable at a macroscopic anatomical scale (for recent review see Harper, 1998). Di Sclafani et al. (1995), however, did find a stronger association between ventricular dilation and age in the alcoholics than in the controls.

INTERMANUAL DIFFERENCES AND LATERALIZED SENSORY PRESENTATION

The efficacy of the measuring instruments for assessing cognitive functions – hemispheric laterality in particular – is critical. Tasks where distinct stimuli are presented either simultaneously or asynchronously to sense organs on one or the other side of the body, or that require separate responses by the left or right hands, are important tools for assessing hemispheric asymmetries (for review see Ellis & Oscar-Berman, 1989). In such tasks, stimuli are processed (and motor responses are made) by neural events controlled mainly by the cerebral hemisphere contralateral to the side of sensory input (or response effector). Because of the decussation (crossing) of neuronal transmission fibers within the central nervous system, stimuli presented to the sensory field on one side of the body (e.g., the Left Visual Field [VF]) proceed first to the opposite side of the brain (i.e., the right hemisphere) before crossing over to the other side of the brain. Similarly, motor responses are made by the limb opposite to the hemisphere of interest (e.g., the left hand is controlled by the right hemisphere).

From these organizational principles comes a relatively straightforward test of the right-hemisphere hypothesis of alcoholism; that is, to contrast performance of each hand. Since there is asymmetric cerebral dominance of motor control, performance should be better for the preferred over the nonpreferred hand. In the case where the preferred hand is disproportionately better than the nonpreferred hand, this may be taken as evidence for damage to the nondominant hemisphere controlling the nonpreferred hand. Specifically, for right-handed people (i.e., left-hemisphere dominant), alcoholics should perform disproportionately better than nonalcoholic controls with their right hand than their nonpreferred left hand (controlled by the right hemisphere), according to the right-hemisphere hypothesis.

There are several reports of disproportionate impairment of alcoholics when they use their left hands (i.e., right hemisphere) compared to controls (for a review see Ellis & Oscar-Berman, 1989), particularly on the Tactual Performance Test (TPT) of the Halstead-Reitan Neuropsychological Test Battery (Reitan & Davison, 1974). It would thus seem that right-hemisphere control of motor behavior may be especially vulnerable to alcoholism. In a recent study, however, this possibility was evaluated in a relatively large sample of long-term, abstinent alcoholics and nonalcoholic controls (mean ages 42 years and 46 years, respectively). Participants performed several subtests of the Halstead-Reitan Battery with each hand separately. Contrary to the right-hemisphere account of alcoholism, there were no differences in handedness patterns between alcoholics and controls on any of the tasks, even the TPT (Kwon, Rourke, & Grant, 1997).

As with the motor end of behavior, research using lateralized sensory presentation also has provided conflicting evidence for the right-hemisphere hypothesis, as well as for the premature aging model of alcoholism (see reviews by Ellis & Oscar-Berman, 1989; Oscar-Berman, 1992; Parsons & Nixon, 1993). For example, Ellis (1990) used a dichotic listening technique to measure hemispheric asymmetries for perceiving two types of stimuli presented simultaneously to the two ears: linguistic (words) and musical (strings of piano notes). In most people, word perception is accomplished principally by the left hemisphere, whereas musical perception is accomplished principally by the right hemisphere (Lezak, 1995). Therefore, with linguistic stimuli, accuracy for words heard by the right ear would normally be greater than when heard by the left ear, whereas, with musical patterns, accuracy for notes heard by the left ear would normally be greater than when heard by the right ear. The main subject groups in the Ellis (1990) study were abstinent alcoholics and nonalcoholic controls (from ages of 25 years and 74 years). However, it is important that Ellis (1990) also included a group of nonalcoholic stroke patients with focal lesions in the right hemisphere. The focal lesion group served to establish performance baselines that result from confirmed damage to the right hemisphere (for comparison with the predicted right-hemisphere dysfunction in the alcoholics).

The right-hemisphere stroke patients showed a general *rightward shift*, that is, they showed a magnified superiority of the right ear (left hemisphere) for words but also an atypical right ear advantage for the tones. This abnormal pattern did not emerge with the other groups, however. The alcoholics and age equivalent controls performed similarly, whether the stimuli were linguistic or musical; specifically, alcoholics and nonalcoholic controls of all ages obtained typical right ear advantages for words and typical left ear advantages for tonal patterns. Despite the normal performance on dichotic listening by the alcoholics, on Performance subtests of the WAIS-R, Ellis (1990) found that the right-hemisphere stroke patients and the older alcoholics (ages 48 years to 74 years) but not the younger alcoholics (ages 25 years to 47 years) performed significantly worse than same age nonalcoholic controls. In other words, like the right-hemisphere stroke patients, the older alcoholics showed an abnormal Verbal-Performance WAIS-R IQ discrepancy. Thus, the results of the dichotic listening experiments did not support any of the hypotheses, whereas the neuropsychological findings with the same participants were supportive of the right-hemisphere hypothesis of both alcoholism and of aging, in particular the increased vulnerability model.

SPATIAL COGNITION

As just noted, Performance subtests of the WAIS, such as Digit Symbol and Block Design, have been sensitive to the cognitive changes associated with alcoholism and normal chronological aging (Ellis & Oscar-Berman, 1989; Kaplan, 1988). While the Digit Symbol and Block Design subtests are considered to provide measures of visuospatial function and right-hemisphere integrity, performance on the subtests depends upon many diverse functional capacities and many brain areas. Functions tapped include: processing-speed/accuracy, motor-speed/accuracy, working memory, paired associate learning, visual perception, spatial cognition, attention, and visual scanning ability (Wechsler, 1997). Each of these cognitive abilities, in turn, engages multiple brain areas. By tapping diverse functions, clinical neuropsychological tests carry the advantage of exquisite sensitivity to brain injury. By virtue of their sensitivity, the subtests have been useful for demonstrating diminished cognitive abilities in a variety of neurological populations, including alcoholics (Beatty, Blanco, Hames, & Nixon, 1997; for recent research see Beatty, Hames, Blanco, Nixon, & Tivis, 1996; Ciesielski, Waldorf, & Jung, 1995; Di Sclafani et al., 1995; for review see Milberg, Hebben, & Kaplan, 1996). Their sensitivity also diminishes the utility of the subtests toward defining the integrity of focal brain areas. Their lack of specificity is partly responsible for the elusive nature of consistent findings of cognitive compromise in alcoholism. Indeed, normal standardized scores have been achieved by alcoholics (e.g., Beatty, Katzung, Moreland, & Nixon, 1995; Kwon et al., 1997; Volkow et al., 1997) as well as by focal lesion patients (see review by Kaplan, 1988; Kaplan, Palmer, Weinstein, & Baker, 1981).

The sensitivity of clinical neuropsychological tests to brain injury does, nonetheless, make them potentially useful, especially when they supplement studies employing experimental cognitive tasks. Besides providing broad indications of cognitive deficits, when different laboratories use the same neuropsychological assessment procedures comparisons among studies are facilitated. Further, neuropsychological tests can help address whether, for example, the sample size was sufficiently large or the selected population was sufficiently uniform to detect differences among alcoholic and control groups. This is especially important in cases where experimental tests do not show group differences. A *Process approach* to neuropsychological assessment is helpful in this regard (as described by Milberg et al., 1996).

PROCESS APPROACH

Measurements from neuropsychological tests administered in a process-oriented manner not only have the advantage of sensitivity, as for any neuropsychological test, but they have the added advantage of greater specificity regarding cognitive impairments and locus of damage (Kaplan, 1988). This is accomplished by altering the administration or response recording procedures to enable a wide spectrum of measurements to be derived from each clinical test. The Process approach is akin to the extra measurements taken and further data permutations carried out in experimental research.

A process-oriented neuropsychological assessment was combined with administration of experimental tasks in an exemplary study by Beatty, Hames, Blanco, Nixon, and Tivis (1996), and to some extent, also by Beatty, Blanco, Hames, and Nixon (1997). The aim of the Beatty et al. (1996) study was to use competing models of spatial information processing to test theories of spatial impairment in alcoholism. The three models conceptualized spatial ability as focused upon: (1) egocentric (self as reference; frontal lobe) versus allocentric space (object located with reference to another object; right parietal lobe); (2) categorical (relative positions of features to each other; left hemisphere) versus coordinate spatial representation (absolute distance between features; right hemisphere); or (3) featural (local level; left hemisphere) versus configural analysis (global configuration; right hemisphere), with the last applied often to understanding processing of hierarchical visual objects (see later section on this topic). Accordingly, Beatty et al. (1996) noted that the right-hemisphere hypothesis would predict marked impairments by alcoholics on visuospatial tasks engaging coordinate and configural brain functions; note, while not mentioned as such by the authors, the right parietal lobe's role in allocating attention to allocentric space suggests that allocentric tasks may also provide an appropriate test of right-hemisphere functioning. By contrast, a model that posits diffuse bilateral damage (e.g., in frontal or limbic systems) (see Table 1 and Rourke & Løberg, 1996) would predict measurable impairments on visuospatial tasks engaging egocentric functions and, possibly, on frontal lobe components of categorical and featural tasks as well. Beatty et al.'s results, however, were inconsistent with both accounts of alcoholism-related brain damage.

Beatty et al. (1997; 1996) tested young male and female alcoholics and controls (mean ages 40 years and under) on numerous tasks that were each designed to assess aspects of spatial abilities (Beatty et al., 1997; Beatty et al., 1996). Beatty and his colleagues evaluated the featural versus configural analytical model with clinical neuropsychological tests. The alcoholics attained lower scores on both the Block Design and Object Assembly subtests of the WAIS-R. More importantly, because these subtests were administered and scored with the process-oriented approach of the WAIS-RNI (Kaplan, Fein, Morris, & Delis, 1991), they also yielded more data relevant to the question of asymmetries of featural analysis (left hemisphere) and configural analysis (right hemisphere). Specifically, the process-oriented analysis of Block Design performance showed that alcoholics made more configural errors; that is, the error type found in patients with right- but not left-hemisphere lesions (Kaplan et al., 1981). This was not, however, the case for performance on the additional Object Assembly puzzles advocated by the Process approach. The speed of puzzle completion and pattern of impaired performance by alcoholics (Beatty et al., 1997; Beatty et al., 1996) most closely resembled those found in patients with left-hemisphere lesions (Kaplan, 1988). This then suggests an alcoholic impairment in featural processing. Taken together, the Block Design and Object Assembly results did not support the right-hemisphere hypothesis. Instead, because damage in one or the other hemisphere may dominate performance in different tasks, the finding that alcoholics were impaired at both featural and configural analyses was suggestive of bilateral damage.

The other models were evaluated by Beatty et al. (1997; 1996) using experimental tests alone (categorical versus coordinate) or both neuropsychological and experimental tests (egocentric versus allocentric). Alcoholics were impaired on the test of categorical but not coordinate relations, and they were indistinguishable from controls on remote memory for the same information, contrary to the right-hemisphere hypothesis. Alcoholics performed normally on the egocentric task (a clinical test) and on one out of three allocentric tasks (clinical and experimental tests). This is the opposite of the pattern predicted by a frontal-limbic account (Tarter, 1975), and the mixed allocentric task results, as measures of right parietal function, provide conflicting evidence regarding the right-hemisphere hypothesis.

The above studies (Beatty et al., 1997; Beatty et al., 1996; Ellis, 1990) illustrate how experimental tests of cognitive function can supplement standard clinical neuropsychological evaluation of neurobehavioral deficits in alcoholism and aging. Clinical tests have been used widely in alcoholism research because they sensitively reveal patterns of impairment and sparing across many overlapping and contrasting functional domains by engaging multiple perceptual, cognitive, and response-related functions. To enhance specificity, tests developed by cognitive psychologists can often serve as critical additions to the investigative arsenal in alcoholism research. Among these, the tasks that are especially informative are those employed in cognitive neuroscientific investigations to index a restricted set of brain functions. Besides being well suited for pinpointing the cognitive domains disrupted, they provide a functional neurobiological background against which a richer explanation of cognitive deficits in alcoholism (and aging) may be rendered. To further illustrate the role that such experimental tests play in alcoholism research, let us first take a closer look at the two types of experimental tests, mental rotation and imagery, that were used in the two studies by Beatty and colleagues (1997; 1996) in the context of the egocentric versus allocentric space account.

MENTAL ROTATION AND MENTAL IMAGERY

In the mental rotation task used by Beatty et al. (1997; 1996), people saw two-dimensional (2-D) depictions of three-dimensional objects constructed of cubes. From four 2-D pictures, they chose the two depictions that, when rotated mentally, matched the target picture. For the mental imagery task people were required to report whether or not there were curves in the capitalized form of each lower case letter presented (Beatty et al., 1997; Beatty et al., 1996). While mental representations may be formed in both tasks, a spatial transformation of the representation is entailed by mental rotation but probably not by mental imagery.

For evaluation of the right-hemisphere account of alcoholism, these tasks were aptly pitted against each other. Mental rotation is dependent predominantly upon the right hemisphere, whereas mental imagery is dependent predominantly upon the left hemisphere. The specific brain areas activated during mental rotation of objects are inferior and superior parietal cortices and angular gyrus and some premotor areas in the frontal lobes (e.g., Kosslyn, DiGirolamo, Thompson, & Alpert, 1998). These brain areas are distinct from those activated during mental imagery, namely, occipital, occipitotemporal, or inferior temporal cortices (Beatty et al., 1996; Corballis & Sergent, 1989; D'Esposito et al., 1997; Ditunno & Mann, 1990; Loverock & Modigliani, 1995). Therefore, in addition to considering the right-hemisphere hypothesis, the Beatty et al. studies also spoke to the effects of alcoholism on the anterior-posterior axis (and the dorsal-ventral dichotomy) (Mishkin, Ungerleider, & Macko, 1983) of the brain. This is important because the frontal and parietal areas (i.e., anterior and dorsal) implicated in mental rotation have been found to be more compromised by alcoholism than the occipital and temporal areas (i.e., far posterior and ventral) implicated in mental imagery. Thus, impairments by alcoholics were expected on mental rotation but not on mental imagery tasks.

As expected, mental rotation performance was impaired in alcoholics compared to controls (Beatty et al., 1997; Beatty et al., 1996), confirming earlier findings (Glenn & Parsons, 1991; Tarter, 1975). In contrast, mental imagery performance was similar between alcoholic and control groups in one study (Beatty et al., 1997) but not in the other (Beatty et al., 1996), although both studies showed the same small trend toward impairment. The latter tendency may reflect cognitive functions that are common to mental imagery and mental rotation tasks, with degree of involvement differing between tasks. For instance, the spatial analysis and/or attentional functions predominantly controlled by areas of the right parietal lobe may be more strongly engaged during mental rotation than mental imagery. Further, while there is evidence for hemispheric dominance in both tasks, there is also evidence of bilateral involvement in mental rotation and mental imagery (Kosslyn et al., 1998; Loverock & Modigliani, 1995).

Regardless, the Beatty et al. (1997; 1996) findings indicate that the cognitive functions engaged predominantly during mental rotation (e.g., spatial transformation) are vulnerable to the effects of alcoholism, and they are more vulnerable than those engaged predominantly during mental imagery. If consistency across studies is taken as an indicator, the mental rotation and mental imagery results support the right-hemisphere account of alcoholism; they suggest that both right- and left-hemisphere functions (i.e., mental rotation and mental imagery processes, respectively) are compromised by alcoholism, but the right hemisphere is disproportionately impaired. This conclusion, however, depends upon the presumption of mental rotation as a right-hemisphere dominant task and mental imagery as left-hemisphere dominant, an idea that may not hold as evidence for bilateral involvement accumulates. Rather, the clearest finding of these studies is that alcoholism impairs visuospatial function more than some other visual functions, as indicated by the greater spatial demands of mental rotation over mental imagery.

While these tasks have not been used with alcoholic groups of different ages, there is research on how aging affects mental rotation and mental imagery. The studies suggest that there is impairment with increasing age. In particular, with aging, mental rotation accuracy decreases (e.g., Herman & Bruce, 1983), and mental image activation and maintenance accuracy decrease (e.g., Dror & Kosslyn, 1994). The impaired performance of alcoholics and elderly on both tasks (Herman & Bruce, 1983) provides little support for the right-hemisphere hypothesis of alcoholism and aging.

LATERALIZED CUED ATTENTION

Another cognitive domain that is useful for evaluating the right-hemisphere hypothesis is that of attention, where the right hemisphere plays a specialized role (see for recent reviews Friedrich, Egly, Rafal, & Beck, 1998; Heilman & Valenstein, 1993; Ivry & Robertson, 1998). In a recent study of visual attention, Evert and Oscar-Berman (submitted) measured the abilities of alcoholics and nonalcoholic controls between the ages of 29 years and 76 years to respond to targets processed by the two cerebral hemispheres. The methods they used were directly relevant to evaluating not only the right-hemisphere hypothesis but also the premature aging hypothesis. Moreover, lateralized presentation of the stimuli in the left and the right VFs further accentuated the ability of this study to evaluate the role of the right hemisphere in alcoholism and aging. Evert and Oscar-Berman (submitted) measured the effects of increased attentional demands in a visual cued-detection task, first, to establish right-hemispheric specialization in young healthy controls (under age 50) and then to assess right-hemispheric functional decline in the alcoholic and aging individuals. In the cued-detection task, a precue provided information about the most probable location of a subsequent target letter (i.e., in the left and the right VFs).

The young nonalcoholic controls showed a VF asymmetry. In particular, there was a specific disruption when an invalid cue was presented to the right VF (i.e., the left hemisphere), but the target appeared instead in the left VF (i.e., the right hemisphere). Thus, there was a right-hemisphere advantage in this task, since there was no disruption on trials where there were invalid cues to the Left VF and targets in the opposite VF. Unlike the younger controls, the alcoholics in both age groups (and the older nonalcoholic controls) showed no evidence of a right-hemisphere (left VF) advantage on the task; they were influenced by the validity of the cue regardless of the visual field where it appeared. In sum, the results from this experiment provided support for the accelerated aging model of premature aging and for the right-hemisphere models of alcoholism and aging.

HIERARCHICAL PATTERN PERCEPTION AND ATTENTION

While recent research with alcoholic participants using hierarchical stimuli is lacking (to our knowledge), there are recent findings from cognitive neuroscientific studies with healthy nonalcoholic people that elucidate earlier work on global versus local processing in alcoholics. In hierarchical visual patterns, a global shape is formed from the spatial configuration of many local elements (e.g., local level small triangles forming a global level square). Global-local tasks engage asymmetrically organized brain processes, with certain (global) functions carried out predominantly by the right hemisphere and other (local) functions carried out predominantly by the left hemisphere.

Evidence for this comes from studies such as that of Robertson and Delis (1986) who asked patients with lesions of the right or left hemisphere to make similarity judgments about hierarchical visual patterns. On each trial, a sample image (e.g., a square made of squares) was shown above two possible matching items. One item matched the form of the sample only at the global level (e.g., a square made of triangles), while the other matched only at the local level (e.g., a triangle made of squares). Patients with right-hemisphere lesions tended to choose the local match, whereas those with left-hemisphere lesions tended to choose the global match.

Using a similar paradigm, Kramer, Blusewicz, Robertson, and Preston (1989) found that alcoholics performed as predicted by the right-hemisphere hypothesis of alcoholism. Specifically, alcoholics chose the global match less often than nonalcoholic controls. The altered global bias of alcoholics reflected a quantitative rather than qualitative change because the influence of other variables, such as stimulus size and position, on hierarchical task performance was similar in alcoholics and controls. The degree of salience is thus reduced at the global level with chronic alcoholism, but the way hierarchical stimuli are processed seems to be similar in alcoholics and nonalcoholic controls. Interestingly, alcohol administered to young nonalcoholic people resulted in a global processing impairment resembling that seen in chronic alcoholics (Lamb & Robertson, 1987).

A standard clinical neuropsychological test was also administered in the Kramer et al. (1989) study. On the WAIS-R Block Design subtest, alcoholics showed a higher incidence of configural errors relative to the controls. This finding is consistent with that from another study showing that configural errors on Block Design were similar for alcoholics and patients with circumscribed brain lesions in the right hemisphere (Akshoomoff, Delis, & Kiefner, 1989). Thus, alcoholics appeared to have a right-hemisphere dysfunction of configural analysis. An advantage of Kramer et al.'s (1989) concurrent use of both clinical and experimental tests was that they could then perform correlational analyses on the two data pools. Block Design configural errors, however, were not significantly correlated with the increased local response bias on hierarchical stimuli. This suggests that, while both global processing of hierarchical images and Block Design configural errors may assess the efficiency of global level analysis, damage to somewhat distinct brain areas may be responsible for altered performance in each task. Indeed, other evidence suggests that either right parietal dysfunction or altered hemispheric dominance from callosal atrophy may affect performance on both tasks, whereas right frontal dysfunction (as in alcoholics) may be more important for errors on Block Design than for reduced global bias on hierarchical patterns (Chase, Fedio, Foster, et al., 1984; Kaplan, 1988; Pfefferbaum et al., 1996; Robertson, Lamb, & Knight, 1988; Robertson, Lamb, & Knight, 1991).

Findings from another experimental task with hierarchical stimuli were also consistent with the right-hemisphere hypothesis of alcoholism (Robertson, Stillman, & Delis, 1985). In this case, a simple geometric figure was shown alone (e.g., a triangle) or in the context of other figures with the same form and orientation (e.g., three upright triangles in a row). On each trial, the orientation of the shape or row of shapes changed, and participants reported the orientation of the stimuli. When a figure was shown in context, its perceived orientation could change compared to when it was presented alone; in other words, the global context (the *perceptual reference frame*) alters the perceived orientation of the local elements. Alcoholics were found to be less influenced by the global context of the shapes than nonalcoholic controls. Specifically, with an isolated figure, controls and alcoholics showed a right alignment bias. In contrast, when a central figure was shown in the global context of two abutting figures, controls no longer showed the right-sided bias, whereas alcoholics continued to do so, as if they were ignoring the global reference frame.

While the premature aging hypothesis of alcoholism was not addressed in the Robertson et al. (1985) study, it was addressed in the Kramer et al. (1989) study but was not supported. There were no reliable correlations between age and either hierarchical task performance or Block Design configural errors in alcoholics or controls (Kramer et al., 1989), consistent with related research on Block Design (e.g., Libon et al., 1994). The null finding with aged nonalcoholic controls stands in contrast to a positive finding from another study that aging impairs memory for hierarchical stimuli (Akshoomoff, Delis, & Haist, 1993). This impairment, however, affected memory for local but not global level information, running counter to the right-hemisphere hypothesis of aging. In particular, elderly people (ages 60 years to 78 years) recalled and recognized fewer local level forms than young (21 years to 39 years) or middle aged (44 years to 57 years) people, but aging did not affect memory for global form. Since the integrity of memory depends upon processing capacity, findings from both studies suggest that aging does not impair global level processing (Akshoomoff et al., 1993; Kramer et al., 1989). Further research, however, needs to assess processing capacity directly to determine whether local processing is instead compromised with aging.

Recent studies using neuropsychological, brain imaging (PET and functional MRI), and electrophysiological (e.g., event-related brain potential; ERP) techniques provide fine-grained neuroanatomical and temporal information regarding brain areas important for hierarchical pattern perception. Studies where a task is performed while measuring brain activity (with functional brain imaging or other brain sensing techniques) are especially important, as they provide the most direct way to link cognitive function (or dysfunction) in a brain region to behavioral task performance. Of course, direct links are also provided by neuropsychological studies where high resolution brain scans (e.g., MRI) reveal the loci of neural injury. For example, since patients with right or left prefrontal lesions perform normally on tasks with hierarchical stimuli, whereas those with right or left posterior lesions do not, anterior regions seem less important than posterior brain regions for attending to global and local levels of objects (Robertson & Delis, 1986; Robertson et al., 1988; Robertson et al., 1991).

On a still finer scale, neuropsychological and brain imaging studies converge upon the superior-temporal gyrus and inferior parietal lobe as critical for analysis and selective attention of hierarchical patterns. Areas in the right hemisphere dominate global processing and those in the left hemisphere dominate local processing (Fink et al., 1996) (for review of neuropsychological studies see Robertson & Lamb, 1991). Brain imaging studies (PET and fMRI) have also indicated that right and left ventral posterior visual cortices (i.e., inferior occipital and lingual gyri) are differentially modulated by globally versus locally directed perception. However, the hemispheric dominance is a top-down effect from the parietal lobe, and the direction of the hemispheric dominance depends upon the stimulus category. Specifically, in the ventral posterior region, the left (language) hemisphere analyzes local letter-like forms, whereas the right (visuospatial) hemisphere analyzes local objects. In contrast, the global forms (e.g., local teacups forming a global anchor) are analyzed by the corresponding region in the hemisphere opposite the one specializing in the local form (Fink et al., 1996; Fink et al., 1997; Martinez et al., 1997). The fine temporal information from ERPs combined with PET reveals that the hemispheric dominance of hierarchical pattern perception is primarily the consequence of later brain functions (after 260 msecs). This high-order processing is in the asymmetrically organized temporal-parietal region that controls visuospatial attention to global or local levels of objects (Heinze, Hinrichs, Scholz, Burchert, & Mangun, 1998).

Recent cognitive neuroscientific findings thus provide a precise description of the neural systems responsible for patterns of hemispheric dominance with hierarchical visual patterns. This new knowledge, in turn, indicates that the altered patterns of performance with hierarchical patterns in alcoholic and aging individuals may principally reflect damage to the right parietal region, although callosal dysfunction is also a possibility. It should be noted that ventral posterior regions of the brain (i.e., the inferior occipital and lingual gyri) have not been implicated in alcohol-related brain damage as much as frontal brain systems (e.g., Pfefferbaum et al., 1997; Sullivan et al., 1998), and in at least one study, metabolic activity of posterior regions was normal (e.g., Volkow et al., 1997). Thus, posterior ventral regions are unlikely to be responsible for altered laterality patterns in alcoholics, based on current understanding from both cognitive neuroscientific investigations and neuroanatomical examination of alcoholic brain abnormalities.

A recently developed model of perceptual lateralization (*double filtering by frequency* theory or *DFF*) suggests that both hemispheres are important for global and local information processing but differ in how they analyze complex information (Ivry & Robertson, 1998). In particular, the right hemisphere specializes in low frequency information, whereas the left hemisphere specializes in high frequency information. Thus, depending upon the spatial frequencies present in a visual image and whether they are the attended frequencies, either the right or left parietal lobe may be more important.

Based on this model from cognitive neuroscience, Ivry and Robertson (1998) recently offered two accounts of impaired global level performance from alcoholism. The first is consistent with the right-hemisphere hypothesis of alcoholism and suggests that disproportionate damage to the right hemisphere would disrupt the asymmetrically organized low spatial frequency filters therein. The second contradicts the right-hemisphere hypothesis of alcoholism and suggests that alcoholism would impair the functioning of left-hemisphere dominant systems that enable attention to switch from the local to global level.

Predictions from DFF theory, however, cannot be easily distinguished from those based on a competing model from cognitive neuroscience (Ivry & Robertson, 1998). Consequently, Ivry and Robertson (1998) also suggested an account of alcoholism based on this other model, according to which the right hemisphere normally emits a wider spotlight of spatial attention than the left hemisphere. By this third account, alcohol may affect processes that determine the size of the attentional spotlight, reducing the region over which attention is spread. This may impair the ability of alcoholics to attend to and analyze the global level of hierarchical patterns (Brown & Kosslyn, 1995). Evidence for this last account is the finding that intoxicated nonalcoholic individuals are better at detecting a foveal target but worse at detecting a peripheral target, as compared to sober controls. It is as if the attentional spotlight is focused narrowly on foveal information at the expense of peripheral coverage when people are under the influence of alcohol (Post, Lott, Maddock, & Beede, 1996). Which of the above three accounts is best cannot be determined presently; one reason is that there is controversy surrounding whether a distinction can be made between (a) allocating attention to a spatial region of varying size (the spotlight account) versus (b) attending to different spatial resolutions (DFF theory).

OTHER VISUAL TASKS

There has been renewed interest in evaluating early sensory function in neurological populations with the recent emergence of well-honed techniques to do so. After all, certain aspects of visuospatial impairments could be a function of decreased early visual sensory functions rather than a function of visual cognition. Indeed, psychophysical evaluations have revealed that alcoholics show a reduction in visual contrast sensitivity over all spatial frequencies as compared to controls (Roquelaure et al., 1995). Consistent with this, alcohol intake reduces the contrast sensitivity function (Nicholson, Andre, Tyrrell, Wang, & Leibowitz, 1995), suggesting that extensive alcohol intake (as in alcoholism) eventually produces long-lasting reductions in contrast sensitivity. Thus, early visual abnormalities may account for at least some of the behavioral impairments in alcoholism on visual tasks.

Indeed, recent cognitive neuroscientific investigations of early sensory processing in alcoholics indicates that this is the case. Damage to earlier sensory processing (before 150 msecs) may contribute to alcoholics' deficits in performance, if not to hemispheric asymmetry. Early visual, as well as auditory, ERPs seem to differ between alcoholic and control groups, with neurophysiological dysfunction indicated by ERP prolongation and size reduction (Nicolás et al., 1997). Further evidence for low-level damage is a decrease in estimated scalp surface energy observed by Cohen, Porjesz, Begleiter, and Wang (1997) while alcoholics performed a visual task at a time when extrastriate processing still fulfills primarily perceptual functions (Allison, McCarthy, Nobre, Puce, & Belger, 1994; Heinze et al., 1998; Schendan, Ganis, & Kutas, 1998).

Taken altogether, the preceding findings show fairly strong support for the idea that visual functions are abnormal in alcoholic and aging individuals. There are visual processing deficits from early sensory to later visuospatial cognitive processes, as assessed, for example, by spatial frequency, contrast sensitivity, and backward masking (see also, Oscar-Berman, Goodglass, & Cherlow, 1973; Schlotterer, Moscovitch, & Crapper-McLachlan, 1984). Still, the degree to which the abnormalities are tied to right-hemisphere dysfunction remains to be clarified.

Regardless, an important implication of abnormal visual functions in alcoholism and aging follows from the inherent relationship between processing and memory. The success of prior processing is an important factor in determining the efficacy of learning and memory encoding and retrieval (for discussion of this idea see a review by Miyashita, 1993). Once processing is sufficiently advanced, memory for the processed information can be encoded and related knowledge retrieved (e.g., Allan & Rugg, 1997; Paller, Kutas, & Mayes, 1987; Paller, Kutas, & McIsaac, 1995; Schendan, 1998). It is thus likely that learning and memory for spatial information is impaired in alcoholics and the elderly.

A number of studies have explored the conditions under which alcoholics do and do not show normal spatial learning and memory, despite impaired visuospatial abilities. In contrast to their intact premorbid geographic memory, alcoholics are impaired on tests of memory for recently acquired spatial information, such as the *New Map Test*, where they learn and remember the locations of 15 imaginary cities in three fictional states (Beatty et al., 1997; Beatty et al., 1996). Aspects of maze learning and memory are also impaired by alcoholism. In a push-button maze task, alcoholics differed from the controls (Bowden & McCarter, 1993). In that study, alcoholics failed to show equi-availability of spatial memory representations when learning and remembering shortcut movements, which were considered to depend upon explicit memory systems. In contrast, alcoholics and controls were equivalent in learning and remembering retrace movements that were considered to depend upon procedural memory, a component of implicit memory systems (i.e., memory without awareness) (for recent review see Schacter & Buckner, 1998). Thus, alcoholics showed mildly impaired explicit (but not implicit) learning and memory for spatial information. It is noteworthy that, to some extent, deficits in spatial learning may reflect premorbid deficiencies in spatial learning. Evidence for this comes from the demonstration that visuospatial learning is also impaired in nonalcoholic individuals with a family history of alcoholism compared to those without such a family background (e.g., Garland, Parsons, & Nixon, 1993).

At this point, it should be emphasized that alcoholics and healthy aging people have difficulty with memory for other materials besides visuospatial stimuli (Bates & Convit, in press; Rourke & Løberg, 1996). There are, for example, recent reports of impaired delayed explicit recall of both verbal and nonverbal materials in alcoholic and aging populations (e.g., Craik & Jennings, 1992; Di Sclafani et al., 1995), although not all studies have shown deficits (e.g., Sullivan et al., 1995). In addition, chronic alcoholics and patients with left-hemisphere brain damage recalled less essential and detailed verbal material than patients with right-hemisphere brain damage (Tivis & Parsons, 1997), a finding not consistent with the right-hemisphere hypothesis. However, alcoholics and left-hemisphere patients also were more depressed than the right-hemisphere patients (Tivis & Parsons, 1997). Further, in another study with the same verbal memory tests, alcoholics did not differ reliably from controls when affective state was accounted for in the statistical analyses (Nixon, Hallford, & Tivis, 1996). Clearly, additional research is needed to determine the pattern of memory deficits, especially since other factors (e.g., emotional abnormalities) may account for poor memory performance.

ADDITIONAL FINDINGS FROM COGNITIVE NEUROSCIENCE

One of the few techniques of cognitive neuroscience, namely ERPs, that has been applied to issues of neurobehavioral changes with alcoholism and aging has yielded evidence for changes in brain systems engaged late in information processing, besides the evidence for early sensory changes described earlier. For example, certain findings based on ERP examinations of alcoholic and aged brains are consistent with the idea that changes in brain regions involved in attentional modulation that are activated late in processing (after 260 msecs) (Heinze et al., 1998) may be responsible for the visuospatial changes. The preponderance of ERP findings indicates that alcoholic brains differ neurophysiologically during later (after 300 msecs) cognitive processing (e.g., Cohen et al., 1997). The main electrophysiological marker of brain changes from alcoholism is the same one that prominently indexes brain changes in aging, that is, the P300 component. The size of the P300 is often found to be smaller in alcoholic and aged individuals than in control groups (e.g., Cohen et al., 1997; Polich, 1997; Porjesz et al., 1998).

More importantly for the right-hemisphere hypothesis, some studies report greater P300 reduction on the right than left side of the head. As a recent example, the results of a P300 study of visual perceptual fusion support the right-hemisphere hypothesis (Tsagareli, 1995). When the two parts of a whole geometric shape are rapidly and sequentially presented under conditions of backward masking, the parts can fuse perceptually to form a single shape. Using such a task, Tsagareli (1995) found that alcoholics discriminated the parts from the whole more slowly than control participants. In particular, alcoholics were slower to decide whether a complete and closed geometric figure had been shown, rather than two open fragments of geometric figures. What is more important is that alcoholics did not show the right-hemisphere advantage that controls demonstrated (i.e., with left VF presentation). This behavioral finding was mirrored in the P300 brain electrical potential, which was reduced in alcoholics, especially over the right hemisphere (Tsagareli, 1995). The late emergence of this effect indicates that the problem occurred at a high-order processing stage.

In a related study that emphasized working memory processes, ERPs after 250 msecs over right posterior scalp regions also differed between alcoholics and controls, with novel geometric figures that fit or did not fit to create a whole when conjoined with a preceding sample stimulus (Zhang, Begleiter, & Porjesz, 1997). Working memory functions in the frontal lobes are thought to affect posterior processing, thereby influencing posterior activity. Therefore, vulnerable frontal neural systems that support working memory in alcoholics may exert an impaired influence on right posterior regions of the brains as well. Alternatively, posterior – as well as frontal – neural systems may be impaired in alcoholics. The participants in these ERP studies were too young (mean ages 35 years or less) to evaluate the premature aging hypothesis. Regardless, this study indicates that short-term, working memory for visuospatial information is impaired in alcoholics. This finding also has implications for the issue of long-term memory impairment in alcoholism, given cognitive neuroscientific suggestions of a neuroanatomical link between short- and long-term memory functions (e.g., Gabrieli et al., 1996). Long-term memory for visuospatial information may thus result to some extent from impaired visuospatial working memory, as well as impaired visuospatial processing.

MUSICAL, FACIAL, AND EMOTIONAL COGNITION

Besides spatial cognition, other functions under control of the right hemisphere would be expected to be disrupted according to the right-hemisphere hypothesis of alcoholism. Among the functions with strong right-hemisphere involvement are musical, facial, and affective cognition. Note that while spatial cognition may be related to configural (or global) analysis of faces (Tanaka & Farah, 1993), spatial ability (such as that measured by mental rotation) and emotion are not related (Crucian & Berenbaum, 1998).

As described earlier for music, Ellis (1990) found that dichotically presented tonal patterns were processed similarly by alcoholics and controls but not by patients with right-hemisphere lesions. By contrast, in another study of dichotic perception of melodies and words, Drake et al. (1990) found that alcoholic men did show evidence of right-hemisphere dysfunction: They had a significantly smaller left-ear superiority for melodies and a significantly larger right-ear superiority for words than controls.

Faces are another stimulus material that is dominated by right-hemisphere processing. Moreover, convergent findings in cognitive neuroscience indicate that right-hemisphere specialization for face stimuli takes place in low-level visual perceptual and higher-order semantic and other cognitive systems (e.g., Buckner, 1996; Damasio, Grabowski, Tranel, Hichwa, & Damasio, 1996; Puce, Allison, Asgari, Gore, & McCarthy, 1996). Thus, nearly any task with face stimuli should probe right-hemisphere dominant brain functions, making faces an especially crucial material for testing the right-hemisphere hypothesis of alcoholism and aging. Since cognitive neuroscientific evidence, however, implicates the right posterior ventral region in face perception (Puce et al., 1996), and there is a dearth of evidence for alcoholic brain damage specific to this region, impaired performance by alcoholics is unlikely on tasks that primarily tap early perceptual processing of faces in the posterior ventral region.

It is thus important that alcoholic performance on tasks with face stimuli have typically been assessed using higher-order cognitive tasks assessing explicit memory or emotion (e.g., Cermak et al., 1989; Oscar-Berman, Hancock, Mildworf, & Hutner, 1990). For example, recent studies indicate that alcoholics are impaired at learning to attach names to the faces of unfamiliar people, a kind of cued recall task (Beatty et al., 1995; Tivis, Beatty, Nixon, & Parsons, 1995). On face recognition tasks, however, alcoholic and control performance differs in some studies but not others. While alcoholic Korsakoff patients, who have long-term explicit memory impairments (for recent evidence see Oscar-Berman & Pulaski, 1997), are deficient at perceiving and remembering the emotional information conveyed by faces, non-Korsakoff alcoholics are not (Oscar-Berman et al., 1990). Elderly individuals, however, regardless of alcohol history, perceived and remembered fewer emotional expressions in the faces than younger people (Oscar-Berman et al., 1990). Thus, neither the right-hemisphere nor the premature aging hypotheses of alcoholism was supported. In contrast, another study found that alcoholics correctly recognize fewer inverted faces than nonalcoholic controls (Nixon et al., 1996). Inverted faces, however, are thought be processed by posterior brain areas involved in object perception rather than those critical for face perception; only upright faces benefit from processing in brain areas specialized for face perception (Farah, Wilson, Drain, & Tanaka, 1995). Thus, the impairment by alcoholics on recognition of inverted but not upright faces, suggests that the processing of objects, rather than face processing *per se*, may be impaired in alcoholism, and processing differences between upright versus misoriented face images probably are responsible for the poor memory. However, this study did not find the classic face inversion effect in the control group (where turning an image upside-down impairs face identification disproportionately more than for other objects) (Diamond & Carey, 1986); hence, further research is needed.

Besides functional and neuroanatomical considerations, some of the inconsistency in the results from alcoholics can be explained by affective differences among research populations. For example, when affective properties (e.g., anxiety) were controlled, observed group effects on face recognition and other tasks, including visuospatial ones, were reduced or eliminated (Nixon et al., 1996). Therefore, at least some of the impaired performance of alcoholics on face recognition accuracy and response time may reflect affective characteristics, such as abnormal levels of anxiety, that often accompany alcoholism (Oscar-Berman, 1992; Oscar-Berman, 1998). For that reason, a comprehensive understanding of changes in emotional perception is a fruitful area of research, one that has largely been neglected. Further, the topic of emotional abnormalities in alcoholism and aging is important not just from the standpoint of contributions to cognitive functions (such as perceptual and attentional skills), but also because of the role of the right hemisphere in emotion.

Emotional abnormalities, such as those known to accompany alcoholism (McGue, Slutske, Taylor, & Iacono, 1997; Oscar-Berman, 1992; Oscar-Berman et al., 1990), result from lesions in multiple brain systems (Borod, 1993; Gainotti, Caltagirone, & Zocolotti, 1993; Heller, Nitschke, & Miller, 1998). Modular models of emotion combine concepts from lateral dominance with ideas about cortical-subcortical interactions (Borod, 1993). Many brain centers act to take in emotional cues, evaluate them and execute appropriate reactions. Nonetheless, the right hemisphere's role in emotional functions generally is more relevant than the left's, and the right hemisphere (especially in the right frontal lobe) is more relevant for processing negative emotions than for positive emotions (for reviews, see Borod, 1993; Gainotti et al., 1993). Therefore, tasks that measure emotional functions (especially tasks that include stimuli with a negative valence) can be used to tap right-hemisphere abilities. If alcoholics have deficient right-hemisphere function, they should have more difficulty perceiving emotional materials than non-emotional materials. Moreover, among the emotional materials, alcoholics should have more difficulty perceiving negative than positive emotional stimuli. Likewise, if alcoholism interacts with aging, then deficits should be most pronounced in older alcoholics (compared with their nonalcoholic peers).

In a study of emotional functions in alcoholics in our laboratory, a visual backward-masking and perceptual laterality paradigm was used to assess emotional processing abilities in detoxified alcoholics compared to nonalcoholic controls ages 30 years to 69 years (Hunter & Oscar-Berman, 1996). Emotional and non-emotional words were presented to the left or right VFs, followed by a visual masking stimulus. The research participants were asked to judge the emotional valence of each word (positive, negative, or neutral) and to respond verbally or manually (button presses). The dependent measure was the critical interstimulus interval needed to escape the backward-masking effect. The alcoholics showed a significant right VF (left-hemisphere) advantage in both response modes, whereas the controls did not. Furthermore, older alcoholics showed a selective impairment in processing negative words. Thus, when emotional materials were used, the findings supported the right-hemisphere model of alcoholism, as well as the increased vulnerability version of the premature aging hypothesis.

SUMMARY AND CONCLUSIONS

The right and left halves of the brain process sensory input and motor information differently. While the left hemisphere has a dominant role in linguistic behavior and the right hemisphere plays a dominant role in spatial cognition, the two hemispheres are complementary in their processing modes depending upon context and task demands. The left hemisphere plays a special role in processing piecemeal information analytically and sequentially, and the right hemisphere plays a special role in integrating information holistically. A common observation in work with alcoholics and with normal aging individuals is that both groups show lower scores on Performance IQ subtests (containing many visuospatial tasks) than on Verbal IQ subtests. From these observations, several hypotheses have emerged: (1) alcoholism may affect right-hemispheric functions more than left-hemispheric functions; (2) aging may affect right-hemispheric functions more than left-hemispheric functions; and (3) alcoholism may accelerate normal chronological aging. Research on cognitive capabilities and differences between the two cerebral hemispheres in alcoholics and in nonalcoholic aging individuals has provided limited support for the *premature aging* hypothesis and even less consistent support for the *right-hemisphere* hypothesis.

Since distinct functions and multiple brain areas can underlie different visuospatial tasks, broadly-defined neurobehavioral alterations can occur from injury to only a subset of visuospatial functions. Cognitive neuroscientific research has made notable progress in recent years with the advent of new functional brain imaging and sensing techniques and improvements to traditional approaches toward defining the functional contribution of specific brain systems to human behavior. These findings with populations of neurologically intact and impaired nonalcoholics, coupled with the neuroanatomical, neuropsychological, and cognitive neuroscientific studies of alcoholic and aged individuals, have provided additional means for more precisely testing the right-hemisphere hypothesis and the premature aging hypothesis. To date, the increased-vulnerability model of the premature aging hypothesis has received more support from imaging research than from neurobehavioral research. However, conclusive support still has not been forthcoming for either hypothesis. Nonetheless, with the new techniques available, we anticipate a successful future in understanding the ways the cerebral hemispheres act to integrate and complement their functions, as well as a similar leap in progress at pinpointing precisely the neurobehavioral consequences of long-term chronic alcoholism, normal chronological aging, and the synergism of alcoholism and aging.

AKNOWLEDGMENTS

The writing of this report was supported by NIAAA Grants R37-AA07112 and K05-AA00219 and by funds from the Medical Research Service of the US Department of Veterans Affairs.

REFERENCES

Adams, K. M., Gilman, S., Johnson Greene, D., Koeppe, R. A., Junck, L., Kluin, K. J., Martorello, S., Johnson, M. J., Heumann, M., & Hill, E. (1998). The significance of family history status in relation to neuropsychological test performance and cerebral glucose metabolism studied with positron emission tomography in older alcoholic patients. *Alcoholism-Clinical and Experimental Research*, *22* (1), 105-110.

Adams, K. M., Gilman, S., Koeppe, R. A., Kluin, K. J., Brunberg, J. A., Dede, D., Berent, S., & Kroll, P. D. (1993). Neuropsychological deficits are correlated with frontal hypometabolism in positron emission tomography studies of older alcoholic patients. *Alcoholism: Clinical and Experimental Research*, *17* (2), 205-210.

Akshoomoff, N. A., Delis, D. C., & Haist, F. (1993). Age-related changes in memory for visual hierarchical stimuli. *Developmental Neuropsychology*, *9* (3), 259-269.

Akshoomoff, N. A., Delis, D. C., & Kiefner, M. G. (1989). Block constructions of chronic alcoholic and unilateral brain-damaged patients: A test of the right hemisphere vulnerability hypothesis of alcoholism. *Archives of Clinical Neuropsychology*, *4* (3), 275-281.

Allan, K. & Rugg, M. D. (1997). An event-related potential study of explicit memory on tests of cued recall and recognition. *Neuropsychologia*, *35* (4), 387-397.

Allison, T., McCarthy, G., Nobre, A., Puce, A., & Belger, A. (1994). Human extrastriate visual cortex and the perception of faces, words, numbers, and colors. *Cerebral Cortex*, *4* (5), 544-554.

Banich, M. T. & Heller, W. (1998). Evolving perspectives on lateralization of function. *Current Directions in Psychological Science*, *7* (1), 1-37.

Bates, M. E. & Convit, A. (in press). Neuropsychology and neuroimaging of alcohol and illicit drug abuse. In A. Calev (Ed.), *Neuropsychological functions in psychiatric disorders*. Washington, D.C.: American Psychiatric Press.

Beatty, W. W., Blanco, C. R., Hames, K. A., & Nixon, S. J. (1997). Spatial cognition in alcoholics: Influence of concurrent abuse of other drugs. *Drug and Alcohol Dependence*, *44*, 167-174.

Beatty, W. W., Hames, K. A., Blanco, C. R., Nixon, S. J., & Tivis, R. (1996). Visuospatial perception, construction and memory in alcoholism. *Journal of Studies on Alcohol*, *57* (2), 136-143.

Beatty, W. W., Katzung, V. M., Moreland, V. J., & Nixon, S. J. (1995). Neuropsychological performance of recently abstinent alcoholics and cocaine abusers. *Drug and Alcohol Dependence*, *37*, 247-253.

Belzunegui, T., Insausi, R., Ibanez, J., & Gonzalo, L. M. (1995). Effect of chronic alcoholism on neuronal population in the mammillary body and the anterior thalamic complex of man. *Histology and Histopathology*, *10* (3), 633-638.

Borod, J. C. (1993). Cerebral mechanisms underlying facial, prosodic, and lexical emotional expression: A review of neuropsychological studies and methodological issues. *Neuropsychology*, *7*, 445-463.

Bowden, S. C. & McCarter, R. J. (1993). Spatial memory in alcohol-dependent subjects: Using a push-button maze to test the principle of equiavailability. *Brain and Cognition*, *22* (1), 51-62.

Brown, H. D. & Kosslyn, S. M. (1995). Hemispheric differences in visual object processing: Structural versus allocation theories. In Davidson, R.J. & Hugdahl, K (Eds.), *Brain asymmetry* (pp. 77-97). Cambridge, MA,: MIT Press.

Buckner, R. L. (1996). Beyond HERA: Contributions of specific prefrontal brain areas to long-term memory retrieval. *Psychonomic Bulletin and Review*, *3* (2), 149-158.

Cermak, L. S., Verfaellie, M., Letourneau, L., Blackford, S., Weiss, S., & Numan, B. (1989). Verbal and nonverbal right hemisphere processing by chronic alcoholics. *Alcoholism: Clinical and Experimental Research*, *13* (5), 611-616.

Chase, T. N., Fedio, P., Foster, N. L., & Al, E. (1984). Wechsler Adult Intelligence Scale performance. Cortical localization by fluorodeoxyglucose F18-positron emission tomography. *Archives of Neurology*, *41*, 1244-1247.

Ciesielski, K. T., Waldorf, A. V., & Jung, R. E., Jr. (1995). Anterior brain deficits in chronic alcoholism. Cause or effect? *Journal of Nervous and Mental Disorders*, *183* (12), 756-761.

Cohen, H. L., Porjesz, B., Begleiter, H., & Wang, W. (1997). Neurophysiological correlates of response production and inhibition in alcoholics. *Alcoholism: Clinical and Experimental Research*, *21* (8), 1398-1406.

Corballis, M. C. & Sergent, J. (1989). Hemispheric specialization for mental rotation. *Cortex*, *25* (1), 15-25.

Courville, C. B. (1966). *Effects of alcohol on the nervous system of man*. Los Angeles: San Lucas Press.

Craik, F. I. M. & Jennings, J. M. (1992). Human memory. In F. I. M. Craik & T. A. Salthouse (Eds.), *The handbook of aging and cognition* (pp. 51-110). Hillsdale, NJ: Lawrence Erlbaum Associates, Inc.

Crucian, G. P. & Berenbaum, S. A. (1998). Sex differences in right hemisphere tasks. *Brain and Cognition, 36*, 377-389.

D'Esposito, M., Detre, J. A., Aguirre, G. K., Stallcup, M., Alsop, D. C., Tippet, L. J., & Farah, M. J. (1997). A functional MRI study of mental image generation. *Neuropsychologia, 35* (5), 725-730.

Damasio, H., Grabowski, T. J., Tranel, D., Hichwa, R. D., & Damasio, A. R. (1996). A neural basis for lexical retrieval. *Nature, 380* (6574), 499-505.

Davila, M. D., Shear, P. K., Lane, B., Sullivan, E. V., & Pfefferbaum, A. (1994). Mammillary body and cerebellar shrinkage in chronic alcoholics: An MRI and neuropsychological study. *Neuropsychology, 8*, 433-444.

Di Sclafani, V., Ezekiel, F., Meyerhoff, D. J., MacKay, S., Dillon, W. P., Weiner, M. W., & Fein, G. (1995). Brain atrophy and cognitive function in older abstinent alcoholic men. *Alcoholism: Clinical and Experimental Research, 19* (5), 1121-1126.

Diamond, R. & Carey, S. (1986). Why faces are and are not special: An effect of expertise. *Journal of Experimental Psychology: General, 115*, 107-117.

Ditunno, P. L. & Mann, V. A. (1990). Right hemisphere specialization for mental rotation in normals and brain damaged subjects. *Cortex, 26* (2), 177-188.

Drake, A. I., Hannay, H. J., & Gam, J. (1990). Effects of chronic alcoholism on hemispheric functioning: An examination of gender differences for cognitive and dichotic listening tasks. *Journal of Clinical and Experimental Neuropsychology, 12* (5), 781-797.

Dror, I. E. & Kosslyn, S. M. (1994). Mental imagery and aging. *Psychology and Aging, 9* (1), 90-102.

Eichenbaum, H. (1997). Declarative memory: Insights from cognitive neurobiology. *Annual Review of Psychology, 48*, 547-572.

Ellis, R. J. (1990). Dichotic asymmetries in aging and alcoholic subjects. *Alcoholism, Clinical and Experimental Research, 14* (6), 863-871.

Ellis, R. J. & Oscar-Berman, M. (1989). Alcoholism, aging, and functional cerebral asymmetries. *Psychology Bulletin, 106*, 128-147.

Estruch, R., Nicolas, J. M., Salamero, M., Aragon, C., Sacanella, E., Fernandez-Sola, J., & Urbano-Marquez, A. (1997). Atrophy of the corpus callosum in chronic alcoholism. *Journal of Neurological Sciences, 146* (2), 145-151.

Evert, D. & Oscar-Berman, M. (submitted). Selective attentional processing and the right hemisphere: Effects of alcoholism and aging. *Neuropsychology*.

Evert, D. L. & Oscar-Berman, M. (1995). Alcohol-related cognitive impairments: An overview of how alcoholism may affect the workings of the brain. *Alcohol Health and Research World, 19* (2), 89-96.

Farah, M. J., Wilson, K. D., Drain, H. M., & Tanaka, J. R. (1995). The inverted face inversion effect in prosopagnosia: Evidence for mandatory, face-specific perceptual mechanisms. *Vision Research, 35* (14), 2089-2093.

Fink, G. R., Halligan, P. W., Marshall, J. C., Frith, C. D., Frackowiak, R. S. J., & Dolan, R. J. (1996). Where in the brain does visual attention select the forest and the trees? *Nature, 382* (6592), 626-628.

Fink, G. R., Marshall, J. C., Halligan, P. W., Frith, C. D., Frackowiak, R. S., & Dolan, R. J. (1997). Hemispheric specialization for global and local processing: The effect of stimulus category. *Proceedings of the Royal Society of London - Series B: Biological Sciences, 264* (1381), 487-494.

Friedrich, F. J., Egly, R., Rafal, R. D., & Beck, D. (1998). Spatial attention deficits in humans: a comparison of superior parietal and temporal-parietal junction lesions. *Neuropsychology, 12* (2), 193-207.

Gabrieli, J. D. E., Desmond, J. E., Demb, J. B., Wagner, A. D., Stone, M. V., Vaidya, C. J., Keane, M. M., & Glover, G. H. (1996). Functional magnetic resonance imaging of semantic memory processes in the frontal lobes. *Psychological Science, 7* (5), 278-283.

Gainotti, G., Caltagirone, C., & Zocolotti, P. (1993). Left/right and cortical/subcortical dichotomies in the neuropsychological study of human emotions. *Cognition and Emotion, 7*, 71-93.

Garland, M. A., Parsons, O. A., & Nixon, S. J. (1993). Visual-spatial learning in nonalcoholic young adults with and those without a family history of alcoholism. *Journal of Studies on Alcohol, 54* (2), 219-224.

Gilman, S., Adams, K. M., Johnsongreene, D., Koeppe, R. A., Junck, L., Kluin, K. J., Martorello, S., Heumann, N., & Hill, E. (1996). Effects of disulfiram on positron emission tomography and neuropsychological studies in severe chronic alcoholism. *Alcoholism - Clinical and Experimental Research, 20* (8), 1456-1461.

Glenn, S. W. & Parsons, O. A. (1991). Effects of alcoholism and instructional conditions on speed/accuracy tradeoffs. *Alcoholism: Clinical and Experimental Research, 15* (4), 612-619.

Harding, A. J., Wong, A., Svoboda, M., Kril, J. J., & Halliday, G. M. (1997). Chronic alcohol consumption does not cause hippocampal neuron loss in humans. *Hippocampus, 7* (10), 78-87.

Harper, C. (1998). The neuropathology of alcohol-specific brain damage, or does alcohol damage the brain? *Journal of Neuropathology & Experimental Neurology, 57* (2), 101-110.

Heilman, K. M. & Valenstein, E. (1993). *Clinical Neuropsychology* (3rd ed.). New York: Oxford University Press.

Heinze, H. J., Hinrichs, H., Scholz, M., Burchert, W., & Mangun, G. R. (1998). Neural meachanisms of global and local processing: A combined PET and ERP study. *Journal of Cognitive Neuroscience, 10* (4), 485-498.

Heller, W., Nitschke, J. B., & Miller, G. A. (1998). Lateralization in emotion and emotional disorders. *Current Directions in Psychological Science, 7* (1), 26-32.

Herman, J. F. & Bruce, P. R. (1983). Adults' mental rotation of spatial information: Effects of age, sex and cerebral laterality. *Experimental Aging Research, 9* (2), 83-85.

Hutner, N. & Oscar Berman, M. (1996). Visual laterality patterns for the perception of emotional words in alcoholic and aging individuals. *Journal of Studies on Alcohol, 57* (2), 144-154.

Ivry, R. B. & Robertson, L. C. (1998). *The two sides of perception*. Cambridge, MA: MIT Press.

Jernigan, T. L., Butters, N., DiTraglia, G., Schafer, K., Smith, T., Irwin, M., Grant, I., Schuckit, M., & Cermak, L. S. (1991). Reduced cerebral grey matter observed in alcoholics using magnetic resonance imaging. *Alcoholism: Clinical and Experimental Research, 15* (3), 418-427.

Kaplan, E. (1988). A process approach to neuropsychological assessment. In T. Boll & B. K. Bryant (Eds.), *Clinical neuropsychology and brain function: Research, measurement, and practice* (pp. 129-167). Washington, D. C.: American Psychological Association.

Kaplan, E., Fein, D., Morris, R., & Delis, D. C. (1991). *WAIS-R as a neuropsychological instrument*. San Antonio, TX: The Psychological Corporation, Harcourt Brace Jovanovich, Inc.

Kaplan, E., Palmer, E. P., Weinstein, C., & Baker, E. (1981). *Block design: A brain-behavior based analysis*. Paper presented at the Annual European Meeting of the International Neuropsychological Society, Bergen, Norway.

Kopelman, M. D. (1995). The Korsakoff syndrome. *British Journal of Psychiatry, 166* (2), 154-173.

Kosslyn, S. M., DiGirolamo, G. J., Thompson, W. L., & Alpert, N. M. (1998). Mental rotation of objects versus hands: Neural mechanisms revealed by positron emission tomography. *Psychophysiology, 35* (2), 151-161.

Kramer, J. H., Blusewicz, M. J., Robertson, L. C., & Preston, K. (1989). Effects of chronic alcoholism on perception of hierarchical visual stimuli. *Alcoholism: Clinical and Experimental Research, 13* (2), 240-245.

Kril, J. J., Halliday, G. M., Svoboda, M. D., & Cartwright, H. (1997). The cerebral cortex is damaged in chronic alcoholics. *Neuroscience, 79* (4), 983-998.

Kwon, L. M., Rourke, S. B., & Grant, I. (1997). Intermanual differences on motor and psychomotor tests in alcoholics: No evidence for selective right-hemisphere dysfunction. *Perceptual and Motor Skills, 84* (2), 403-414.

Lamb, M. R. & Robertson, L. C. (1987). The effect of acute alcohol on attention and the processing of hierarchical patterns. *Alcoholism: Clinical and Experimental Research, 11*, 243-248.

Lezak, M. D. (1995). *Neuropsychological assessment* (3rd ed.). Oxford: Blackwell Scientific Publications.

Libon, D. J., Glosser, G., Malamut, B. L., Kaplan, E., Goldberg, E., Swenson, R., & Prouty Sands, L. (1994). Age, executive functions, and visuospatial functioning in healthy older adults. *Neuropsychology, 8* (1), 38-43.

Loverock, D. S. & Modigliani, V. (1995). Visual imagery and the brain: A review. *Journal of Mental Imagery, 19* (1-2), 91-132.

Martinez, A., Moses, P., Frank, L., Buxton, R., Wong, E., & Stiles, J. (1997). Hemispheric asymmetries in global and local processing: Evidence from fMRI. *Neuroreport, 8* (7), 1685-1689.

Mayes, A. R. (1995). Memory and amnesia. *Behavioural Brain Research, 66* (1-2), 29-36.

McGue, M., Slutske, W., Taylor, J., & Iacono, W. G. (1997). Personality and substance use disorders: Effects of gender and alcoholism subtype. *Alcoholism: Clinical and Experimental Research, 21* (3), 513-520.

Milberg, W. P., Hebben, N., & Kaplan, E. (1996). The Boston Process Approach to neuropsychological assessment. In I. Grant & K. M. Adams (Eds.), *Neuropsychological assessment of neuropsychiatric disorders* (2nd ed., pp. 58-80). New York: Oxford University Press.

Mishkin, M., Ungerleider, L. G., & Macko, K. A. (1983). Object vision and spatial vision: Two cortical pathways. *Trends in Neurosciences, 6* (10), 414-417.

Miyashita, Y. (1993). Inferior temporal cortex: Where visual perception meets memory. *Annual Review of Neuroscience, 16*, 245-263.

NIAAA. (1997). *Ninth special report to the US Congress on alcohol and health*. Bethesda, MD: NIAAA.

Nicholson, M. E., Andre, J. T., Tyrrell, R. A., Wang, M., & Leibowitz, H. W. (1995). Effects of moderate dose alcohol on visual contrast sensitivity for stationary and moving targets. *Journal of Studies on Alcohol, 56* (3), 261-266.

Nicolás, J. M., Catafau, A. M., Estruch, R., Lomeña, F. J., Salamero, M., Herranz, R., Monforte, R., Cardenal, C., & Urbano-Marquez, A. (1993). Regional cerebral blood flow-SPECT in chronic alcoholism: Relation to neuropsychological testing. *Journal of Nuclear Medicine, 34* (9), 1452-1459.

Nicolás, J. M., Estruch, R., Salamero, M., Orteu, N., Fernandez-Sola, J., Sacanella, E., & Urbano-Marquez, A. (1997). Brain impairment in well-nourished chronic alcoholics is related to ethanol intake. *Annals of Neurology, 41* (5), 590-598.

Nixon, S. J., Hallford, H. G., & Tivis, R. (1996). Neurocognitive function in alcoholic, schizophrenic, and dually diagnosed patients. *Psychiatry Research, 64*, 35-45.

Oscar-Berman, M. (1992). The contribution of emotional and motivational abnormalities to cognitive deficits in alcoholism and aging. In L. Squire & N. Butters (Eds.), *Neuropsychology of memory* (2nd ed., pp. 81-94). New York: Guilford Press.

Oscar-Berman, M. (1998). *Cognitive, behavioral, and structural deficits: Neuropsychological sequelae of chronic alcoholism*. National Institute on Alcohol Abuse and Alcoholism neuroscience and behavior portfolio review of issues related to vulnerability, National Institute on Alcohol Abuse and Alcoholism, Washington, D. C.

Oscar-Berman, M., Goodglass, H., & Cherlow, D. G. (1973). Perceptual laterality and iconic recognition of visual materials by Korsakoff patients and normal adults. *Journal of Comparative and Physiological Psychology, 82* (2), 316-321.

Oscar-Berman, M., Hancock, M., Mildworf, B., & Hutner, N. (1990). Emotional perception and memory in alcoholism and aging. *Alcoholism: Clinical and Experimental Research, 14* (3), 383-393.

Oscar-Berman, M. & Pulaski, J. L. (1997). Associative learning and recognition memory in alcoholic Korsakoff patients. *Neuropsychology, 11* (2), 282-289.

Paller, K. A., Kutas, M., & Mayes, A. R. (1987). Neural correlates of encoding in an incidental learning paradigm. *Electroencephalography and Clinical Neurophysiology, 67* (4), 360-371.

Paller, K. A., Kutas, M., & McIsaac, H. K. (1995). Monitoring conscious recollection via the electrical activity of the brain. *Psychological Science, 6* (2), 107-111.

Parsons, O. (1987). Neuropsychological consequences of alcohol abuse: Many questions-some answers. In O. Parsons, N. Butters, & P. Nathan (Eds.), *Neuropsychology of alcoholism* (pp. 153-175). New York: Guilford Press.

Parsons, O. A. & Nixon, S. J. (1993). Neurobehavioral sequelae of alcoholism. *Behavioral Neurology, 11* (1), 205-218.

Pfefferbaum, A., Lim, K. O., Desmond, J. E., & Sullivan, E. V. (1996). Thinning of the corpus callosum in older alcholic men: A magnetic resonance imaging study. *Alcoholism: Clinical and Experimental_Research, 20* (4), 752-757.

Pfefferbaum, A. & Rosenbloom, M. J. (1993). In vivo imaging of morphological brain alterations associated with alcoholism. In W. A. Hunt & S. J. Nixon (Eds.), *Alcohol-induced brain damage* (Vol. 22, pp. 71-87). Rockville, MD: USDHHS, National Institutes of Health.

Pfefferbaum, A., Sullivan, E. V., Mathalon, D. H., & Lim, K. O. (1997). Frontal lobe volume loss observed with magnetic resonance imaging in older chronic alcoholics. *Alcoholism: Clinical and Experimental Research, 21* (3), 521-529.

Pfefferbaum, A., Sullivan, E. V., Rosenbloom, M. J., Shear, P. K., Mathalon, D. H., & Lim, K. O. (1993). Increase in brain cerebrospinal fluid volume is greater in older than in younger alcoholic patients: a replication study and CT/MRI comparison. *Psychiatry Research, 50* (4), 257-274.

Polich, J. (1997). EEG and ERP assessment of normal aging. *Electroencephalography and Clinical Neurophysiology, 104* (3), 244-256.
Porjesz, B., Begleiter, H., Reich, T., VanEerdewegh, P., Edenberg, H. J., Foroud, T., Goate, A., Litke, A., Chorlian, D. B., Stimus, A., Rice, J., Blangero, J., Almasy, L., Sorbell, J., Bauer, L. O., Kuperman, S., O' Connor, S. J., & Rohrbaugh, J. (1998). Amplitude of visual P3 event-related potential as a phenotypic marker for a predisposition to alcoholism: Preliminary results from the COGA project. *Alcoholism: Clinical and Experimental Research, 22* (6), 1317-1323.
Post, R. B., Lott, L. A., Maddock, R. J., & Beede, J. I. (1996). An effect of alcohol on the distribution of spatial attention. *Journal of Studies on Alcohol, 57,* 260-266.
Puce, A., Allison, T., Asgari, M., Gore, J. C., & McCarthy, G. (1996). Differential sensitivity of human visual cortex to faces, letterstrings, and textures: A functional magnetic resonance imaging study. *Journal of Neuroscience, 16* (16), 5205-5215.
Reitan, R. M. & Davison, L. A. (Eds.). (1974). *Clinical neuropsychology: Current status and applications.* Washington, D. C.: V. H. Winston & Sons.
Robertson, L. C. & Delis, D. C. (1986). "Part-whole" processing in unilateral brain-damaged patients: Dysfunction of hierarchical organization. *Neuropsychologia, 24* (3), 363-370.
Robertson, L. C. & Lamb, M. R. (1991). Neuropsychological contributions to theories of part/whole organization. *Cognitive Psychology, 23* (2), 299-330.
Robertson, L. C., Lamb, M. R., & Knight, R. T. (1988). Effects of lesions of temporal-parietal junction on perceptual and attentional processing in humans. *Journal of Neuroscience, 8* (10), 3757-3769.
Robertson, L. C., Lamb, M. R., & Knight, R. T. (1991). Normal global-local analysis in patients with dorsolateral frontal lobe lesions. *Neuropsychologia, 29* (10), 959-967.
Robertson, L. C., Stillman, R., & Delis, D. C. (1985). The effect of alcohol abuse on perceptual reference frames. *Neuropsychologia, 23* (1), 69-76.
Roquelaure, Y., Le Gargasson, J. F., Kupper, S., Girre, C., Hispard, E., & Dally, S. (1995). Alcohol consumption and visual contrast sensitivity. *Alcohol and Alcoholism, 30* (5), 681-685.
Rourke, S. B. & Løberg, T. (1996). The neurobehavioral correlates of alcoholism. In I. Grant & S. J. Nixon (Eds.), *Neuropsychological assessment of neuropsychiatric disorders* (2nd ed., pp. 423-485). New York: Oxford University Press.
Schacter, D. L. & Buckner, R. L. (1998). Priming and the brain. *Neuron, 20* (2), 185-195.
Schendan, H. E. (1998). *The timecourse of activation of the neural operations and representations supporting visual object identification and memory.* Unpublished doctoral dissertation, University of California, San Diego, La Jolla, CA.
Schendan, H. E., Ganis, G., & Kutas, M. (1998). Neurophysiological evidence for visual perceptual categorization of words and faces within 150 ms. *Psychophysiology, 35,* 240-251.
Schlotterer, G., Moscovitch, M., & Crapper-McLachlan, D. (1984). Visual processing deficits as asessed by spatial frequency, contrast sensitivity and backward masking in normal ageing and Alzheimer's disease. *Brain, 107,* 309-325.
Shear, P. K., Sullivan, E. V., Lane, B., & Pfefferbaum, A. (1996). Mammillary body and cerebellar shrinkage in chronic alcoholics with and without amnesia. *Alcoholism: Clinical and Experimental Research, 20* (8), 1489-1495.
Sullivan, E. V., Deshmukh, A., Desmond, J. E., Shear, P. K., Lim, K. O., & Pfefferbaum, A. (1996). Volumetric MRI analysis of cerebellar hemispheres and vermis in chronic alcoholics: Relationship to ataxia (abs). *Journal of the International Neuropsychological Society, 2,* 34.
Sullivan, E. V., Marsh, L., Mathalon, D. H., Lim, K. O., & Pfefferbaum, A. (1995). Anterior hippocampal volume deficits in nonamnesic, aging chronic alcoholics. *Alcoholism: Clinical and Experimental Research, 19* (1), 110-122.
Sullivan, E. V., Mathalon, D. H., Lim, K. O., Marsh, L., & Pfefferbaum, A. (1998). Patterns of regional cortical dysmorphology distinguishing schizophrenia and chronic alcoholism. *Biological Psychiatry, 43* (2), 118-131.
Sullivan, E. V., Rosenbloom, M. J., & Pfefferbaum, A. (1998). *Brain vulnerability to alcoholism: Evidence from neuroimaging studies.* National Institute on Alcohol Abuse and Alcoholism neuroscience and behavior portfolio review of issues related to vulnerability, National Institute on Alcohol Abuse and Alcoholism, Washington, D. C.
Tanaka, J. W. & Farah, M. J. (1993). Parts and wholes in face recognition. *Quarterly Journal of Experimental Psychology: Human Experimental Psychology, 46A* (2), 225-245.
Tarter, R. E. (1975). Psychosocial deficit in chronic alcoholics: A review. *International Journal of Addition, 10,* 327-368.

Tivis, L. J. & Parsons, O. A. (1997). Assessment of prose recall performance in chronic alcoholics: Recall of essential versus detail propositions. *Journal of Clinical Psychology, 53* (3), 233-242.

Tivis, R., Beatty, W. W., Nixon, S. J., & Parsons, O. A. (1995). Patterns of cognitive impairment among alcoholics: Are there subtypes? *Alcoholism: Clinical and Experimental Research, 19* (2), 496-500.

Tsagareli, M. G. (1995). The interhemispheric functional organization of human visuo-spatial perception. *Neuroreport, 6* (6), 925-928.

Volkow, N. D., Hitzemann, R., Wang, G. J., Fowler, J. S., Burr, G., Pascani, K., Dewey, S. L., & Wolf, A. P. (1995). Monitoring the brain's response to alcohol with positron emission tomography. *Alcohol Health and Research World, 19*, 296-299.

Volkow, N. D., Wang, G. J., Overall, J. E., Hitzemann, R., Fowler, J. S., Pappas, N., Frecska, E., & Piscani, K. (1997). Regional brain metabolic response to lorazepam in alcoholics during early and late alcohol detoxification. *Alcoholism: Clinical and Experimental Research, 21* (7), 1278-1284.

Wang, G. J., Volkow, N. D., Roque, C. T., Cestaro, V. L., Hitzemann, R. J., Cantos, E. L., Levy, A. V., & Dhawan, A. P. (1993). Functional importance of ventricular enlargement and cortical atrophy in healthy subjects and alcoholics as assessed with PET, MR imaging, and neuropsychologic testing. *Radiology, 186* (1), 59-65.

Wechsler, D. (1981). *Wechsler Adult Intelligence Scale-Revised: Manual*. New York: The Psychological Corporation.

Wechsler, D. (1997). *WAIS-III and WMS-III Technical Manual* (3rd ed.). San Antonio, TX: Harcourt Brace & Company.

Wechsler, D. & Stone, C. P. (1945). *Wechsler Memory Scale*. New York: The Psychological Corporation.

Zhang, X. L., Begleiter, H., & Porjesz, B. (1997). Is working memory intact in alcoholics? An ERP study. *Psychiatry Research, 75* (2), 75-89.

COGNITIVE PERSPECTIVES ON HUMOR COMPREHENSION AFTER BRAIN INJURY

Hiram Brownell and Andrew Stringfellow

INTRODUCTION

All humans have the ability to appreciate humor; everyone can laugh and experience mirth. Indeed, humor itself is ubiquitous in human societies. In different forms, it is used in happy situations as well as in awkward and sad situations, and, accordingly, the social functions of humor are varied. The diverse character of humor appreciation makes it a promising but also challenging topic that can be addressed from a number of perspectives. In this chapter, we take a neuroscientific approach to understanding some major facets of humor and responses to it. Although an exhaustive treatment of this complex topic is obviously beyond the scope of any one paper, we discuss a few different lines of research that provide a foundation for a neurological account of humor appreciation. We begin with a brief review of some structural and psychological components of selected types of humor. We next identify different pathologies of humor appreciation and laughter. A sketch of a neurological framework is then used to summarize many features of humor appreciation and its dissolution as a result of brain injury. We, in addition, identify issues that invite closer examination as researchers attempt to understand humor appreciation as the sum of many parts.

OVERVIEW OF HUMOR

Humor appreciation has many effects on the organism, mainly beneficial. Initially, heart rate, blood pressure and circulation, respiration, muscle contraction, immune system activity, and electrochemical activity in the brain all increase; this stimulation period is followed by a refractory period where heart rate, blood pressure, and muscle tension decrease, while immune system activity continues at a higher rate (Fry, 1992; 1994). It may be surprising, but humor appreciation is not unique to humans. Other primates (chimpanzees, gorillas, and orangutans) also "laugh" (Fry, 1994; Provine, 1996). This suggests that some capacity for humor appreciation may have first appeared over six million years ago, before the respective evolutionary paths diverged (Fry, 1994). In humans, however, the capacity for humor has certainly evolved far beyond that of the other primates who only laugh in response to tickling. And humor and humor appreciation certainly occupy essential roles in human social interaction.

STRUCTURAL AND SITUATIONAL COMPONENTS OF HUMOR

A host of reviews (e.g., Forabosco, 1992; Hillson & Martin, 1994; Katz, 1993; McGhee, Ruch, & Hehl, 1990; Ruch & Rath, 1993; Staley & Derks, 1995, among many others) discuss the same two basic ingredients for humor: *incongruity* and *resolution*. Incongruity is typically defined as a discrepancy between expectation and experience. Resolution is defined as making sense of the expectations altered by incongruity, for example, inferring how the punch line in fact fits with the body of a joke. It has been suggested (Nerhardt, 1976, as cited in Katz, 1993) that incongruity without any obvious resolution can lead to an experience of humor. For example, when a person lifts a series of weights and then lifts a weight that is much lighter or heavier than those preceding, the usual response is laughter or smiling, which are taken as indicators of humor appreciation. Thus, a person can, in some settings, experience humor in the absence of a clearly defined resolution component. However, most reviews, such as those cited above, stress the importance of both incongruity and resolution for something to be found humorous. The position taken in this chapter is to examine the components that often contribute to humor comprehension rather than to argue for the absolute necessity of any one component such as resolution, especially because the neuropsychological literature on humor appreciation is based largely on the incongruity-resolution model.

A related caveat concerns the generalizability of the work done to date. Provine (1996) reported that among a corpus of over a thousand occurrences of naturally occurring laughter in conversation overheard in public places, more than 80% were in response to quips and remarks (e.g., "You don't have to drink, just buy us drinks" and "Do you date within the species?") rather than in response to formal, structured jokes or stories. However, the stimulus items in most studies of normal and pathological humor are structured jokes and cartoons; thus, the processes implicated in appreciating humor in experimental settings may not be entirely representative of the processes most often implicated in appreciating humor in natural settings. The generalizability of findings from structured stimulus items remains an open question.

In the context of a short story joke, a punch line is incongruous in that it differs in some relevant way from a listener's expectations. The punch line normally supports resolution to the degree that the listener can infer a logical fit between the punch line and the joke despite any incongruity. Consider the following example:

> A man went up to a lady in a crowded square. "Excuse me," he said. "Do you happen to have seen a policeman anywhere around here?" "I'm sorry," the woman answered, "but I haven't seen a sign of one." Then the man said, "All right, hurry up and give me your watch and pocketbook then."[1]

---

[1] The jokes used as examples in this paper and in the research cited were taken from a number of different sources and do not reflect the creative efforts of the authors.

A typical schema for dealing with a request for help finding a policeman centers on the requester's (the man) needing assistance of some kind, possibly for directions to some address. In this example, after the hearer (the woman) apologizes for not being able to satisfy the request for a policeman, the man would, canonically, be expected to thank the woman, or, perhaps, ask her for assistance. The punch line is incongruous in that the man introduces a whole new topic into the discussion: theft. The surprising command to hand over the watch and pocketbook can be integrated with the context by appreciating that the man's true goal was achieved by means of deception: He needed to find out whether or not a policeman was nearby. Never having wanted to make contact with an officer, the man assessed the potential for theft without raising the suspicions of the woman. Everything fits on this interpretation of the man as a psychologically sophisticated criminal.

Hillson and Martin (1994) offer an elegant discussion of incongruity and resolution in humor processing using the domains-interaction approach associated with metaphor research (e.g., Tourangeau & Sternberg, 1981). This work is noteworthy because it considers *degrees* of incongruity and resolution rather than just their presence or absence. Metaphors involve comparisons between two concepts drawn from disparate semantic domains such as "Sylvester Stallone is the Trans Am of actors." Once the initial discrepancy (or incongruity) is apprehended, problem solving is used to identify potential bases of similarity. An apt metaphor is one that forces a listener to bridge two very dissimilar domains and then appreciate the close equivalence between the two concepts once their initial discrepancy is acknowledged. Greater semantic distance or discrepancy between domains reflects greater incongruity: actors and cars are more different than, for example, actors and world leaders. The resolution component of humor corresponds to the similarity of the concepts to each other with respect to the position each occupies within its respective domain: Stallone is large and strong, and perhaps a little threatening, and the Trans Am car, made by Pontiac, is usually equipped with a large, strong engine and is advertised in a way to encourage a degree of threat, or *machismo*. Thus, the Trans Am and Sylvester Stallone can be found in roughly the same semantic space within their respective domains.

Hillson and Martin used nouns from six different domains in their study: actors, world leaders, birds, cars, foods, and newspapers/magazines. Participant ratings identified two semantic dimensions that reflected the amount of perceived difference between the domains from which the nouns were drawn: human-nonhuman, and a combination of beauty and speed. Actors and cars are dissimilar on the humanness dimension while actors and world leaders are not. Hillson and Martin also identified two semantic dimensions that were applied to exemplars in all domains and, as such, could be used to locate exemplars within their respective domains: size and evaluation. Cars and actors can be large or small and can be seen as positive or negative. When participants rated the funniness of stimuli ("Sylvester Stallone is the Trans Am of actors"), their humor ratings were positively related to the size of the between-domain semantic distance. That is, actors compared to vehicles were funnier than actors compared to world leaders. Additionally, ratings reflected the within-domain equivalence: Big actors (Stallone) compared to large cars (Trans Am) were funnier than big actors compared to small cars (Volkswagen beetle). However, this relationship only held when there was large between-domain discrepancy, resulting in an interaction between- and within-domain semantic distance. In sum, the degree of incongruity predicted whether something was funny or not funny; the degree of resolution possible predicted whether an incongruous combination was simply funny or funnier. This work provides empirical support for the importance of gradations of incongruity and resolution for rated funniness. Considerable research by others, particularly Ruch and his colleagues, has similarly supported the psychological reality of these two components of humor (Ruch, 1981; 1984; Ruch & Hehl, 1986b, all as cited in McGhee et al., 1990).

Another contributing factor to humor is content. Recently, Katz (1993) offered a useful analysis of what he terms *tendentious humor* (that is, humor including sexual, scatological, or disparaging content) and how variation in content fits within a larger view of humor. In his model, Katz focused on the increase in arousal level brought about by humorous stimuli. He posited that stimuli containing an incongruous element would produce a surfeit of stimulation: both the expected concept and the incongruous concept would be simultaneously activated to varying extents. This activation would sum, producing excess arousal in the organism that could be interpreted as a sensation of humor appreciation or amusement. In the absence of resolution, incongruity alone can produce the arousal necessary for the appreciation of a humorous stimulus. (However, as Katz states, incongruity in and of itself is not necessarily funny: no matter how surprising, finding that one's car has been towed is not funny due to the negative emotion associated with the towing.) Katz suggested that tendentious content also affects the arousal level of the perceiver: aggressive or taboo content can boost arousal, just as does perceived incongruity. Taboo content, perhaps due to its exciting, aggressive, or dangerous nature, could raise the background level of arousal in the organism. Thus, less incongruity would be required from a stimulus to cross the arousal threshold necessary for the sensation of amusement.

Another aspect of content that affects appreciation concerns the identity of any victims of the humorous situation. The role of a joke's victim is complex in that identification with the victim can alter the perceived humorousness of a stimulus. ("Tragedy is when I cut my finger; comedy is when you walk into an open sewer and die," attributed to Mel Brooks, as cited in Larson, 1989.) The audience may experience a higher arousal level when a standard victim is introduced. However, casting someone or something as an object of derision may receive less-than-universal cultural acceptance: which joke features work to influence humorousness will be tied to one's group identity. For example, many Americans today do not identify closely with Bill Clinton or Newt Gingrich. Upon hearing an aggressive joke with Clinton or Gingrich as the victim, the aggressive content will likely facilitate humorousness by raising a listener's arousal level. If a listener, perhaps a member of the Clinton or Gingrich families, identifies with the victim, no facilitation will be experienced. Similarly, women rate jokes with aggressive sexual content less funny if the victim is female, whereas men rate jokes with aggressive sexual content less funny if the victim is male (Mundorf et al., 1988).

The setting in which one encounters humor will also affect the experience, in particular because humor is, in large a measure, a social phenomenon. For most people, the act of attending a night club to hear a comedian will lower their threshold for what is worth laughing at because they are primed for humor. And, accordingly, attending a funeral would be expected to raise the threshold for humor. Olson and Roese (1995) compared average funniness ratings to a humorous monologue from a control group and a group of participants who had been informed that the laboratory setting tended to inhibit laughter. The groups displayed equivalent amounts of mirth during testing, but the group warned about inhibition associated with laboratory settings rated the monologue as significantly funnier than the control group. Laughter is also contagious. One truly bizarre report (Black, 1982, as cited in Shaibani et al., 1994; see also Provine, 1996) describes an epidemic of contagious, hysterical laughter that affected girls and women in East Africa; the fits of laughing spread first among adolescent girls at a school, then to their mothers, and then to different villages. Some victims required hospitalization for exhaustion. Laugh tracks, which are used to convince a home audience that the material in a situation comedy is funny, seem to work (e.g., Martin & Gray, 1996; see also Provine, 1996, for discussion) though individual differences such as a listener's degree of self awareness can have an impact (e.g., Porterfield et al., 1988). Even a laugh box purchased at a novelty store can elicit laughter or at least a smile from most people (Provine, 1996).

Finally, and importantly, there are cultural frames for jokes. A person's awareness that an utterance is intended to be funny will influence his or her appreciation of humor. There are, for example, culturally accepted joke signs: "Knock, knock...," "A dog walks into a bar and orders a martini...," and "There were three (fill in the blank) seated together on an airplane...." A person will experience a higher level of arousal, or perhaps a lowered threshold for amusement, upon hearing a familiar joke setup. There are, then, several ways to alter one's threshold for interpreting an utterance or event as humorous.

In summary, some frames (settings, victims, standard setups, etc.) will be potent enough to guarantee that at least some listeners find humor; others will be sufficiently offensive to destroy any humor for most people; and, finally, many less extreme settings will serve to enhance or detract from the success of the core joke for a majority of listeners. Thus, the experience of humor can be facilitated or inhibited by inclusion of types of content or linguistic frames, quite apart from the amount of incongruity or resolution.

PERSONALITY VARIABLES RELATED TO HUMOR APPRECIATION

As suggested above in the context of the effectiveness of laugh tracks, individual differences can provide much insight into humor comprehension. In particular, Ruch and his colleagues have documented in several cultures (e.g., Forabosco & Ruch, 1994; Ruch & Hehl, 1993; Ruch, McGhee, & Hehl, 1990) that personality traits are linked to preferences in humor. For example, Ruch and Hehl (1993) reported a positive correlation between liking humor that allows complete resolution to a joke and a need for order. Other studies suggest that conservatism, or an intolerance for ambiguity, is negatively correlated with liking nonsense humor (humor that offers incongruity without complete resolution). A sensation-seeking approach to life, on the other hand, is positively correlated to liking nonsense humor. McGhee et al. (1990) incorporated this body of work into a developmental model of humor. In brief, while there is a consistent preference for resolution, the degree of preference changes over the life span. For example, from 14 years old to 66 years old (the range measured in the Ruch et al., 1990 study), increasing age was correlated with increasing conservatism and an increasing fondness (higher average funniness ratings) of humor that allowed complete resolution, and increasing age is associated (in relative terms) with decreasing fondness for nonsense humor.

INDICES OF HUMOR APPRECIATION

A subjective experience of humor can be measured in a variety of ways with potentially important differences. The most common dependent variable in the studies cited above is a subjective rating of funniness in which a participant assigns a stimulus an appropriate value on a single dimension. Worth noting is that a single measure such as a funniness rating may or may not reflect the complexity of a person's psychological experience. Ruch and Rath (1993), for example, recorded people's responses to three sets of stimuli that represented, respectively, incongruity-resolution humor, nonsense humor, and sexual humor. Participants' rated the items along several scales such as (translated from German) *tastelessness*, *funniness*, and *simplicity*, and they rated their own feeling states along other scales such as *exhilaration, boredom,* and *anger*. A single positive evaluation dimension emerged from factor analysis of all scales and all types of stimuli. This positive factor was labeled *funniness/exhilaration* by Ruch and Rath and loaded on individual scales such as *funniness* and *exhilaration*. The positive dimension corresponds well to intuitive notions of what high values on a joke funniness scale could mean in psychological terms: A funny joke leaves a listener feeling exhilarated and amused. Ruch and Rath also identified two negative dimensions; one reflected a negative emotional response to an item and was labeled *offensive/indignation*. This factor was based on the *tastelessness* and *anger* scales, among others, and was not correlated with the positive dimension. The other negative dimension reflected intellectual dissatisfaction and was labeled *simple/boredom*. It was based on, among others, the *simplicity* and *boredom* scales. This dimension demonstrated a reliable negative correlation with exhilaration. Specifically, as exhilaration increased, boredom decreased. There are, then, different reasons why a listener might not enjoy a joke or cartoon and give it a low funniness rating: it may be unsurprising, or it may be offensive.

Though not used as often in empirical research as a measure of a person's response to a joke, laughter, of course, is universal among humans and, intuitively, provides an appealing metric for amusement. (See Provine, 1996, for a list of laughter features that make identification easy.) One cautionary note is the weakness of the link between laughter together with other overt responses such as smiling and the more commonly used funniness ratings. LaPointe, Katz, and Kraemer (1995), for example, examined funniness ratings and spontaneous mirth responses in groups of left-hemisphere-damaged aphasic (LHD) patients and non-brain-damaged controls and found only moderate correlations ($r = 0.32$ for LHD and $r = 0.37$ for controls). Although the mirth responses were recorded on a first presentation of items and the funniness ratings on a second exposure to the same items, the point remains that a person's spontaneous laughter or smiling (i.e., mirth) may diverge from ratings obtained as part of a laboratory procedure, suggesting that different measures of humor can reflect different components of the experience.

PATHOLOGY RELATED TO HUMOR APPRECIATION

Humor appreciation is a complicated process, itself comprised of several processes that are also extremely complex and that each implicate diverse brain regions. For the purposes of this discussion, we will consider three processes necessarily intrinsic to humor appreciation. The order of presentation is not intended to reflect a processing sequence. Humor must be comprehended: A stimulus must be perceived and represented by the brain, and the incongruity (and resolution, if present) must be detected. This process will draw heavily on cerebral representations and prefrontal processing. Emotional valence must be assigned to the stimulus; this process must evaluate the type and degree of emotion evoked, involving somatic, cerebral, and limbic processing. Finally, a response congruent to the emotion experienced may be produced, typically laughter. Laughter is a motor process that involves the brainstem, the neocortex and its corticobulbar connections, as well as neocortical pathways.

Several different patient populations exhibit altered responses to humor stimuli. The deficits are diverse, reflecting, for example, cognitive problems in understanding some components of a stimulus, altered emotional responses, or exhibiting inappropriate expressions of amusement such as laughter. Each of the above systems may suffer dysfunction due to brain damage. Studies measuring participants' understanding of the cognitive or structural basis of humor are important but incomplete in that the emotional facets of humor responsiveness are not as often studied. Brain damage or dysfunction can produce emotional deficits, as in a lack of awareness of somatic and/or emotional states. Emotional lability, which we will not discuss, may also accompany brain damage or dysfunction: A patient may respond to a slight provocation with a disproportionate emotional outburst. Some neurological disorders can also produce laughter in the absence of humorous stimuli, which is termed *pathological laughter*. It should be noted that pathological laughter is generally considered distinct from the affective outbursts seen in the emotionally labile patient (Shaibani et al., 1994; Starkstein et al., 1995): pathological laughter is mood-incongruent – the victims are aware they are laughing, but report no feelings of mirth, nor can they name any stimulus in particular that is provoking the laughter – whereas the outbursts of the emotionally labile patient are mood-congruent – the expressed emotion typically mirrors the emotion experienced internally by the patient. With neither pathological laughter nor emotional lability is the behavior viewed by others as appropriate to the situation.

These impairments, because they are so different, contribute to a broad view of what portions of the brain are critical for the normal appreciation of humor. We present brief discussions of the resolution portion of verbal humor and a cognitive perspective on empathy and its role in humor, and we then proceed to a discussion of the roles of emotion and laughter.

DEFICITS IN RESOLUTION

Several previous reviews (e.g., Brownell & Gardner, 1988; Brownell et al., 1995; Brownell & Martino, 1998; Brownell et al., in press; Joanette et al., 1990; Molloy et al., 1990; Shammi, 1997) (see also Shammi & Stuss, 1999) have outlined the basic finding that brain damage can selectively impair a patient's appreciation of the resolution component of verbal humor. Bihrle et al. (1986) (see also Brownell et al., 1983) tested patients with unilateral right-hemisphere brain damage (RHD) resulting, for the most part, from middle cerebral artery lesions due to stroke. They presented RHD patients with incomplete jokes and asked them to select the correct, standard punch line from a set of alternatives. The alternatives varied with respect to which of two basic components – incongruity and resolution – were represented. For example, in what follows, the *straight forward* alternative represented a conventional continuation of the schema begun in the body of the joke and, as such, contained no incongruity. The various *nonsequitur* alternatives all contained incongruity; some were superficially related to the joke content but none provided a basis for satisfying resolution.

Stimulus
A man went up to a lady in a crowded square. "Excuse me," he said. "Do you happen to have seen a policeman anywhere around here?" "I'm sorry," the woman answered, "but I haven't seen a sign of one." Then the man said,...

Correct Punch line Containing Incongruity and Resolution
"All right, hurry up and give me your watch and pocketbook then."

Straightforward Alternative Containing Resolution but Not Incongruity
"Damn, I've been looking for a half hour and can't find one."

Neutral Nonsequitur Alternative Containing Incongruity but Not Resolution
"Baseball is my favorite sport."

Associated Nonsequitur Alternative Containing Incongruity but Not Resolution
"My uncle is a cop."

Humorous Nonsequitur Alternative Containing Incongruity but Not Resolution
"All of the wheels fell off of my car."

On each trial in the study, a patient saw the beginning of a joke and had to select the correct punch line from among the alternative types listed above.

One major result which has been replicated in different studies was that RHD patients were drawn to incongruous nonsequitur endings that provided no satisfying resolution. The interpretation offered was that the patients retained a sense of the structure of a joke as a narrative form in that they knew to pick an ending that was surprising in some way; however, the RHD patients were impaired in their ability to infer how a punch line might fit with the body of the joke. Thus, they were relatively unsuccessful at discriminating between the correct punch line which contained both incongruity and resolution, and nonsequitur endings, which contained incongruity but not resolution. Indeed, RHD patients have difficulty performing roughly analogous types of resolution inferences even when the items are not humorous (e.g., Brownell et al., 1986).

As illustrated above, the stimulus items used in the Bihrle et al. (1986) study included an alternative type labeled *humorous nonsequitur*. These were defined as having a slapstick element that could be considered funny in and of itself, purely on the basis of incongruity. In addition, though this was not discussed in the Bihrle et al. paper, the humorous nonsequitur endings were also aggressive in that the slapstick humor typically specified a victim. Other examples of humorous nonsequiturs used in the study include: "Then the tenant's pants fell down and his plaid boxer shorts were exposed," "The butcher takes a pie and throws it in her face," and "Slipping on a banana peel, he split his pants." RHD patients showed a particular inclination to select humorous nonsequiturs over correct punch lines. The marked difficulty choosing between correct punch lines and humorous nonsequiturs suggests, in addition to a difficulty with resolution, an awareness that slapstick is an accepted type of humor.

Bihrle et al. (1986) also developed a humor comprehension task based on four-frame captionless cartoons. The basic design was improved over that used in the verbal task. Alternative endings were drawn for each cartoon strip. In addition to the correct ending intended by the artist, there was a straightforward ending and various types of nonsequitur endings described above. The cartoon task also differed from the verbal task in other respects: On a single trial in the verbal task, a participant had to choose the correct punch line from among a set of five alternatives; on a single trial in the cartoon task, a participant had to make a binary choice between the correct punch line and just one incorrect alternative. Correct punch lines were paired with the different types of incorrect endings over different trials in the study. The results corroborated that RHD patients were impaired with the resolution component of humor in that they fared worse discriminating nonsequitur endings from correct endings than they did discriminating straightforward endings from correct endings. And the RHD patients performed worst when they had to choose between humorous nonsequitur endings and correct endings.

Another feature of the cartoon task was that its nonverbal nature allowed testing of patients who were aphasic as a result of unilateral left-hemisphere damage (LHD) resulting from a stroke, most often in the territory of the middle cerebral artery. The LHD patients showed a markedly different pattern of results: overall, they performed better than the RHD patients. More specifically, they performed worse in discriminating straightforward endings from correct endings, and they performed best in discriminating humorous nonsequitur endings from correct endings. LHD patients, apparently, were not at all drawn to the same elements of the stimuli as were the RHD patients. LHD patients may be particularly sensitive to the need for resolution in narrative. Another possible contributing factor is that LHD patients found the humorous nonsequiturs unpleasant due to their aggressive content. Gillikin and Derks (1991) reported that LHD patients objected to several aggressive stimulus items, whereas the RHD and the non-brain-damaged controls found those items funny. Although there are several factors that might contribute to

LHD patients' performances, the effects of left-hemisphere- and right-hemisphere-damage are very different. Additional support for the difference is provided by Shammi (1997) who has more recently tested groups of nonaphasic left prefrontal patients, right prefrontal patients, bilateral prefrontal patients, left posterior patients, and right posterior patients on an extensive battery of humor tasks. Shammi's general result is that the right prefrontal and bilateral prefrontal groups, but not the left prefrontal group, showed the general pattern of deficit described above (from Bihrle et al., 1986) for patients with RHD damage due to middle cerebral artery stroke. In particular, the right prefrontal group was drawn toward humorous nonsequitur endings and the bilateral prefrontal group was drawn toward all types of endings.

DEFICITS IN THEORY OF MIND

A new line of research has added another perspective on how right-hemisphere damage might impact humor comprehension: A disrupted *theory of mind*, or ability to attribute beliefs and intentions to other people in order to explain or predict their behavior, may limit RHD patients' performance on a number of tasks including some related to humor comprehension. Happé, Brownell, and Winner (1999) tested groups of RHD patients, LHD patients, and non-brain-damaged control participants on two types of humor: single-frame cartoons that *did* and *did not* require a sophisticated theory of mind in order to appreciate the humor fully. The humor in the theory of mind cartoons used in the study rested on one character's deception of another or on a single character's mistaken belief about something. (The short story joke presented above, though not used in the Happé et al. study, involves theory of mind in the form of one character's deception of another character.) In contrast, the humor of non-theory of mind cartoons was often based on physical impossibilities, such as a skier's ski tracks going around each side of a tree (as though the skier had simply split him-/herself in half in order to pass the tree). For each cartoon, the original was paired with an altered version that was changed to render the cartoon not funny. Participants were asked to select the correct member of each pair and to explain why their choice was funny. The general result was that RHD patients showed a selective deficit in interpreting cartoons based on theory of mind: The control participants and the LHD patients performed equally well on both item sets when selecting the humorous member of each pair whereas the RHD patients fared significantly worse on the theory of mind stimuli. Also, the RHD patients presented a similar deficit in the quality of their explanations of why a cartoon was funny (LHD patients were unable to provide free responses in the explanation condition). It is important to note, just as for RHD patients' impairments in resolution, similar impairments have been documented in other studies using ironic materials and also using nonhumorous materials. Winner et al. (1998), for example, reported that participants' ability to understand a type of theory of mind question (what one person thinks about another person's beliefs, which is a second order mental attribution) predicts their success discriminating deceptive lies from ironic comments.

Because RHD appears to disrupt a person's theory of mind and, presumably, related abilities, these patients perform poorly in a number of social settings. It is not entirely clear how much overlap exists between the impairment of resolution described in earlier papers and the theory of mind impairment outlined by Winner et al. and Happé et al. Both clearly represent cognitive sequelae of right-sided brain damage that limits patients' abilities to understand many instances of humor. One possible integration of the theory of mind and resolution deficits derives from differences between types of humor: Humor that rests on theory of mind (e.g., deception, trickery, and ignorance) is more likely to require resolution than is humor that does not involve mental states (e.g., physical humor, slapstick humor, and bizarre incongruity). If true, this speculation suggests that a portion of middle-aged and older RHD patients' theory of mind impairment may reflect a decreased ability to carry out resolution. On this view, the Happé et al. humor study fits well within the existing body of work on humor deficits.

CHANGES IN EMOTIONAL RESPONSIVENESS AND PERSONALITY

In comparison to the large body of work focused on participants' understanding of the cognitive or structural basis of humor, there has been relatively little research examining the emotional facets of humor responsiveness. When humor is appreciated, it is a positive emotional experience; this is distinct from when humor is understood, but not appreciated, as when a joke is either boring or offensive. Accordingly, a listener's mood might be expected to influence his or her evaluation of a joke's funniness, and/or a good joke could improve one's mood. Ruch & Rath (1993), for example, demonstrated a tight link between people's ratings of their own positive reactions to jokes and cartoons (e.g., feelings of amusement and exhilaration) and their evaluations of the stimuli themselves (e.g., funniness). While funniness ratings and outright laughing may not always correlate highly (e.g., LaPointe et al., 1994), emotional reactions to humorous stimuli, either positive or negative, play a major role in our experience of humor.

There is a rich literature documenting the role of the right hemisphere in mediating emotion (e.g., Banich, 1997; Kolb & Whishaw, 1996; Liotti & Tucker, 1995; Tucker & Frederick, 1989). More specifically, three hypotheses are offered. Many reports support the *valence hypothesis* that the right-hemisphere is more involved with negative emotion and the left hemisphere with positive emotion (e.g., Davidson, 1993; Robinson et al., 1984; Sackeim et al., 1982). Alternatively, a host of other studies favor the *right hemisphere hypothesis* that the right hemisphere is more involved with all emotional processing, regardless of valence (see Wittling & Roschmann, 1993, for one recent study supporting this position). Ross, Homan, and Buck (1994) integrate the two positions, suggesting that the right hemisphere supports both positive and negative primary emotions and that the left hemisphere at times inhibits the right hemisphere and is by itself capable of generating positive social emotions for social displays (e.g., Buck & Duffy, 1980, as cited by Ross et al., 1994).

Finally, Tucker and his colleagues (e.g., Liotti & Tucker, 1995) offer a different and thorough analysis of the laterality of emotion that emphasizes links between subcortical and cortical regions and includes evolutionary, cyto-architectural, and neurochemical considerations. One aspect of this overview of emotion is that the right hemisphere is intimately involved in positive emotions.

Lesions to the right cortical areas, or lesions that disconnect cortical from subcortical regions, work to disinhibit right subcortical structures, resulting in a nonchalant, hypomanic, or inappropriately positive affect. Lesions to left cortical areas, or lesions that disconnect cortical and subcortical regions, similarly disinhibit subcortical regions intimately involved in more negative emotion. More generally, Liotti and Tucker (1995) describe the neocortices in the two hemispheres as extensions of limbic structures, and hemispheric asymmetries as tied to differential elaborations of *ventral* and *dorsal* processing. The right-hemisphere (particularly the posterior parietal region) is closely connected with the cingulate gyrus and hippocampal structures. Functionally, the right-hemisphere has elaborated dorsal processing in that it coordinates spatial with hedonic processing, facilitates attention to emotionally significant events, and integrates arousal with holistic attention.

While there is inconsistency across the views expressed by different researchers working in this field, one generalization is secure: cortical and subcortical regions within the right hemisphere are heavily involved in mediated emotional responses. Less clear are the ways in which this apparent dominance for emotional processing relates directly to humor appreciation, though there are intriguing suggestions. One famous paper by Gainotti (1972) (see also Robinson et al., 1984, and Sackeim et al., 1982), for example, reported a higher incidence of an inappropriately positive demeanor (described as *nonchalance*) and inappropriate laughter following lesions to the right, or nondominant, hemisphere than to the left, or dominant, hemisphere. While there is not always a link between laughter and underlying experience of humor, as discussed below (e.g., Shaibani, Sabbagh, & Doody, 1994), Gillikin and Derks (1991) report that some RHD patients in their study, though no LHD patients, laughed inappropriately at their own explanations of unfunny stimuli in a humor test, which is consistent with other descriptions of RHD patients' behavior (e.g., Gardner et al., 1983). This heightened tendency to laugh may be conceptualized in different ways. If RHD leaves a person with a generally more positive mood state due to some disinhibition, he or she may not have to experience very much of an increase in exhilaration or amusement from a joke to start laughing. Alternatively, the laughter response can be considered as separate from the inner experience of amusement: An RHD patient may be no more amused than most people by a joke, but may have a *hair trigger* for initiating a mood-incongruent laughter response.

The impact of RHD damage on patients' mood cannot be the entire story. Gillikin and Derks, in the study cited above (1991), present relevant information. Participants in their study were assessed on a geriatric depression inventory before participation. There were no group differences, and the averages fell in the mild depression range. No individuals scored in the moderate or severe ranges. As part of the study, participants gave self-ratings for mood both before and after taking the humor evaluation test. The RHD patients were, on average, slightly lower than the LHD patients in self-rated mood before starting the test, though this group difference was not described as statistically reliable. The RHD patients produced approximately equal improvements in self-rated mood before and after completing the joke evaluation test. Thus, RHD due to stroke does not uniformly render patients happier as assessed by self-ratings. What remains is a complicated set of goals: gaining a better understanding of what precisely humor appreciation and mood measures tell us and exploring the links between mood, amusement, and expressions of mirth.

RHD patients' increased tendency to laugh may also reflect different preferences for humor. As suggested in the Bihrle et al. study (1986), RHD may render a person more appreciative of simple incongruity humor and relatively less appreciative of incongruity-resolution humor, which is the opposite pattern of preferences reported for middle-aged and older adults by Ruch et al. (1990). As a result, RHD patients may laugh at things that other adults don't find funny. We think this latter possibility is an important factor. As mentioned above, Ruch and Rath (1993) have outlined one positive dimension (funniness/exhilaration) and two negative dimensions (offensive/indignation and simple/boredom) to account for normal listeners' responses to humor. If brain damage curtails or changes a person's sense of what is boring or distasteful, that person may find some things funny that most others do not. Specifically, descriptions of RHD patients often report a lack of empathy, disinhibition, and a diminished appreciation of appropriate behavior in different contexts (e.g., Gardner, 1975; Gardner et al., 1983) (see Alexander, Benson, & Stuss, 1989 and McDonald, 1993, for a discussion of similar characteristics manifested by frontal patients). RHD patients, particularly right prefrontal patients as reported by Shammi (1997), may be less sensitive to who among their listeners might identify with a joke's victim. What is offensive for some may not be offensive for patients with significant amounts of damage to specific regions of the brain. Further, a lack of self-awareness and ability to self-monitor and inhibit may result in RHD patients' expressing enjoyment that most others would not dare admit. RHD patients may place less importance on the offensive aspects of a stimulus, which, perhaps, renders the presence of incongruity relatively more salient. By itself, the incongruity provides a more effective cue for RHD patients than it does for other listeners which is consistent with RHD patients' reduced ability to infer a resolution for jokes and cartoons (Bihrle et al., 1986; Brownell et al., 1986).

PATHOLOGICAL LAUGHTER

Spontaneous laughter is one, and arguably the only, universal indicator of humor appreciation. It occurs in natural settings and is a direct reflection of underlying amusement. Nonetheless, there is clearly a dissociation between underlying humor appreciation and laughter because, after all, people can find something quite funny without laughing. Further, people can produce non-spontaneous (e.g., polite) laughter; however, this type of laughter is measurably different in quality from spontaneous laughter (Provine, 1996). Spontaneous laughter is complex – it involves the contraction of fifteen facial muscles, changes in the respiration pattern, spasmodic contractions of skeletal muscles, tachycardia, and increased catecholamine production, among other actions (Fry, 1992). In spontaneous laughter, all of these components are mediated autonomically.

Many cases of pathological (spontaneous) laughter in the absence of perceived humorous stimuli have been reported; patients exhibiting pathological laughter have typically suffered lesions in the hypothalamus or the brainstem, regions regulating and controlling autonomic function. Cascino et al. (1993) (see also Dark, McGrath,

& Ron, 1996; Shaibani et al., 1994) review several cases of hypothalamic hamartoma linked to gelastic seizures, where laughter occurs as part of the seizures. Pathological laughter may also be observed as an indicator of a brainstem stroke (Wali, 1993) or tumor (Lal & Chandy, 1992). Kim (1997) reported three cases of pathological laughter following ischemic damage to the pons. Also, Doorenbos et al. (1993) reported a patient who exhibited a goal-directed intention tremor in his left arm and leg subsequent to a (unilateral) hemorrhage in the cerebellum. The patient would laugh with the onset of the tremor even though he was not experiencing amusement; he could control the laughter by controlling the tremor (for example, by grabbing his left arm).

The neocortex is connected to the brainstem via white matter pathways that form part of the internal capsule. Unsurprisingly, then, lesions that damage the internal capsule may also produce pathological laughter, perhaps releasing brainstem nuclei from neocortical modulation. Kim (1997) reports nine cases of pathological laughter following damage to the posterior limb of the internal capsule after a unilateral stroke (five cases involving the left hemisphere and four cases involving the right). Ceccaldi et al. (1994) report three cases of patients who exhibited pathological laughter in the absence of pathological crying subsequent to unilateral lesions in left (one case) or right (two cases) striatocapsular regions. The internal capsule is surrounded laterally by the basal ganglia; it should be noted that disinhibition or dismodulation of brainstem nuclei following damage to the basal ganglia may also be partially responsible for the pathologic laughter in patients (Grumet, 1989). In most of the above cases (both Kim, 1997 and Ceccaldi et al., 1994) the condition resolved after several months duration.

The presence of pathological laughter (and crying) is also associated with less-discrete lesions. Sufferers of Angelman's Syndrome, a chromosomal-deletion syndrome where brainstem damage is implicated, experience episodes of pathological laughter (Nirenberg, 1991). Such episodes begin in childhood and still occur in many adult sufferers (Laan et al., 1996; Nirenberg, 1991). Shaibani et al. (1994) report that demyelinating diseases, such as multiple sclerosis and amyotrophic lateral sclerosis, can result in pathological laughter and crying, and state that lesions in and around the third ventricle and lesions in the pontine region can lead to this disorder. Feinstein et al. (1997) confirmed that nearly ten percent of multiple sclerosis patients did in fact suffer episodes of pathological laughter and/or crying and that these patients tended to be in later stages of the disease, presenting more subcortical damage. Starkstein et al. (1995) discuss pathological laughing and crying in substantial percentages of Alzheimer patients with extensive subcortical atrophy as well as with involvement of the internal capsule and hypothalamus. And Zeilig et al. (1996) found pathological laughter or mixed laughter and crying in five percent of closed head traumatic brain injury (TBI) patients. The TBI patients did not present any consistent location of damage, but they were on average more severely injured than those patients who did not manifest pathological laughter; this profile is not inconsistent with diffuse axonal damage (Zeilig et al., 1996) which would affect white matter pathways including the capsular regions.

The general picture that emerges is that the motoric components of laughing can be released or triggered by a neurological abnormality that is divorced from any psychological experience of amusement. What is left undefined is exactly how the cortical and subcortical regions normally function together to initiate laughter and, more generally, to explain the experience of finding something funny.

CONCLUSION

Humor is a wonderful facet of human existence. The complexity of humor suggests that it draws on a huge array of neurological structures and cognitive processes. As does almost every point in the following summary, evidence suggests participation of both cortical and subcortical structures within the right and left. hemispheres. Left-hemisphere structures are, of course, critical because so many common humor genres (e.g., short story jokes and quips) are linguistic, and, as pointed out by Liotti and Tucker (1995), the left-hemisphere certainly contributes to emotion. On balance, though, we think that the study of humor appreciation will reveal more about the right hemisphere and the many connections between cortical regions and limbic structures, including the orbital frontal regions.

A person has some varying degree of receptivity to humor. The neurology of mood as a stable personality trait or as a transient state is beyond our purview, but a person's readiness for amusement is critical to humor's success. The links between mood and humor in brain-damaged patients is an important factor that requires better understanding. Apart from mood, the listener probably relies on several cues to the nature or valence of a setting to increase or decrease the anticipation of amusement. If a speaker is laughing or smiling at his or her own joke he or she must be in a good mood, or at least trying to convey that impression. A speaker may also use prosody appropriate for humor. Finally, the speaker and listener should be together in a location suitable for humor. Right-hemisphere structures have been implicated for prosodic comprehension (e.g., Ross, 1981; Ross et al., 1994) and facial expression (e.g., Banich, 1997; Kolb & Whishaw, 1996), and there is some evidence that an intact right hemisphere is needed for good appreciation of the affective value of situations (e.g., Cicone, Wapner, & Gardner, 1980).

On encountering a stimulus, the listener evaluates it in terms of what was expected. By comparing what is expected with what occurs, the listener can detect incongruity and then decide whether or not it can be resolved. Incongruity detection, which involves the evaluation of novel events in the environment and matching representations of what was expected with what actually happened, implicates structures within the right hemisphere (e.g., Liotti & Tucker, 1995). The cognitive assessment of resolution requires participation of posterior cortical (e.g., Bihrle et al., 1986) and prefrontal structures (McDonald, 1993; Shammi, 1997). Outstanding goals include defining the role(s) of subdivisions within prefrontal areas of both hemispheres, evaluating the significance of the emotion resulting from perceived incongruity (surprise), and explaining how and where surprise combines with the cognitive product of resolution to produce humorousness.

Another issue is whether the arousal brought about by an intended joke (Katz, 1993) is interpreted either as amusing; offensive due perhaps to its aggressive, scatological, sexual, or gross content; or boring due to its simplicity/predictability (Ruch & Rath, 1993). Limbic structures and cortical association areas will figure prominently in marking some topics as not at all conducive to humor and others as pleasant and good fodder for fun and in marking some resolutions as intellectually enjoyable or boring.

Finally, if a joke, remark, or event of any sort is deemed sufficiently funny the motor sequences involved in smiling and perhaps laughing may be initiated. Brainstem nuclei and hypothalamic structures are intimately involved with mediating laughter and will complete a neural humor circuit. It is not yet clear what factors allow or disinhibit laughter as a response to successful humor. Variation in susceptibility to laughter may reflect degrees of a listener's ability (or desire) to use cortical structures to inhibit these sequences (Liotti & Tucker, 1995).

Humor appreciation as an area of inquiry within cognitive neuroscience demands and offers a great deal. As illustrated by the range of sources cited in this chapter, even a preliminary overview will require that researchers take into account different perspectives that range in scope from detailed descriptions of anatomical structures to statements about cognitive factors and extending even to consideration of cultural norms. Crossing disciplinary boundaries and levels of analysis in this way can only add to the sophistication of our efforts to understand cognition.

ACKNOWLEDGMENTS

This was a collaborative effort. Authors are listed alphabetically. Preparation of this chapter was supported by grants R01 NS27894 and P01 DC00102.

REFERENCES

Alexander, M. P., Benson, D. F., & Stuss, D. T. (1989). Frontal lobes and language. *Brain and Language, 37*, 656-691.

Banich, M. T. (1997). *Neuropsychology*. Boston: Houghton Mifflin.

Bihrle, A., Brownell, H., Powelson, J., & Gardner, H. (1986). Comprehension of humorous and nonhumorous materials by left- and right-brain-damaged patients. *Brain and Cognition, 5*, 399-411.

Brownell, H. H. & Gardner, H. (1988). Neuropsychological insights into humour. In J. Durant & J. Miller (Eds.), *Laughing matters: A serious look at humour* (pp. 17-34). London: Longman.

Brownell, H. H., Gardner, H., Prather, P., & Martino, G. (1995). Language, communication, and the right hemisphere. In H. S. Kirshner (Ed.), *Handbook of neurological speech and language disorders* (pp. 325-349). New York: Marcel Dekker.

Brownell, H. H., Michel, D., Powelson, J., & Gardner, H. (1983). Surprise but not coherence: Sensitivity to verbal humor in right-hemisphere patients. *Brain and Language, 18*, 20-27.

Brownell, H. H., Potter, H., Bihrle, A., & Gardner, H. (1986). Inference deficits in right brain-damaged patients. *Brain and Language, 27*, 310-321.

Brownell, H. & Martino, G. (1998). Deficits in inference and social cognition: The effects of right hemisphere brain damage on discourse. In M. Beeman & C. Chiarello (Eds.), *Right hemisphere language comprehension: Perspectives from cognitive neuroscience* (pp. 309-328). Mahwah, NJ: Erlbaum.

Brownell, H., Griffin, R., Winner, E., Friedman, O., & Happe, F. (in press). Cerebral lateralization and theory of mind. To appear in S. Baron-Cohen, H. Tager-Flusberg, & D. Cohen (Eds.), *Understanding other minds: Perspectives from autism and developmental cognitive neuroscience* (2nd ed.). Oxford: Oxford University Press.

Cascino, G. D., Andermann, F., Berkovic, S. F., Kuzniecky, R. I, Sharbrough, F. W., Keene, D. L., Bladin, P. F., Kelly, P. J., Olivier, A., & Feindel, W. (1993). Gelastic seizures and hypothalamic hamartomas: Evaluation of patients undergoing chronic intracranial EEG monitoring and outcome of surgical treatment. *Neurology, 43*, 747-750.

Ceccaldi, M., Poncet, M., Milandre, L., & Rouyer, C. (1994). Temporary forced laughter after unilateral strokes. *European Neurology, 34*, 36-39.

Cicone, M., Wapner, W., & Gardner, H. (1980). Sensitivity to emotional expressions and situations in organic patients. *Cortex*, *16*, 145-158.

Dark, F. L., McGrath, J. J., & Ron, M. A. (1996). Pathological laughing and crying. *Australian and New Zealand Journal of Psychiatry*, *30*, 472-479.

Davidson, R. J. (1993). Parsing affective space: Perspectives from neuropsychology and psychophysiology. *Neuropsychology*, *7*, 464-475.

Doorenbos, D. I., Haerer, A. F., Payment, M., & Clifton, E. R. (1993). Stimulus-specific pathological laughter: A case report with discrete unilateral localization. *Neurology*, *43*, 229-230.

Feinstein, A., Feinstein, K., Fray, T., & O'Connor, P. (1997). Prevalence and neurobehavioral correlates of pathological laughing and crying in multiple sclerosis. *Archives of Neurology*, *54*, 1116-1121.

Forabosco, G. (1992). Cognitive aspects of the humor process: The concept of incongruity. *Humor*, *5*, 45-68.

Forabosco, G. & Ruch, W. (1994). Sensation seeking, social attitudes and humor appreciation in Italy. *Personality and Individual Differences*, *16*, 515-528.

Fry, W. (1994). The biology of humor. *Humor*, *7*, 111-126.

Fry, W. F. (1992). The physiologic effects of humor, mirth, and laughter. *Journal of the American Medical Association*, *267*, 1857-1858.

Gainotti, G. (1972). Emotional behavior and hemispheric side of the lesion. *Cortex*, *8*, 41-55.

Gardner, H. (1974). *The shattered mind*. New York: Random House.

Gardner, H., Brownell, H. H., Wapner, W., & Michelow, D. (1983). Missing the point: The role of the right hemisphere in the processing of complex linguistic materials. In E. Perecman (Ed.), *Cognitive processes in the right hemisphere* (pp. 169-191). New York: Academic Press.

Gillikin, L. S. & Derks, P. L. (1991). Humor appreciation and mood in stroke patients. *Cognitive Rehabilitation*, *9*, 30-35.

Grumet, G. W. (1989). Laughter: Nature's epileptoid catharsis. *Psychological Reports*, *65*, 1059-1078.

Happé, F. G. E., Winner, E., & Brownell, H. (1998). The getting of wisdom: Theory of mind in old age. *Developmental Psychology*, *34*, 358-362.

Happé, F., Brownell, H., & Winner, E. (1999). Acquired 'theory of mind' impairments following right hemisphere stroke. *Cognition*, *70*, 211-240.

Hillson, T. & Martin, R. (1994). What's so funny about that: The domains-interaction approach as a model of incongruity and resolution in humor. *Motivation and Emotion*, *18*, 1-29.

Joanette, Y., Goulet, P., & Hannequin, D. (1990). *Right hemisphere and verbal communication*. New York: Springer-Verlag.

Katz, B. F. (1993). A neural resolution of the incongruity-resolution and incongruity theories of humour. *Connection Science*, *5*, 59-75.

Kim, J. S. (1997). Pathologic laughter after unilateral stroke. *Journal of the Neurological Sciences*, *148*, 121-125.

Kolb, B. J. & Whishaw, I. Q. (1996). *Fundamentals of human neuropsychology* (4th ed.). San Francisco: W. H. Freeman.

Laan, L. A. E. M., den Boer, A. T., Hennekam, R. C. M., Renier, W. O., & Brouwer, O. F. (1996). Angelman syndrome in adulthood. *American Journal of Medical Genetics*, *66*, 356-360.

Lal, A. P. & Chandy, M. J. (1992). Pathological laughter and brain stem glioma. *Journal of Neurology, Neurosurgery, and Psychiatry*, *55*, 628-629.

LaPointe, L. L., Katz, R. C., & Kraemer, I. (1985). The effects of stroke on appreciation of humor. *Cognitive Rehabilitation*, *3*, 22-24.

Larson, G. (1989). *The prehistory of the Far Side: A tenth anniversary exhibit*. Kansas City: Andrews and McMeel.

Liotti, M. & Tucker, D. M. (1995). Emotion in asymmetric corticolimbic networks. In R. J. Davidson & K. Hugdahl (Eds.), *Brain asymmetry* (pp. 389-423). Cambridge, MA: MIT Press.

Martin, G. N. & Gray, C. D. (1996). The effects of audience laughter on men's and women's responses to humor. *Journal of Social Psychology*, *136*, 221-231.

McDonald, S. (1993). Viewing the brain sideways? Frontal versus right hemisphere explanations of non-aphasic disorders. *Aphasiology*, *7*, 535, 549.

McGhee, P. E., Ruch, W., & Hehl, F. J. (1990). A personality-based model of humor development during adulthood. *Humor*, *3*, 119-146.

Molloy, R., Brownell, H. H., & Gardner, H. (1990). Discourse comprehension by right hemisphere stroke patients: Deficits of prediction and revision. In Y. Joanette & H. H. Brownell (Eds.), *Discourse ability and brain damage: Theoretical and empirical perspectives* (pp. 113-130). New York: Springer-Verlag.

Mundorf, N., Bhatia, A., Zillman, D., Lester, P., & Robertson, S. (1988). Gender differences in humor appreciation. *Humor, 1,* 231-243.
Nirenberg. S. A. (1991). Normal and pathologic laughter in children. *Clinical Pediatrics, 30,* 630-632.
Olson, J. M. & Roese, N. J. (1995). The perceived funniness of humorous stimuli. *Personality and Social Psychology Bulletin, 21,* 908-913.
Porterfield, A. L., Mayer, F. S., Dougherty, K. G., Kredich, K. E., Kronberg, M. M., Marsee, K. M., & Okazaki, Y. (1988). Private self-consciousness, canned laughter, and responses to humorous stimuli. *Journal of Research in Personality, 22,* 409-423.
Provine, R. R. (1996). Laughter. *American Scientist, 84,* 38-45.
Robinson, R. G., Kubos, K. L., Starr, L. B., Rao, K., & Price, T. R. (1984). Mood disorders in stroke patients: Importance of location of lesion. *Brain, 107,* 81-93.
Robinson, R. G., Parikh, R. M., Lipsey, J. R., Starkstein, S. E., Price, T. R., comments: Ivan, T. M., Franco, K., Allman, P., & Robinson, R. G. (1993). Pathological laughing and crying following stroke: validation of a measurement scale and a double-blind treatment study. *American Journal of Psychiatry, 150,* 286-293; comments: *151,* 290-292.
Ross, E. D. (1981). The aprosodias: Functional and anatomical organization of the affective components of language in the right hemisphere. *Archives of Neurology, 38,* 561-569.
Ross, E. D., Homan, R. W., & Buck, R. (1994). Differential hemispheric lateralization of primary and social emotions: Implications for developing a comprehensive neurology for emotions, repression, and the subconscious. *Neuropsychiatry, Neuropsychology, and Behavioral Neurology, 7,* 1-19.
Ruch, W. & Hehl, F. (1993). Humour appreciation and needs: Evidence from questionnaire, self-, and peer-rating data. *Personality and Individual Differences, 15,* 433-445.
Ruch, W. & Rath, S. (1993). The nature of humor appreciation: Toward and integration of perception of stimulus properties and affective experience. *Humor, 6,* 363-384.
Ruch, W., McGhee, P., & Hehl, F. (1990). Age differences in the enjoyment of incongruity-resolution and nonsense humor during adulthood. *Psychology and Aging, 5,* 348-355.
Sackeim, H. A., Greenberg, M. S., Weiman, A. L., Gur, R. C., Hungerbuhler, J. P., & Geschwind, N. (1982). Hemispheric asymmetry in the expression of positive and negative emotions. *Archives of Neurology, 39,* 210-218.
Shaibani, A. T., Sabbagh, M. W., & Doody, R. (1994). Laughter and crying in neurologic disorders. *Neuropsychiatry, Neuropsychology, and Behavioral Neurology, 7,* 243-250.
Shammi, P. (1997). *Humor in brain-damaged patients.* Unpublished doctoral dissertation, University of Toronto, Canada.
Shammi, P. & Stuss, D. T. (1999). Humour appreciation: A role of the right frontal lobe. *Brain, 122,* 657-666.
Staley, R. & Derks, P. (1995). Structural incongruity and humor appreciation. *Humor, 8,* 97-134.
Starkstein, S. E., Migliorelli, R., Tesón, A., Petracca, G., Chemerinsky, E., Manes, F., & Leiguarda, R. (1995). Prevalence and clinical correlates of pathological affective display in Alzheimer's disease. *Journal of Neurology, Neurosurgery, and Psychiatry, 59,* 55-60.
Tourangeau, R. & Sternberg, R. J. (1981). Aptness in metaphor. *Cognitive Psychology, 13,* 27-55.
Tucker, D. & Frederick, S. (1989). Emotion and brain lateralization. In H. Wagner & T. Manstead (Eds.), *Handbook of social psychophysiology: Emotion and social behaviour.* New York: John Wiley.
Wali, G. M. (1993). "Fou rire prodromique" heralding a brainstem stroke. *Journal of Neurology, Neurosurgery, and Psychiatry, 56,* 209-210.
Winner, E., Brownell, H., Happé, F., Blum, A., & Pincus, D. (1998). Distinguishing lies from jokes: Theory of mind deficits and discourse interpretation in right hemisphere brain-damaged patients. *Brain and Language, 62,* 89-106.
Wittling, W. & Roschmann, R. (1993). Emotion-related hemisphere asymmetry: Subjective emotional responses to laterally-presented films. *Cortex, 29,* 431-448.
Zeilig, G., Drubach, D. A., Katz-Zeilig, M., & Karatinos, J. (1996). Pathological laughter and crying in patients with closed traumatic brain injury. *Brain Injury, 10,* 591-597.

ANOSOGNOSIA

Kenneth M. Heilman,
Anna M. Barrett,
and John C. Adair

INTRODUCTION

Patients with a severe hemiplegia may be unaware of their deficit. Babinski (1914) called this lack of awareness *anosognosia*. The term anosognosia derives from the Greek word *gnosis*, which means knowledge, *noso*, which means disease, and *a*, which means without. After Babinski's description of this disorder, many other forms of unawareness of illness have been described. For example, patients with cortical blindness may be unaware that they cannot see (Anton, 1896) and patients with hemianopsia, especially of the left side, may be unaware that they are blind on one side. Patients with amnesia, especially associated with basal forebrain or thalamic lesions such as Korsakoff's Syndrome, may be unaware that they have any deficit, and patients with Alzheimer's disease often are unaware that they are demented. Wernicke's aphasics often appear unaware that they are speaking in jargon, and, on occasion, may become irritated with the person to whom they are speaking because that person does not understand them. Patients with other forms of aphasia may be unaware of the paraphasic errors they produce. Even some patients with ideomotor apraxia appear unaware that they can no longer perform skilled movements correctly.

Some patients will acknowledge that they have a disability, but appear to demonstrate little concern about either their illness or disability. Critchley (1953) called this state of unconcern *anosodiaphoria*. Anosodiaphoria may be a mild form of anosognosia. For example, patients who are initially unaware of their hemiplegia after being told multiple times that they are hemiplegic may finally acknowledge that there is a problem. However, they may appear to be unconcerned because they have not gained this knowledge through self-discovery, but rather through another individual's observation. Brain injury may also reduce emotional expressions (see Heilman, 1993) and therefore, in some cases, anosodiaphoria may be related to an emotional communication disorder.

Failure to be aware of a neurological deficit may interfere with medical treatment. For example, patients with anosognosia are less likely to present for early intervention with agents such as tPA, and limiting their access to this urgent treatment may increase the disability associated with a stroke. Unawareness of disability may also interfere with rehabilitation, and patients who do not recognize their disability may engage in activities, such as driving, that could endanger people's lives. Therefore, anosognosia, from a clinical perspective, is not a trivial problem. The study of anosognosia may also provide knowledge as to how the brain mediates self-awareness. In this article, we will briefly review some of the major hypotheses that have been advanced to explain this disorder. In this last decade, we have performed a series of experiments in our laboratory that attempt to elucidate the mechanism underlying this disorder. Some of these have been summarized in a previous article (Heilman et al., 1998). We will review several of these studies and update our discussion with some new observations. Although there are many forms of anosognosia, we will focus on what Babinski termed *anosognosia*, namely, unawareness of hemiplegia.

PSYCHOLOGICAL DENIAL

In their book *Denial of Illness*, Weinstein and Kahn (1955) suggested that the motivation to deny illness and disability is a natural phenomenon. Therefore, Weinstein and Kahn postulated that patients with diseases that induced disabilities, such as hemiplegia, hide their illness because this denial is a psychological defense mechanism that helps attenuate the distress of a catastrophic event such as a hemiplegia. To test this hypothesis, Weinstein and Kahn studied the pre-morbid personality characteristics of those individuals who demonstrated denial of their illness and found that the patients who demonstrated anosognosia used denial as a coping strategy even before their illness more frequently than did patients who appeared to be aware of their deficits.

Many clinicians have noted that denial of hemiplegia appears to be more frequently associated with right- than with left-hemisphere lesions. Some investigators thought that denial or unawareness of illness, which as defined by Babinski must be explicit, was asymmetrical because many patients with left-hemisphere disease are aphasic, and therefore cannot explicitly verbally deny their hemiplegia. If denial of illness or unawareness of illness is more frequently associated with right- than with left-hemisphere lesions and this asymmetry is not an artifact related to the confounding variable of aphasia, this asymmetry would not be consistent with Weinstein and Kahn's psychological denial theory. It would not support the denial theory because the coping strategies that a person uses should not be influenced by the side of the brain that is damaged by a stroke.

Selective hemispheric anesthesia is given to patients undergoing evaluation for possible seizure surgery (Wada study). We wanted to use this selective hemispheric anesthesia procedure to learn if unawareness of hemiplegia may be more frequently associated with right- than with left-hemisphere dysfunction. Unfortunately, during left-hemisphere anesthesia, patients who are left-hemisphere dominant for language may be unable to communicate. Therefore, we assessed our subjects for anosognosia by asking them if their arm was weak after they recovered from the hemispheric anesthesia. In our initial study (Gilmore et al., 1992), we studied eight patients who became globally aphasic with left-hemisphere anesthesia. All these patients developed right hemiplegia associated with their global aphasia. After recovery, all eight patients were aware that during this procedure their right arm was weak. In contrast, when their right hemisphere was anesthetized, although all eight patients developed a left hemiplegia after they recovered from anesthesia, none of the patients were aware that their left arm was weak. During this Wada procedure, none of our patients lost consciousness, and, at the time they were questioned, none of the patients appeared to be confused. In subsequent studies in our laboratory, we replicated our results; however, the replications were not quite as robust as our initial pilot study. Although Dywan, McGlone, and Fox (1995) were unable to replicate our findings, other investigators, including Carpenter et al. (1995) and Durkin et al. (1994), were able to replicate our findings.

In the Wada study for anosognosia it was the same people who were tested after right- and left-hemisphere anesthesia. Therefore, premorbid personality differences could not account for the asymmetries we found. In addition, during the time patients were asked questions about their hemiplegia, they were no longer hemiplegic and, therefore, there was no reason for these subjects to have psychologically motivated denial as a defense mechanism for a catastrophic event. Although our findings appear to refute the denial hypothesis, they do not preclude the possibility that there are individuals who deny their disabilities for psychological purposes. Because we asked our subjects if they were weak after they recovered from hemispheric anesthesia, it remains possible that the asymmetries we describe were related not to asymmetries of anosognosia, but rather to selective amnesia. For example, it is possible that during the time our patients had right-hemisphere dysfunction, when asked about weakness, they may have been aware of and acknowledged their weakness, but that when they recovered they were amnesic for this weakness.

To test this *hemisphere selective amnesia hypothesis*, we asked patients during right-hemisphere anesthesia, when they were hemiparetic, if they were weak (Adair et al., 1995a). We also asked the same subjects after the hemispheric anesthesia wore off if they had been weak. We found that the proportion of our patients who had anosognosia during anesthesia were the same as the proportion of patients who demonstrated unawareness of weakness after they recovered from anesthesia. These results suggest that asymmetries of anosognosia that we observed after hemispheric anesthesia were not related to selective (right-hemisphere) amnesia.

During Wada testing, we made another observation that is inconsistent with Weinstein and Kahn's psychological denial hypothesis. In some of our subsequent studies, we found that there were individuals with left-hemisphere anesthesia who would deny their hemiplegia. If they were denying their hemiplegia because of psychologically motivated denial, one could certainly expect that these patients should also deny language deficits or aphasia associated with hemispheric anesthesia. We studied patients who had selective anesthesia of the left hemisphere and noted that some patients were unaware of the hemiplegia but were aware of their aphasia (Breier et al., 1995). There were other patients who were aware of the hemiplegia but unaware of their aphasia. To postulate that anosognosia is a psychologically motivated denial used by subjects as a defense mechanism certainly cannot explain this dissociation.

CONFUSION

Hécaen and Albert (1978) suggested that anosognosia may be related to confusion. Mesulam and his colleagues (1976) demonstrated that acute confusional states may be more frequently associated with right- than left-hemisphere strokes.

In some of our testing protocols, we asked subjects about weakness after their hemispheric anesthesia resolved. Therefore, confusion could not explain these patients' unawareness of hemiplegia. However, it remains possible that during the hemisphere anesthesia they did not become aware of the hemiplegia because they were confused. Whereas there are some patients who, during right-hemisphere anesthesia, appear to be confused at the time of initial testing, many of our patients did not appear to have a confusional state.

IMPAIRED SENSORY FEEDBACK

Levine and his co-workers (1991) suggested that patients with anosognosia for hemiplegia may be unaware of their hemiplegia because they do not get sensory feedback that the limb is weak. In order to detect a hemiparesis, one may either view the limb to see if it is working or use proprioceptive systems to note that there is movement. To test this *feedback hypothesis*, we placed numbers in our experimental subjects' left hands during the time they were undergoing hemispheric anesthesia. We then brought their left hands into their right visual fields and right head and body hemispace. To make certain that they visualized the left hand, we asked them to identify the number that was placed in the hand. After our subjects named the number correctly, we asked if their arm and hand were weak. We did have some subjects who, upon seeing their hand and being asked if that hand was weak, attempted to move their left hand and discovered that their hand was weak. In these subjects, we cannot rule out the possibility that a sensory deficit may have been contributing to their anosognosia. However, other patients even after seeing their hand had anosognosia.

Patients with a hemianopsia, and even a somatosensory defect, should be able to explore the left side and, based on this exploration, be able to visualize the left hand in their right visual field. Therefore, hemianopsia, in the absence of left-sided exploratory defect that is often associated with unilateral hemispatial neglect, cannot, by itself, explain unawareness of hemiplegia.

HEMISPATIAL NEGLECT

It has been well established that neglect is more commonly associated with right- than left-hemisphere dysfunction (see Heilman et al., 1993). It is possible that the patients who discovered that the hand was weak when it was brought from left to right hemispace were suffering from hemispatial neglect. Unfortunately, we did not test these individuals for hemispatial neglect and, therefore, cannot be certain that the lack of feedback, secondary to spatial neglect, induced their anosognosia. In addition, if hemispatial neglect accounts for these patients' unawareness, neglect would explain anosognosia for hemiplegia in only a small proportion of subjects. Most subjects remained unable to recognize that their hand was weak when it was brought to the right visual field and right hemibody.

PERSONAL NEGLECT OR ASOMATOGNOSIA

Patients with right-hemisphere dysfunction may not only demonstrate a unilateral or hemispatial neglect, they also may demonstrate personal neglect, or *asomatognosia*. The patients who were able to name the number in their hand may not have been able to determine that their hand and arm were weak because they did not recognize that the hand with the number was their own hand. To determine if patients undergoing hemispheric anesthesia had asomatognosia and if this disorder was related to their anosognosia, we performed another experiment (Adair et al., 1995b). After barbiturate injection and the onset of hemiparesis, the examiner either moved the subjects' hands into a restrictive viewing space where the patients could see their hands or moved the subjects' hands to a position that was outside the viewing space. In this latter condition, the examiner positioned his or her own hand in the subjects' viewing space and asked the patients if the hand that they were viewing was the examiner's or their own hand. To make certain that the examiner's hand looked similar to the patient's hand, we selected an examiner who was approximately the same age as the subject and also the same gender and race. We found a small group of subjects with anosognosia associated with right-hemisphere anesthesia who were unable to discriminate between their own versus the examiners' hands (Adair et al., 1997). However, the overwhelming majority of our subjects, in spite of being unaware of their hemiparesis, were able to recognize their own versus the examiners' hands. These results suggest that although there are some subjects whose anosognosia may be related to personal neglect or asomatognosia, these self-recognition disorders cannot entirely account for anosognosia.

PHANTOM MOVEMENTS

Patients who have an extremity amputated often have the sensation that the extremity is still present. Some patients, when attempting to move this *phantom limb*, can have the feeling that the extremity is moving. We wanted to learn if this phantom limb movement could account for anosognosia (Lu et al., 1997a). We again used the Wada procedure to learn if patients with right-hemisphere anesthesia were experiencing phantom movement. We tested for phantom movement by asking our blindfolded patients to attempt to lift their left upper extremity and then to demonstrate their left limb's position by placing their right upper extremity in the same position as the left. To learn if phantom movement was associated with a loss of proprioceptive feedback we also tested proprioception of this left limb during right-hemispheric anesthesia by lifting the paretic arm and having the blindfolded patients demonstrate the position of the left limb by raising their right upper extremity to the same position as the left limb. Using this procedure, we found that only one subject with anosognosia had experienced phantom movement. There were other subjects who had phantom movement but these subjects were without anosognosia. The patient with the phantom movement and anosognosia also had impaired proprioception. However, the two other subjects with phantom movement appeared to have normal proprioception, suggesting that a loss of position sense is not a necessary condition for experiencing a phantom movement. Our results also suggest that phantom movement in the absence of visual and proprioceptive feedback may contribute to anosognosia. However, this mechanism would appear to play only a minor role.

CONFABULATION

Patients with neurological disorders may confabulate responses. By the term *confabulation* we mean a response that is not rooted in reality and is not motivated by a desire to mislead. Although anosognosia may be considered to be a form of confabulation, Feinberg and colleagues (1994) wanted to learn if patients with anosognosia have a propensity to confabulate in other domains. To investigate confabulation these investigators studied patients who had and did not have anosognosia for hemiplegia. In order to assess confabulation, they tested the patients' ability to identify stimuli rapidly presented in the visual field, contralateral to their hemispheric lesion. These investigators found that patients with anosognosia were significantly more likely to confabulate seeing objects in this contralateral visual field than those subjects without anosognosia. In order to further study the relationship between anosognosia and confabulation, we again studied patients who had intractable epilepsy and were undergoing selective hemispheric anesthesia (Lu et al., 1997b). During hemispheric anesthesia, when the subjects had a contralateral hemiparesis, we applied one of three different tactile stimuli to our patient's fingertips. During the time the stimulus was being applied, the subjects were prevented from directly viewing these materials. In some trials, no stimulus was applied. After the subjects were or were not stimulated, they were presented with a response card. This response card had three different textured materials with which the subjects may have been touched. The response card also had a question mark to indicate if they were uncertain whether or not they had been touched or what texture they had touched. If the subjects pointed to a texture when they were not touched it was considered a confabulatory response. If they pointed to a blank or question mark when touched with the textured material it was considered a failure to perceive. If they pointed to the wrong texture when touched it was considered a perceptual error. On this test we found no significant relationships between anosognosia and confabulation. There were subjects who were aware of the hemiparesis but confabulated their response, and there were other subjects with anosognosia who did not confabulate in this task. There were some subjects who did have both anosognosia and confabulation, but in these subjects the mechanism of confabulation was unknown.

DISCONNECTION

Geschwind (1965) suggested that confabulation may be related to hemispheric disconnection. He also suggested that anosognosia may be related to hemispheric disconnection. According to Geschwind's *disconnection hypothesis*, lesions of the right hemisphere may not only destroy primary sensory areas as well as sensory association areas but these lesions may also involve associative fibers that disconnect the sensory association areas in the right hemisphere from the language-speech centers, situated in the left hemisphere. In the absence of information from the right hemisphere, induced by this disconnection, the undamaged left hemisphere fabricates responses to functions subserved and monitored by the injured right hemisphere. Geschwind's disconnection hypothesis for anosognosia may not only explain the mechanisms of confabulation and anosognosia, but also may provide an explanation of why anosognosia is more frequently associated with right- than left-hemisphere lesions. To test the disconnection hypothesis, using the Wada technique, we examined patients undergoing right-hemisphere anesthesia by moving their left paretic hand into their right visual field, such that the left hemisphere could be made aware of the left arm. Even if there was left-hemisphere disconnection from the right hemisphere, the left hemisphere should be able to directly view the left-hemiparetic extremity. We found that only five of fifteen subjects were helped with this maneuver (Adair et al., 1997).

Although, as we have discussed, anosognosia for hemiplegia is more commonly associated with right- than left-hemisphere anesthesia, we have seen subjects who became hemiparetic and were unaware of their paresis with left-hemisphere anesthesia. Unfortunately, an interhemispheric disconnection syndrome could not account for these findings. That these five subjects discovered weakness when their left hand was brought in to their right body space and visual field may have not been entirely related to bypassing the hemispheric disconnection. The discovery of weakness when the arm is moved to the right may have been related to bypassing hemispatial neglect and faulty feedback.

INTENTIONAL FEED-FORWARD HYPOTHESIS

In the experiment we described above, when the patient's hand was brought into the right body space and the right visual field, the patients who discovered that they were paretic only discovered their paresis after they were asked to move their left hand and found that it would not move. This observation may suggest that some patients' anosognosia is related to a motor activation or an intentional feed-forward deficit (Heilman, 1991). The *feed-forward theory* of anosognosia deals with expectations. If a person has no expectation of movement and then does not detect movement, that person may not realize that he or she is weak. This feed-forward hypothesis suggests that there may exist, some place in the brain, a comparator. The plan for a movement's execution sets the comparator, and, if feedback comes into the comparator that does not match the expectation, the subject is alerted that there may be a performance failure. In the case of weakness, paresis is detected when there is a mismatch between the expectancy of movement and the perception of movement. In the clinic, one can see patients who have intentional motor deficits. These patients have no intention or desire to move. If the patient has no intention or desire to move, that person does not set the comparator and does not develop the expectation of movement. When there is a failure of movement, no mismatch is generated, and there is no recognition of disability. We tested this motor expectancy model by measuring the activation of proximal muscles, using electromyogram (EMG) in brain-damaged and control subjects during the time they squeezed a dynamometer with their right and left hands (Gold et al., 1994). We found that when the patient with anosognosia squeezed the dynamometer with his normal ipsilateral hand, that both the pectoralis on the left and right sides contracted. However, when asked to squeeze with the contralateral paretic hand, the patient with anosognosia barely contracted either pectoralis muscle. Control patients with hemiplegia who did not have anosognosia, and even a patient with spatial neglect, all contracted both pectoralis muscles when asked to squeeze with both right and left hands. These observations suggest that in this patient with anosognosia and hemiplegia there was a loss of motor intention. In the absence of motor intention there was no expectancy to move and, therefore, no mismatch when there was a failure to move.

INTENTION IN RIGHT AND LEFT SPACE

The feedback or motor intention hypothesis of anosognosia may also help to account for the observation that anosognosia for hemiplegia is more frequently associated with right- than left-hemisphere lesions. Coslett and co-workers (1989) examined patients for a *limb akinesia*, an intentional deficit, and found that limb akinesia was more often associated with right- than with left-hemisphere lesions. Heilman and Van Den Abell (1979) demonstrated that warning stimuli directed to the right hemisphere of normal subjects reduced reaction times for both hands but warning stimuli directed to the left hemisphere primarily reduced the reaction time of the right hand. These results in normal subjects suggest that the right hemisphere's intentional systems can help activate motor systems for both the right and left hands. However, the left-hemisphere intentional motor systems primarily activate the motor systems that control the right hand. Left-hemisphere injury may induce a less severe intentional deficit because the right hemisphere can compensate for the left but with right-hemisphere injury, the left hemisphere cannot compensate for the right. This asymmetry results in a higher frequency of motor intentional deficits with right- than with left-hemisphere damage.

In a prior section we discussed failures of feedback that were induced by sensory and attentional deficits. A detection failure may also be related to deficits in exploration. The exploration of right and left hemispace may also be asymmetrically controlled by the right and left hemispheres. We recently examined exploratory eye movements in patients while they were asked to make repeated precise movements of either their right or their left hand (Lu et al., 1999). Although the subjects were aware that they were being videotaped they did not know that one of the behaviors the raters would be measuring was eye movements during this task. We found that the eye movements associated with left-hand activity were significantly different than those associated with right-hand activity. When moving the fingers of the left hand the subjects looked leftward, but during right-hand movements the subjects would look in both directions. Each hemisphere is responsible primarily for moving the eyes into the opposite hemispace. These results suggest that movement in left space by the left hand primarily activates the right hemisphere, but movement in right space with the right hand activates both hemispheres. These patients with exploratory asymmetries were subsequently given selective hemisphere anesthesia (the Wada test) and these subjects became anosognosic with right-hemisphere anesthesia. Previous studies have demonstrated that the right hemisphere may monitor both right and left space, but the left hemisphere primarily monitors right space (Heilman & Van Den Abell, 1980; Pardo et al., 1991). This exploratory asymmetry of eye movements provides further evidence that attentional and intentional asymmetries may contribute to anosognosia associated with right-hemisphere dysfunction, because an isolated left hemisphere will not explore the limbs in left space.

CONCLUSIONS

Based on our work, primarily using the Wada procedure, we have not identified a single mechanism that can entirely account for anosognosia for hemiplegia. Certainly, for psychological reasons, people do deny disabilities; however, this hypothesis cannot explain why anosognosia of hemiplegia is more frequently associated with right- than with left-hemisphere dysfunction. It also cannot explain why patients may be aware of one deficit such as aphasia and be unaware of another deficit such as a hemiparesis. We also provided evidence that some patients with anosognosia may improve when feedback is improved by moving the paretic hand into the right body hemispace and the right visual field. Therefore, the lack of feedback from both sensory defects and spatial neglect may also play a role in anosognosia. If patients do not recognize that an extremity belongs to them, they certainly will not recognize that there is a deficit, and asomatognosia may be another important factor in anosognosia. When deprived of feedback, some patients with a left hemiparesis feel that they are moving their paralyzed arm. However, this phantom movement is only rarely associated with anosognosia. Although right-hemisphere dysfunction may induce a confusional state, many patients with anosognosia are without confusion. The isolated left hemisphere may confabulate, but confabulation and hemispheric disconnection appear to play only a minor role in anosognosia. People must have the intention to move and develop expectations before they can discover that there is a failure to move. Some patients may be unaware of their failure to move because they do not try to move. We again suspect that this explanation of anosognosia cannot be the entire explanation. Based on our studies of anosognosia for hemiplegia we would suggest that normal self-awareness depends on several parallel processes. We must have feedback systems that allow us to monitor our body and be able to attend to different parts of space and to our own bodies. We must develop accurate representations of our body, and these representations must be continuously modified by both expectations and knowledge of results.

REFERENCES

Adair, J. C., Gilmore, R. L., Fennell, E. B., Gold, M., & Heilman, K. M. (1995a). Anosognosia during intraoperative barbiturate anesthesia: Unawareness or amnesia for weakness. *Neurology, 45,* 241-243.
Adair, J. C., Na, D. L., Schwartz, R. L., Fennell, E. M., Gilmore, R. L., & Heilman, K. M. (1995b). Anosognosia for hemiplegia: Test of the personal neglect hypothesis. *Neurology, 45,* 2195-2199.
Adair, J. C., Schwartz, R. L., Na, D. L., Fennell, E. M., Gilmore, R. L., & Heilman, K. M. (1997). Anosognosia: Examining the disconnection hypothesis. *Journal of Neurology, Neurosurgery and Psychiatry, 63,* 798-800.
Anton, G. (1896). Blindheit nach beiderseitiger Gehirnerkrankung mit Verlust der Orienterung in Raume. *Mitteilungen des Vereines der Ärzte in Steiermark, 33,* 41-46.
Babinski, J. (1914). Contribution a l'étude des troubles mentaux dans hemiplegie organique cerebrale (anosognosie). *Revue Neurologique, 27,* 845-847.

Breier, J. I., Adair, J. C., Gold, M., Fennell, E. B., Gilmore, R. L., & Heilman, K. M. (1995). Dissociation of anosognosia for hemiplegia and aphasia during left-hemisphere anesthesia. *Neurology, 45*, 65-67.

Carpenter, K., Berti, A., Oxbury, S., Molyneux, A. J., Bisiach, E., & Oxbury, J. M. (1995). Awareness of and memory for arm weakness during intracarotid sodium amytal testing. *Brain, 118*, 243-251.

Coslett, H. B. & Heilman, K. M. (1989). Hemihypokinesia after right-hemisphere strokes. *Brain and Cognition, 9*, 267-278.

Critchley, M. (1953). *The parietal lobes*. London: Hafner Press.

Durkin, M. W., Meador, K. J., Nichols, M. E., Lee, G. P., & Loring, D. W. (1994). Anosognosia and the intracarotid amobarbital procedure (Wada test). *Neurology, 44*, 978-979.

Dywan, C. A., McGlone, J., & Fox, A. (1995). Do intracarotid barbiturate injections offer a way to investigate hemispheric models of anosognosia? *Journal of Clinical and Experimental Neuropsychology, 17*, 431-438.

Feinberg, T. E., Roane, D. M., Kwan, P. C., Schindler, R. J., & Haber, L. D. (1994). Anosognosia and visuoverbal confabulation. *Archives of Neurology, 51*, 468-473.

Geschwind, N. (1965). Disconnexion syndromes in animals and man. *Brain, 88*, 237-294, 585-644.

Gilmore, R. L., Heilman, K. M., Schmidt, R. P., Fennell, E. M., & Quisling, R. (1992). Anosognosia during Wada testing. *Neurology, 42*, 925-927.

Gold, M., Adair, J. C., Jacobs, D. H., & Heilman, K. M. (1994). Anosognosia for hemiplegia: An electrophysiologic investigation of the feed-forward hypothesis. *Neurology, 44*, 1804-1808.

Hécaen, H. & Albert, M. (1978). *Human neuropsychology*. New York: Wiley.

Heilman, K M. (1991). Anosognosia: Possible neuropsychological mechanisms. In G. P. Prigatano & D. L. Schacter (Eds.), *Awareness of deficit after brain injury* (pp. 53-62). New York: Oxford University Press.

Heilman, K. M. & Van Den Abell, T. (1979). Right-hemispheric dominance for mediating cerebral activation. *Neuropsychologia, 17*, 315-321.

Heilman, K. M. & Van Den Abell, T. (1980). Right-hemispheric dominance for attention: The mechanisms underlying hemispheric asymmetries of inattention (neglect). *Neurology, 30*, 327-330.

Heilman, K. M., Bowers, D., & Valenstein, E. (1993a). Emotional disorders associated with neurological disease. In K. M. Heilman & E. Valenstein (Eds.), *Clinical neuropsychology* (pp. 462-498). New York: Oxford University Press.

Heilman, K. M., Watson, R. T., & Valenstein, E. (1993b). Neglect and related disorders. In K. M. Heilman & E. Valenstein (Eds.), *Clinical neuropsychology* (pp. 279-336). New York: Oxford University Press.

Heilman, K. M., Barrett, A. M., & Adair, J. C. (1998). Possible mechanisms of anosognosia: A defect in self-awareness. *Philosophical Transactions Royal Society of London, B 353*, 1903-1909.

Levine, D. N., Calvanio, R., & Rinn, W. E. (1991). The pathogenesis of anosognosia for hemiplegia. *Neurology, 41*, 1770-1781.

Lu, L., Barrett, A. M., Cibula, J., Gilmore, R. L., & Heilman, K. M. (1997a). Phantom movement during the Wada test [abstract]. *Epilepsia, 38* (8), 156.

Lu, L., Barrett, A. M., Schwartz, R. L., Cibula, J., Gilmore, R. L., & Heilman, K. M. (1997b). Anosognosia and confabulation during the Wada test. *Neurology, 49*, 1316-1322.

Lu, L., Barrett, A. M., Gilmore, R. L., & Heilman, K. M. (1999). Exploration as measured by eye movements [abstract]. *Neurology, 52* (2), A488.

Mesulam, M. M., Waxman, S. G., Geschwind, N., & Sabin, T. D. (1976). Acute confusional states with right middle cerebral artery infarctions. *Journal of Neurology, Neurosurgery and Psychiatry, 39*, 84-89.

Pardo, J. V., Fox, P. T., & Raichle, M. E. (1991). Localization of a human system for sustained attention by positron emission tomography. *Nature, 349*, 61-64.

Weinstein, E. A. & Kahn, R. L. (1955). *Denial of illness: Symbolic and physiological aspects*. Springfield, IL: Charles C. Thomas.

DOCTOR FRANÇOIS: A CASE-STUDY OF DEEP DYSLEXIA

André Roch Lecours,
Marie-Josèphe Tainturier,
and Sonia Lupien

Dès l'âge de dix ans, j'ai été sujet à une esquinancie tonsillaire... Tout marcha ainsi jusqu'à quelques années après la culmination de ma force vitale[1]*.... Je m'aperçus qu'en voulant parler je ne trouvais pas les expressions dont j'avais besoin: ce symptôme me surprit et me rendit méditatif.... Lorsque je voulus jeter un coup d'oeil sur le livre que je lisais quand la maladie m'avait atteint, je me vis dans l'impossibilité d'en lire le titre... J'eus l'occasion de sentir toute l'absurdité de l'orthographe de notre langue.*

-Jacques Lordat (1843)

INTRODUCTION

In the early 1960s, at the Salpêtrière Hospital in Paris XIII, it was standard teaching that school-educated right-handed adults with acquired aphasia due to left brain damage sometimes present a reading disorder such that, although voicing single (written) words aloud remains in part possible, the syllables constituting the same words can no longer be read one by one if not lexicalized as open-class items. This behaviour was thus locally labeled as *aphasic alexia*, and it was emphasized that patients with this disorder had greater difficulty in naming letters than reading words: "l'alexie littérale est ici plus importante que l'alexie verbale" (Alajouanine, L'hermitte, & de Ribaucourt-Ducarne, 1960). It is no doubt in view of this dissociation between letters and words that, a few years later, this condition was recognized as *literal alexia* at Sainte-Anne Hospital in Paris XIV where it was further specified (A) that patients with literal alexia encounter great difficulties when requested to read phonologically legal non-words and also closed-class as opposed to open-class words, and (B) that such patients more or less often produce verbal paralexias, in particular, substitutions of target words by semantically and formally related ones: "la lecture des mots... se fait approximativement d'après la forme graphique... les paralexies se produisent dans la sphère... sémantique"

---

[1] The events narrated by Lordat begin in July 1825, when he was 52 years of age.

(Hécaen, 1972). An exceptionally well-documented observation had been published across the Channel a few years earlier (Marshall & Newcombe, 1966), and the condition was soon thereafter re-baptized as *deep dyslexia* (Marshall & Newcombe, 1973), a label that now prevails although it had for a short while been in competition with *phonemic dyslexia* (Shallice & Warrington, 1975).

Spectacular cases of deep dyslexia had been reported, albeit infrequently, as of the early 1930s (Hécaen, 1972; Marshall & Newcombe, 1973; 1980). Renewed interest in this disorder has resulted from the 1966 case report by John Marshall and Freda Newcombe, and it culminated in 1980 with the monograph edited by Coltheart, Patterson, and Marshall. As a matter of fact, the full syndrome of deep dyslexia remains exceptional, and it usually, if not always, occurs in patients with Broca's aphasia with "favorable" evolution toward agrammatism. According to Kaplan and Goodglass (1981), fractional manifestations of it are not uncommon "in aphasia of all types" but more so in the Broca type.

Current teachings, founded to a large extent on the observation of left brain-damaged readers of the English language, are that the full syndrome of deep dyslexia includes (A) gross anomalies in graphophonemic conversion, of which the clearest clinical manifestation is an incapacity to read legitimate non-words, (B) a greater difficulty in reading function (closed-class) as opposed to content (open-class) words, and (C) a production of various types of verbal paralexias, including semantic ones, with a predilection for uncommon and/or longer words, more so if they are non-picturable (Coltheart, 1980a; Marshall & Newcombe, 1973). This is an interesting description but we doubt it would entirely fit deep dyslexia in China, where languages are "isolating" for both mouth and hand, or in a native speaker-writer of a "polysynthetic" language (Hjelmslev, 1966; Lecours, in press).

In the next section of this chapter, we will report on a patient with a spectacular deep dyslexia in French. We will thereafter discuss the semiological profile of this syndrome for French and present a cognitivist model that can explain the semiological profile of this particular case.

DR. FRANÇOIS

Case Report

Dr. François was right-handed, born in France (1919), and residing there, obstetrician by profession and archaeologist by fascination. Until the age of 47 he enjoyed good health, read a lot, felt great pride at observing the growth of his many children, enthusiastically practiced his profession, and devoted his leisure hours to the discovery and reconstruction of antique clay vases. At the end of June, 1966, he consulted for persistent headaches and was diagnosed as having a Foster-Kennedy syndrome (Adams & Victor, 1985). Surgery led to removal of an apricot-size meningioma above his left olfactory groove, but he woke up with right hemiplegia and a maximal Broca's aphasia with speech suppression and total alexia and agraphia (spoken speech comprehension was spared – at least with regard to bed-side interactions).

In November of the same year, Dr. François was transferred to the Centre du Langage created at the Salpêtrière by Alajouanine, Ducarne, and L'hermitte, Jr. Neurological examination then revealed severe bracchio-facial right hemiplegia (paresis of the leg was less severe). Somesthesia was normal from the exteroceptive point of view or nearly so. There existed no auditory deficit and visual fields were full. A very mild buccofacial apraxia (which was nearly never manifest in speech) was observed. But for anosognosia concerning certain types of reading errors, no agnosia of any type was documented to exist.

Although Dr. François indeed had become talkative at this point and was an excellent communicator, one who often resorted to mimicry, gesture, and onomatopoeia when lexicons failed him, his spontaneous speech production was reduced, with severe word-finding difficulties and, as we have just hinted, almost imperceptible phonetic disintegration. As illustrated below in (1), where the patient is answering a question about the two halves of a plot of land where he and a colleague had made archaeological findings, prototypical agrammatic behaviour (Lecours, L'hermitte, & Bryans, 1983) was present:

(1) Ah! Mon vieux! L'archéologie! Oh! Attention, parce que moi, euh, trois ou quatre mois... Et la... euh la région euh Périgueux, trouver les... les pots et caetera.... Alors, deux médecins. Deux médecins: comme ça: alors, portion, là, moi, et l'autre médecin, l'autre. Oui. Après: zut! Parce que moi, je peux pas, là. Euh, euh, le mé... le... le... Là, rien du tout. Moi, rien du tout. Là à côté, euh, là, comme ça, médecin, bon!

(1) Ah! Old chap! Archeology! Oh! Look, because I, uh, three or four months... And the... uh the Périgueux, uh, region, to find the... the vases et cetera.... Then, two physicians. Two physicians: like this: then, part, there, me, and the other physician, the other. Yes. After: dash it! Because me, I can't, there. Uh, uh, the phy... the... the... Here, nothing at all. I, nothing at all. Here, beside, here, like this, physician, OK!

Systematic assessment of the patient's language abilities was done using the Ducarne Aphasia Battery (1964). Although they were far less obvious than in spontaneous speech, word-finding difficulties were observed in oral naming tasks. Not taking into account the very mild phonetic disorder, repetition of syllables and isolated words was normal (given the location of his left brain lesion it is possible that Dr. François' repetition abilities at least partially depended at this point on right hemisphere takeover). A few phonemic paraphasias and syntactic deviations, typically closed-class word deletions, were noted to occur in sentence repetition. One of us (ARL) anecdotally observed at this point that Dr. François could regroup the allographic forms of letters which he was unable to name, a fact to be kept in mind below.

Reading aloud was strikingly impaired. Isolated letters were sometimes misnamed and non-words were never read correctly (including monosyllabic ones). On the whole, the patient's attempts at reading aloud were limited to single words or locutions. Verbal paralexias were common and, from a descriptive standpoint, a large proportion of them could be attributed to one of three categories: either there existed immediately obvious semantic but no formal kinship between target and response (2), or there existed immediately obvious formal but no obvious semantic kinship between target and response (3), or else there was both semantic identity and formal identity (4a) or near identity (4b) between the root component of the target and that of the response, and the error was restricted to one or more than one closed-class bound morpheme (agrammatism in reading):

(2) *autrefois* (formerly) ⇒ *demain* (tomorrow)
(3) *parcelle* (small fragment) ⇒ *pucelle* (virgin)
(4a) *prenant* (taking) ⇒ *prenons* (we take)
(4b) *bruyant* (noisy) ⇒ *bruit* (noise)

Consistent with the terminology that prevailed in Paris when Dr. François was observed, his reading disability was labeled as aphasic alexia[2] (Alajouanine, L'hermitte, & de Ribaucourt-Ducarne, 1960). As acknowledged above, this type of disability is now known as deep dyslexia (Marshall & Newcombe, 1973), and this is the term we will keep using in most of this context. Also consistent with current terminology (Coltheart, Patterson, & Marshall, 1980; Lecours, Lupien, & Bub, 1990): (A) we will use the terms *semantic error* or *paralexia* as synonyms to qualify deviations such as (2) above, and (B) we will use the terms *visual error* and *formal verbal paralexia* as synonyms to qualify deviations such as (3) above. On the other hand, (C) we will avoid using the term *derivational error* to qualify deviations such as (4) above and replace it by *morphological error* or *morphological paralexia*, the reason for this choice being that such errors can be described not only by reference to derivational morphology, as in (4b), but also by reference to inflectional morphology as in (4a) (Badecker & Caramazza, 1987; Job & Sartori, 1984).

Motorwise, written production was entirely dependent on the patient's left hand. Spontaneous writing was reduced to his signature. Single word copying was normal and not slavish (for familiar concrete items; other word types were not tested). As is obvious in (5), where *il* (it) is transformed into *le* (the), where *fait* (is) is deleted, and *beau* (nice) transformed into a potentially homophonic non-word, *bo*, writing to dictation was severely impaired:

(5) *il fait beau* (the weather is nice)   ⇒   *le bo* (the nice)

Oral comprehension was at this point normal: the Ducarne word-picture and sentence-picture matching tasks were executed flawlessly, and Pierre-Marie's three-papers test[3] was completed rapidly, without hesitation or error. Written comprehension was normal for word-picture matching, and only a few errors occurred in matching series of written sentences to the drawings of comic-strip-like

---

[2] As opposed to agnosic alexia (and although the etymology of the prefix "a" was at that point inaccurate in both the word "aphasic" and the word "alexia").

[3] For instance, "Take the largest paper and drop it on the floor, give me the smallest one, then fold the third one and put it in your pocket."

stimuli. (Incidentally, while at the Salpêtrière, Dr. François was often observed to spend time silently reading newspapers and magazines.)

MATERIAL AND METHOD

Dr. François' reading abilities were tested during the last two months of 1966 as he was pursuing an intensive program of speech therapy with Madame Blanche Ducarne. One of us (ARL) then generated and administered him a reading test comprising 1400 stimuli. Because record of the last 94 items was lost, the data to be presented below bear on the first 1306 items.

Reading Test

Each of the 1306 stimuli of the François Reading Test was typed in black at the center of a white card (15 X 10 cm); capital letters were used only at the beginning of proper nouns and the stimuli included the diacritics of French orthography as appropriate. The order of the cards was randomized, and they were presented successively, in free vision and without temporal constraints. Dr. François' responses were tape recorded and transcribed, with any comments included.

In the context of the present study, the 1966 classification of the stimuli was revised with regard to those of the items which had been attributed to a particular word inventory although they were potential homographs of at least one word of another inventory (a far from infrequent situation in French): (A) if the patient's response was correct, or if it did not agree inventory-wise with one of the possibilities inherent in the stimulus, items were segregated under a more general heading (*other word stimuli with an open-class component*); (B) no change was made if the patient's paralexic response was consistent with the initial categorization (for instance, *car* = *because* or *bus* remained among the function words since the patient's response, *donc* (therefore), is an unambiguous function word, and even though *car*, presented out of context, might have been conceived as a legitimate noun); (C) reattribution to another category could also be done, following the same principles, in view of the patient's response (for instance, *ferme* = *farm* or *close*, which was initially attributed to the inventory of nouns, but was reattributed to that of conjugated verbs since the patient's response was *fermer* (to close)).

Conversely, transcription of the patient's responses was done, by reference to corresponding stimuli, in a manner semantically (and formally) as economical as possible. For instance, when the patient uttered /u/ in response to *là* (there) his production was transcribed as *où* (where); that is, homophones such as *ou* (*or*), *houx* (holly), *houe* (hoe), *houes* (hoes) and *hou!* (boo!) were ignored. Semantic economy also guided the English translations of stimuli and paralexic responses that are quoted in this text.

Thus revised, the list of stimuli included 1129 French words, 50 non-words (single letters excluded), and 127 other written entities of various types. The 1129 words included 924 stimuli with at least one open-class component, 165 closed-class words, and 40 interjections. The open-class items consisted of 414 nouns, 240 adjectives, 20 adverbs with the suffix *-ment*, and 250 verbs (50 infinitives, 100 participles, and 100 conjugated verbs). The closed-class items consisted of 50 pronouns, 25 prepositions, 30 conjunctions, 10 determinatives (articles, possessives, and demonstratives), and 50 adverbs without the *-ment* suffix.

A subset of 398 open-class items with an entry in Gougenheim's (1958) dictionary of fundamental French were considered to be "frequent" and opposed to another subset of 352 open-class words – globally matched at best for letter length and syllabic structure – that were considered to be "infrequent" (that is, without a Gougenheim entry). Moreover, two subsets of nouns were opposed as representative of words with high versus low levels of *imageability*; each of these subsets was comprised of 60 items globally matched at best for length, syllabic structure, and frequency. Non-words were of one to three syllables; 40 of them were and 10 were not phonologically legitimate.

It is of importance to note at this point that Dr. François was encouraged, as the assessment of his reading abilities went on, to respond even when he felt uncertain and to provide information about his uncertainties, which he did without reluctance in view of the friendly relationship he and ARL had developed. It was also understood that the latter could challenge his responses, whether they were faulty or correct. Had Dr. François been instructed otherwise, or had the testing situation been more formalized, results to be reported below – and perhaps the interpretations to be proposed as well – might have been appreciably different.

RESULTS

Forty-three per cent of the 1306 stimuli yielded the expected responses, while 46% led to one or several inadequate responses; 11% led to both the production of at least one paralexic response and of the expected one. A total of 2088 responses were noted, 1062 (51%) of which corresponded to conventional responses and 988 (47%) to paralexic responses; absence of response occurred in only 38 cases (2%). Out of 373 monomorphemic stimuli, 88 (23.6%) led to the production of at least one error; this occurred for 370 (69.8%) of the 530 stimuli comprising more than one morpheme.

Let us first underline that, although the patient usually read isolated letters correctly once the early phases of his therapy were behind him, his literal alexia remained severe throughout testing. Indeed, he nearly never could spell words that he had read correctly (6), nor could he passively take orally spelled information into account.

(6) *doigt* (finger)   ⇒   Dr. François: *doigt*
                              ARL: Spell the word.
(In spite of many attempts, the patient cannot name a single letter of the stimulus, whether or not he is looking at the index card.)

More importantly, all but one of the global linguistic characteristics now considered to belong with deep dyslexia were observed in Dr. François' reading productions.

Non-word Effect

When he was presented with non-word stimuli, Dr. François usually made it clear that he recognized them as such, which was to him a source of explicit astonishment (7). Nonetheless and no doubt because of the testing conventions mentioned above, he often produced verbal paralexias when shown such items.

(7) *trubir* ⇒ ...
        Dr. François: Nothing at all there!
        Or else: *bruit* (noise).
        No. Yet...
        Bruiteur? (soundman?)
        Bruitage? (sound effects?)
        Do not know.

Given Dr. François' literal alexia, it was astonishing that he could – when presented with word stimuli including a misspelling (8) – point at erroneous literal components that he was utterly unable to name.

(8) *hngar*[10] ⇒ Dr. François: You're kidding!
        Hangar (shed).
        But a letter, here. There.
(Dr. François points between the *h* and the *n* on the stimulus-card.)

Length Effect

Very short words excepted, a *length effect* (Marshall & Newcombe, 1973) was observed to be present within the François Corpus: for instance, 53 out of 129 four-letter word stimuli (41%), 103 out of 152 eight-letter (67.8%), and 23 out of 25 twelve-letter ones (92%) led to at least one error. In our opinion, this effect is to a large extent related to morphology. On the other hand, 30 out of 51 two-letter word stimuli (58.8%) also led to at least one error and it should be noted that virtually all of them involved function words and interjections.

With regard to the length phenomenon, it was striking how Dr. François could initially strip a polymorphemic stimulus from its affixes (9) and directly excerpt its root.

(9) *embellissant* (embellishing) ⇒ Dr. François: *bel* (beautiful)
        Bel, but better...
        Ah! Yes!
        Embellissement (embellishment)

Word Category Effect

Not taking word length into account, increase in number of errors occurred from nouns (32%), to adjectives (48%), to function words (57%), to infinitives (62%), and to participles and conjugated verbs (74%), a phenomenon labeled as *category effect* (Shallice & Warrington, 1975). It should be kept in mind that paralexias on verbs very often spared the root (i.e., were limited to closed-class bound morphemes) (10).

(10) *tyrannisaient* (they tyrannized) ⇒ Dr. François: *tyranniser*
(to tyrannize)

Frequency Effect

A *frequency effect* was also present. As assessed on a subset of 750 nouns, adjectives and infinitives of comparable length, error production was greater for infrequent (59%) than for frequent (28%) words.

Picturability Effect

As found within a subset of 120 nouns of comparable length and frequency, error production was greater for non-picturable (43%) than for picturable (23%) words (Patterson & Marcel, 1977; Richardson, 1975).

Surprisingly enough, since it is hardly conceivable that this might have been the effect of some previous explicit knowledge, Dr. François' comments also testified to some intuitions concerning relationships of a sort existing between his reading disorder and the frequency and picturability of words (11, 12).

(11) *table* (table) ⇒ Dr. François: *table*.
Here, easy. Difficult, abstraction.
(12) *funeste* (fatal) ⇒ Dr. François: *funeste*.
The words are emerging.
The abstract words.

Class Effect

On the other hand, and if our manner of questioning the François Corpus in this respect corresponds to what has been done by other researchers, the *class effect* (Marshall & Newcombe, 1973) was missing in this case (for words, not for morphemes): 470 out of 924 stimuli with at least one open-class component (51%) and 88 out of 165 (53%) closed-class words led to at least one error.

However, and just as he often identified non-words as such without being asked, it was not uncommon for Dr. François to spontaneously insist that closed-class words (13) – which he often recognized as such and qualified as *petits mots* (little words) – were the source of greater reading difficulties than those of the open-class.

(13) *dont* (of which) ⇒ Dr. François: *donc* (therefore)
No. Can't say. Little word: difficult.

Class And Inventory Transgressions

Paralexic class transgression was most uncommon among Dr. François' paralexias, and it virtually always took the form of a visual error bearing on a closed-class word (14).

(14) *encore* (again) ⇒ *encrier* (inkpot)

Unequivocal inventory transgression for closed-class stimuli was not frequent either, and it took, when it occurred, the form of a semantic and/or formal paralexia. On the other hand, paralexic inventory transgression was frequent for words with an open-class component (62.3% of 650 paralexias). Typically, such errors were of the morphological paralexia type, that is, the error confined itself to closed-class bound-morpheme component(s). Moreover, paralexias were "root-governed" far more often than otherwise. For instance, 46 out of 126 paralexias on conjugated verbs (36.5%) yielded an infinitive, and 34 (27%) a noun; 54 out of 125 paralexias on participles (43.2%) yielded a noun, and 32 (25.6%) an infinitive; and 21 out of the 46 paralexias on infinitives (45.7%) as well as 65 out of the 158 paralexias on adjectives (41.1%) also yielded a noun.

TYPOLOGICAL DATA

The François Corpus included 127 semantic errors (12.9%), 276 formal errors (27.9%), 47 semantic and formal errors (4.8%), and 447 morphological errors (45.2%). Dr. François' paralexias could involve a given word as a whole or else be limited to one of its morphemic components (see below for specific examples). In the former case, errors were nearly always semantic and/or formal; but for a limited number of exceptions, they were more often morphological. In this respect, cumulative data for nouns, adjectives, verbs, and *-ment* adverbs show that, whereas the proportions of semantic and formal paralexias are comparable in response to monomorphemic items and polymorphemic items, that of semantic and formal paralexias is greater in the former and that of morphological ones far greater in the latter (Table 1). Concerning morphological paralexias, one should note that closed-class bound morpheme substitutions (72.2%) were by far more frequent, and additions (4.6%) by far less frequent than deletions (23.1%).

Also as illustrated below, Dr. François' paralexic errors on closed-class words presented out of context could be classified under the same headings as those bearing on single words with at least one open-class morpheme. If one considers in this respect the subset of 205 responses to the 115 pronouns, prepositions, conjunctions and determiners of the François Reading Test, one realizes that 124 (60.5%) of them were erroneous. Out of these 124 paralexias, 12 (9.6%) were clearly of the semantic type, 46 (37%) of the formal type, 13 (10.4%) of the semantic and formal type, and 29 (23.3%) of the morphological type.

Left- Versus Right-sided Errors

Dr. François' morphological paralexias on words with a spared open-class morpheme could be left-sided (involving prefixes) or right-sided (involving suffixes or morphological endings). Considering the subsample of 385 such paralexias in which morpheme deletion, addition or substitution did occur, errors were found to be left-sided in 13 cases (3.4%) and right-sided in 372 cases (96.6%). This huge difference might in part be related to both Dr. François' native tongue and to the fact that the François Reading Test was not based on a theory (Lecours, 1996a). Be

	Total Poly	MONO	DIAC POLY	SYNC POLY
	650/1174 (55.4%)	94/367 (25.6%)	41/92 (44.6%)	515/715 (72%)
SEM	47/650 (7.2%)	chaise ⇒table 11/94 (11.7%)	effluve ⇒marais 3/41 (7%)	perdu ⇒égaré 36/515 (6.9%)
FOR	169/650 (26%)	lieu ⇒lien 38/94 (40%)	banal ⇒banane 10/41 (24%)	concerna ⇒Concarneau 124/515 (24%)
S & F	34/650 (5.2%)	propre ⇒probe 13/94 (13.8%)	bouquet ⇒bosquet 7/41 (17%)	fantaisie ⇒fadaise 14/515 (2.7%)
MOR	314/650 (48.3%)	an ⇒année 14/94 (14.9%)	insolite ⇒solitaire 14/41 (34%)	glorifier ⇒glorieux 286/515 (55.5%)

Table 1. Verbal paralexias on a subset of 1174 responses to single word stimuli comprising at least one open-class morpheme (nouns, adjectives, and verbs). MONO = monomorphemic items. DIAC POLY = diachronic polymorphemic items. SYNC POLY = synchronic polymorphemic items. SEM = Semantic paralexias. FOR = Formal verbal paralexias (visual errors). S&F = Semantic and formal paralexias. MOR = Morphological paralexias. Overall data are given in absolute numbers and in percentages of errors by reference to the total number of responses. Paralexic typology data are given in absolute numbers and in percentages by reference to the total number of errors for each paralexic subtype (66 of Dr François' paralexias were not of the SEM, FOR, S&F, or MOR types).

this as it may, these data do not include 27 morphological paralexias in which the deviation occurred on both the left and right sides.

Surface Typology of the Patient's Paralexic Errors

We will now summarize in a more systematic manner the patient's errors. This subsection focuses on the surface typology of Dr. François' paralexias. Our comments in this respect are formulated by reference to various subsets of stimuli within the test (non-words, single words with various types of morphemic structure, and other entities).

Single Words (Monomorphemic Items)

We considered as belonging to this category a subset of French words including (A) open-class items corresponding to an isolated root, such as *bouc* (male goat) and *dur* (hard), (B) polysyllabic open-class items in which an eventual derived component might have been accessible to well-trained polyglot philologists although not to more standard citizens, for instance *verrat* (boar) and *arôme* (aroma), and (C) closed-class words without an indication of gender or number, such as *qui* (who) and *mais* (but).

Semantically based monomorphemic word substitutions were observed for both open-class and closed-class stimuli. This is portrayed in (15) for the former and in (16) for the latter:

(15) *chaise* (chair) ⇒ *table* (table)
(16) *car* (because) ⇒ *donc* (therefore)

Word substitutions involving monomorphemic items based on visual kinship (formal verbal paralexias) were also observed for both open-class (17) and closed-class (18) stimuli:

(17) *lieu* (place) ⇒ *lien* (link)
(18) *moins* (less) ⇒ *mois* (month)

Beyond the above, a sizeable proportion of Dr. François' paralexias were such that both semantic and formal kinship were apparent between stimulus and response (semantic and formal paralexias). This phenomenon was sometimes observed upon the presentation of monomorphemic stimuli and it occurred for both open-class (19) and closed-class (20) items:

(19) *chandail* (sweater) ⇒ *chaud* (warm)
(20) *sous* (under) ⇒ *sur* (over)

With one or two exceptions, transformation of a monomorphemic item into a polymorphemic one was always done by adding a closed-class bound morpheme (derivation or inflection) to the target. Dr. François produced few such errors.

Given our taxonomy, they are labeled as morphological paralexias although, whether they involved open-class stimuli (21) or closed-class ones (22), all might have also qualified as being semantic and formal:

(21) *ferme* (close) ⇒ *fermer* (to close)
(22) *un* (one – masculine) ⇒ *une* (one – feminine)

Single Words (Diachronic Polymorphemic Items)

We labeled a subset of the Reading Test as *diachronic polymorphemic items*. It includes one type of words with an open-class component and two types of closed-class ones. In the first type, the *root* could exist as a single word but its semantic origin is seldom perceived when it occurs with an affix: for instance, the sense of the root *table* (table) changes in *tablette* (shelf; tablet), *tableau* (blackboard; painting) and *tabler* (to count on). As to the closed-class items, all of the monosyllabic ones were marked for gender and/or number whereas the polysyllabic ones were composed of at least two transparent units, as in *cependant* (nevertheless), which includes *ce* (this) and *pendant* (during).

A few semantically based replacements involving diachronic polymorphemic items were observed in response to both open-class (23) and closed-class (24) stimuli:

(23) *catégorie* (category) ⇒ *arranger* (to set in order)
(24) *la* (the – feminine) ⇒ *une* (one – feminine)

Formal verbal paralexias were also observed for both classes (25;26):

(25) *banal* (commonplace) ⇒ *banane* (banana)
(26) *autant* (as much) ⇒ *alentour* (around)

Paralexic replacements also occurred, for the open-class (27) as well as for the closed-class items (28), with both obvious semantic and formal kinship (semantic and formal errors):

(27) *bouquet* (bouquet) ⇒ *bosquet* (grove)
(28) *les* (the – plural) ⇒ *ses* (his/her – plural)

Diachronic polymorphemic items of all types could also be at the origin of morphological paralexias (29):

(29) *auquel* (to whom) ⇒ *lequel* (whom)

As in (30), closed-class monosyllabic items marked for gender and/or number could also lead to non-transparent although rule-governed morphological paralexias:

(30) *ma* (my – feminine) ⇒ *moi* (me)

Single Words (Synchronic Polymorphemic Items)

Another subset of French words – those composed of at least one open-class morpheme (root) which is shared, without semantic modification, by at least one other French word, and of at least one productive affix and/or morphological ending, was among the randomized stimuli presented to Dr. François. This subset included a number of the nouns and adjectives of the Reading Test, as well as all adverbs with a *-ment* ending and all of its regular infinitives, participles, and conjugated verbs.

Semantic paralexias bearing on synchronic polymorphemic items could, in the case of Dr. François, involve a stimulus globally, without apparent influence of its morphemic structure (31), or else be specific to the root, thus leaving closed-class bound morpheme(s) intact (32). In the latter case, one might talk of a subtype of semantic paralexias in which the error involves a single morpheme (as in many morphological paralexias):

(31) *dînons* (we dine)   ⇒   *manger* (to eat)
(32) *bleuâtre* (bluish)   ⇒   *verdâtre* (greenish)

Likewise, Dr. François' visual errors on this subset could involve an item globally, that is, irrespective of its combined structure (33), and they also could be limited to its root, thus leaving its closed-class bound morpheme(s) intact (34), therefore constituting another subtype of formal paralexia in which the deviation involved a single morpheme (again as in many morphological paralexias):

(33) *aminci* (thinned)   ⇒   *amical* (friendly)
(34) *rager* (to fume)   ⇒   *ramer* (to row)

As illustrated in (35), Dr François' verbal paralexias could seem to be both semantic and formal in polymorphemic as well as in monomorphemic items:

(35) *coloris* (colouring)   ⇒   *colibri* (colibri)

A large majority of Dr François' paralexias on polymorphemic stimuli qualified as morphological paralexias, in which there existed, by definition, semantic and (more or less) formal root identity, the paralexias bearing only on closed-class bound morphemes. Morphological errors could involve prefixes and/or suffixes or both (36) (*derivational paralexias*), morphological endings (37) (*inflectional paralexias*), or both (38). Moreover, such errors could take the form of affix or morphological ending deletion (*stripping*) (39), addition (*filling*) (40) or substitution (*swapping*) (41):

(36) *engourdi* (benumbed)   ⇒   *gourd* (numb)
(37) *écrivant* (writing)   ⇒   *écrivain* (writer)
(38) *utilement* (usefully)   ⇒   *inutile* (useless)
(39) *jardinier* (gardener)   ⇒   *jardin* (gardent)
(40) *chantant* (chanting)   ⇒   *enchantant* (enchanting)

(41) *certainement* (certainly) ⇒ *certitude* (certitude)

With regard to the above type of errors, it should be noted that, in case of suffix or morphological ending substitutions, semantic kinship (42), formal kinship (43), or even both semantic and formal kinship (44) could exist between the replacing and the replaced closed-class bound morphemes:

(42) *recevant* (receiving) ⇒ *receveur* (receiver)
(43) *ignorait* (he ignored) ⇒ *ignorant* (ignorant)
(44) *mercier* (haberdasher) ⇒ *mercerie* (haberdashery)

Semic Extraction Behavior

It was striking that, when experiencing particular difficulty with reading a given stimulus which he recognized as a legitimate word, the patient often engaged in comments having to do with its meaning (*semic extraction behaviour*) (Lecours, Lupien, & Bub, 1990). Behaviour of this sort sometimes amounted to all that the patient could utter (45), or else resulted in the production of either a semantic paralexia (46), of which the patient remained unaware unless it was pointed out to him, or else of the expected response (47). Semic extraction behaviour could also be targeted at a single closed-class bound morpheme within a polymorphemic stimulus (48), and it sometimes ended up with an exhaustive and adequate enumeration of the target's semic properties (49).

(45) *quasi* (almost) ⇒ ...
    Dr. François: I can a little... Then: no.
    ARL: Read the word.
    Dr. François: Don't know.
(46) *tante* (aunt; gay) ⇒ ...
    Dr. François: Dr. François: A man. The woman no.
        The man everything. *Homosexuel* (homosexual).
        That's it!
(47) *perroquet* (parrot) ⇒ ...
(With his left index finger, Dr. François traces on the table the profile of a bird with a big hooked bill; he emphasizes the bird's posture.)
    ARL: *Toucan?* (toucan?)
    Dr. François: No.
    ARL: *Aigle?* (eagle?)
    Dr. François: No.
    ARL: *Paon?* (peacock?)
    Dr. François: No. In Africa.
    At home, warm apartment...
    Perroquet!
(48) *agriculteur* (agriculturist) ⇒ Dr. François: *agricole* (agricultural)
    No, *agriculture* (agriculture).
    No, the gentleman makes agricultural.
    Rats! Too bad!
(49) *grandirez* (you will grow) ⇒ Dr. François: *grande* (tall – feminine)

> *Grande* but...
> Yes.
> Again: *grand* (tall – masculine).
> No.
> Tall but third person?
> Future. Second person. Plural.

A sizeable proportion of Dr. François' reading errors were thus *compounded paralexias*, that is, multiple-step errors. In (50), for instance, the stimulus *hormis* (except) was first read as *jardin* (garden), a transformation which would have remained entirely opaque had not the patient corrected himself and switched to *horticulteur* (horticulturist, gardener), thus suggesting that the initial response was a semantic paralexia related, rather than to the stimulus itself, to a yet to be verbalized formal verbal paralexia. Similar paralexic modes are explicitly there to be observed in (51) and (52).

(50) *hormis* (except) ⇒ ...
 (Dr. François hides the stimulus.)
 Dr. François: To think... *Jardin* (garden).
 No: *horticulteur* (gardener).
 Yes... But... Yes.
(51) *fomenter* (to foment) ⇒ Dr. François: *manger* (to eat).
 No: *boire* (to drink).
 Neither. Dash! To eat, to drink...
 After the meal, the...
 Fromage (cheese).
 That's it!
(52) *équivoque* (equivocal) ⇒ Dr. François: *pédestre* (pedestrian)
 No: *équitation* (equitation).

Utterly opaque paralexias were infrequent among Dr. François' reading errors and it is likely that nearly all of them might have been of the above type (but without actual verbalization of the formal paralexia component). Thus, and although the patient did not himself make this explicit, the three paralexias in (53) somehow become more plausible if one makes inferences about the formal kinship between *craigniez* (you feared) and *saigniez* (you bled), *déchu* (forfeited) and *déchiré* (torn), *écrouler* (to collapse) and *écouter* (to listen):

(53a) *craigniez* (you feared) ⇒ *mouchez* (blow your nose)
(53b) *déchu* (forfeited) ⇒ *cousu* (sewn)
(53c) *écrouler* (to collapse) ⇒ *entendre* (to hear)

As said above and illustrated below, another point that clearly came out of Dr. François' comments was that he could explicitly feel very confident (anosognosic) about semantic paralexias (54). He at times insisted in such cases that his responses were correct and that the expression of doubt by the examiner was unjustified. He could also produce paralexias that were morphologically complex forms of the correct item, and even alter correct responses (55).

(54) *tolérance* (tolerance) ⇒ Dr. François: *libéral* (liberal).
ARL: Look at this word carefully.
Do you really read *libéral?*
Dr. François: Yes. But don't know.
Not read: *tac-tac!*
Libéral
Yes? Ah no!
Libéralité (liberality).
Libéralité? Maybe.
Not *libre* (free).
Here! Now! *Libéral.* Yes!

(55) *ébène* (ebony) ⇒ Dr. François: *ébéniste* (cabinet-maker)
No. Yes?
Afrique (Africa).
No: *ébène?*
Yes: *ébéniste.*

Given his reactions and comments, it was obvious that Dr. François experienced difficulty in becoming aware of certain features of the stimuli that were shown to him versus the responses that he produced. Length incompatibility was one of these characteristics (56), as well as changes in word order (57) and in number of words (58).

(56) *aussitôt* (forthwith) ⇒ Dr. François: *sur* (on)
No: *aussi* (also)
Neither. Don't know.

(57) *ciel gratte* (scraper sky) ⇒ Dr. François: *le gratte-ciel* (the skyscraper)
(With the index card in his hand and his eyes looking at it, and in spite of ARL's explicit indication and questions, Dr. François remains unaware of the verbal metathesis.)

(58) *terre de pomme* (potato[4]) ⇒ Dr. François: *thème* (theme).
No : *pomme de terre* (potato).

Moreover, Dr. François' behaviour indicated on several occasions that interactions between word representations stocked in his input lexicon of visual origin and his semantic knowledge could be flawless although clearly not mediated by graphophonemic conversion. When presented stimuli with one or several homophones (59), he would often, verbally or through explicit gestures (onomatopoeia included) (60), specify the meaning linked to the stimulus itself and mention the other(s).

(59) *sans* (without) ⇒ Dr. François: *cent* (one hundred)
(With his left index finger, Dr. François draws the corresponding number on the table.)
Sang (blood).
(Dr. François points at his heart.)
Sans. As here.

---

[4] At another level of disorder.

(60) *taureau* (bull) ⇒ Dr. François: *Meuh!*
Strength, like tiger, the same thing.
Taureau! Not calf.

It should be clear, at this point, that – whether or not his responses corresponded to targets – Dr. François was absolutely unable to read aloud without matching his utterances to components of his semantic knowledge.

DISCUSSION

The words nowadays attached to deep dyslexia are sometimes of linguistic, sometimes of cognitivist, and sometimes of biological origins, which can make things fuzzy because neuroscience and cognitive science have kept working in parallel (more or less consciously depending on the investigator) since the Paris 1908 debate (Lecours, 1996b; Lecours, Chain, Poncet, Nespoulous, & Joanette, 1992).

At the empirical level, it has been suggested that patients clinically labeled as deep dyslexics have in fact functionally different disorders (Coltheart, 1980a; Rapp & Caramazza, 1991; Shallice, 1988). This notwithstanding, the semiology of deep dyslexia is, nowadays, usually thought to be comprised of an incapacity to read unknown words and non-words, a greater difficulty in reading closed-class than open-class words, and a production of semantic paralexias (considered to be pathognomonic) of formal paralexias and morphological paralexias; this production is said to be greater when stimuli are words of lesser frequency, or else longer ones, or again when they are not picturable and/or belong to certain grammatical categories. Nouns, for instance, are said to be less vulnerable (in English) than any other category (Coltheart, Patterson, & Marshall, 1980).

One might add that the proportion of each paralexic type can vary a great deal from one subject to another, which should not come as a surprise because – whatever the factors inherent in the reading dysfunction itself – these proportions are no doubt constrained by factors such as how one defines each paralexic type, the patient's mother tongue and educational background, the choice of stimuli one makes to test reading abilities, and the instructions one gives to one's patients prior to testing. Be this as it may, studying the François case in detail has led us to reassess – if only a bit – our views regarding the clinical manifestations of deep dyslexia.

The Semantic Paralexia Characteristic

Overall, 12.9% of the François Corpus is comprised of transparent semantic paralexias. They can be classified into three main subtypes, that is, (A) open-class whole-word substitutions, which constitute the prototype, (B) closed-class whole-word substitutions, the existence of which has also been acknowledged by Morton and Patterson (1980), and (C) errors limited to the lexemic root of polymorphemic word-stimuli. In our opinion, the notion of semantic paralexia could be extended to several other entities observed within the François Corpus. These include the replacement of certain closed-class bound-morphemes and the semic extraction behaviour (Lecours, Lupien, & Bub, 1990), whether bearing on whole words, or limited to closed-class bound morphemes. One might also suggest the inclusion of substitution of a closed-class word by another of the same grammatical category. The latter might also be labeled *functional paralexia* since the only relationship is a category one.

If one agrees about the latest entity discussed above, substitutions of closed-class bound-morphemes could also be considered when the only relationship between replaced and replacing (morphemic) units is a linking potential. Let us stress, at this point, that semantic errors have been claimed to constitute the single pathognomonic manifestation of deep dyslexia (Coltheart, 1980a), no doubt in view of the label itself. This might be considered clinically valid because certain patients apparently produce semantic but not visual errors (Célérier, 1991; Caramazza & Hillis, 1990; Hillis, Rapp, Romani, & Caramazza, 1990). Be this as it may, there are cases of deep dyslexia, that of Dr. François for instance, in which the production of semantic errors is there, but they are less copious than the formal and morphological ones (this might of course depend on test content and on the instructions linked to it).

The Formal Paralexia Characteristic

Clear-cut formal paralexias comprised 27.9% of the François Corpus. As with the semantic paralexias, these can be classified into three main subtypes, that is, (A) open-class whole-word substitutions, which constitute the prototype, (B) closed-class whole-word substitutions, and (C) errors limited to the root of polymorphemic items. In our opinion, the notion of visual error could be extended to another form of paralexia which is not uncommon within the François Corpus and which is characterized by the substitution of a closed-class bound-morpheme where an obvious formal relationship can be seen between replaced and replacing morphemes.

The Semantic and Formal Paralexia Characteristic

Like other patients whose reading behaviours have been described in detail (Coltheart, 1980a; Shallice & McGill, 1978), Dr. François' paralexic productions included – not taking into account his 447 morphological paralexias – 47 errors in which one could recognize concomitant semantic and formal relationships between stimulus and response. Other examples (61, 62) are quoted below, if only to further illustrate a fact that potentially bears significance with regard to the functional disorder behind deep dyslexia :

(61) *opaque* (opaque)   ⇒   *opalin* (opaline)
(62) *dernier* (last)   ⇒   *derrière* (behind)

The Morphological Paralexia Characteristic

Forty-four percent of Dr. François' paralexias had to do with closed-class bound morphemes, that is, did not involve the roots of the stimuli. The production of morphological errors is therefore a bona fide semiological characteristic of deep dyslexia (at least in the case of Dr. François, where it dominated the clinical picture, which was not surprising given the patient's agrammatism, his native language of Latin origin, and the stimuli he was shown). Whether or not this semiological characteristic has a significance essentially different from that linked to other paralexic types remains an open question. For Shallice and Warrington (1975), morphological paralexias are essentially semantic errors, given that polymorphemic words can be read as unitary entities and that they are semantically related when the root is indeed shared (with or without formal changes). If so, one might also argue that morphological paralexias are, essentially, visual errors, since polymorphemic words are formally related if they share a root. One might therefore wish to suggest that morphological paralexias are a subtype of semantic and visual errors (Funnel, 1987) akin – up to a point – to other subtypes observed in our patient's productions. As a matter of fact, one might be tempted to agree with this notion, at least in cases of closed-class bound morpheme deletion or addition (23.1% and 4.6% of the morphological paralexias in the Dr. François Corpus).

Nonetheless, as we have argued above, there are – beyond root identity and irrespective of it – reasons to believe that most if not all closed-class bound-morpheme substitutions (72.2% of the morphological paralexias in the François Corpus) are, for their own part, semantically and/or formally based, which has led us to suggest considering them as subtypes of the two paralexic behaviours which we consider to be pathognomonic of Dr. François' deep dyslexia. Of course, this should not be taken to mean that root identity is excluded as a factor favouring the production of morphological paralexia with closed-class bound morpheme substitution. It should be kept in mind, however, that a number of Dr. François' paralexias suggest very strongly – beyond doubt, in our opinion – that there are families of polymorphemic words which are not read as unitary entities.

Importantly, and as previously illustrated, our study of the locus of errors in Dr. François' morphological paralexias revealed an overwhelming predominance of right-sided deviations, especially with regard to substitutions. One cannot avoid considering the possibility that some form of right visual field neglect might have played a role in his reading behaviour (Friedrich, Walker, & Posner, 1985; Shallice & Warrington, 1980), just as a disorder of this sort has been shown to play a role in the sentence-picture matching behaviours of left brain-damaged right-handed aphasics (Lecours, Lupien, & Parente, 1989; Lecours, Mehler, & Parente, 1987; Tyler, 1969). It is likely, given the disease that led to surgery in the case of Dr. François, that his left optic nerve was compressed at one point. If so, this had left no detectable sequelae when the patient was admitted at the Salpêtrière. Moreover, local left optic nerve involvement should obviously not be expected to cause right visual field neglect. On the other hand, detailed neurological examination of our patient, including routine testing for unilateral neglect, was conducted prior to assessment of his reading abilities and it revealed no evidence of a visual field defect of any sort. Thus, it is our impression that the gross imbalance in favour of the right with regard to locus of error in this case might entirely be accounted for (A) on the basis of characteristics inherent to the morphology of the French language and (B) on that of the structure of the Reading Test, which clearly favoured right-sided errors.

The Closed-Class Word Characteristic

Because Dr. François misread 52% of the words with an open-class component and 57% of the closed-class words of the reading test, it seems that his impression of a particular difficulty inherent to processing the latter – although consistent with the claim that deep dyslexia is characterized by greater difficulty in reading function than content words (Coltheart, 1980a; Morton, 1980) – witnessed to his uncertainty rather than to his abilities. On the other hand, given that 45% of the patient's errors were morphological paralexias, one can rightfully assert that 75% of his total paralexic production involved closed-class morphemes. Therefore, at least in the case of French (and no doubt of many other languages of the Indo-European family), one can argue that deep dyslexia is better characterized by stating that it leads to a particular difficulty in reading free or bound closed-class morphemes as opposed to open-class ones.

It should perhaps be emphasized at this point that the open-class/closed-class opposition that one establishes concerning deep dyslexia is not qualitatively related to error types. What we mean is that semantic and/or formal paralexias can occur irrespective of the target's class. Likewise, it should be said that relationships of these types are not limited to whole word substitutions but can also be documented to exist between closed-class bound morphemes in the context of morphological paralexias.

This being said, the semiological validity of the open-class/closed-class opposition cannot be challenged with regard to deep dyslexia among people who speak a language other than an "isolating" one (Hjelmslev, 1966; Lecours, in press). One might then argue that this dissociation, which is a structural characteristic of many natural languages, does have an impact on brain function or dysfunction. The idea we now wish to convey is that, when they "stand alone" (Taft, 1990), some lexical entries retain their semic potential to a large extent (for instance *strawberry*, *walk*, and *think*) and some lose it to some extent (for instance *also*, *of*, and *notwithstanding*); the former remain far more accessible in deep dyslexia than the latter. Indeed, the essential problem observed in cases such as that of Dr. François – in cases where deep dyslexia coexists with agrammatism (which is at least typical and maybe obligatory) – is that syntactically conventional sentences can neither be read aloud nor spontaneously uttered whereas certain roots, words, and coined expressions – those of which the semic potential is less context-dependent – can both be read aloud in isolation and uttered within conversational exchange. Beyond the obvious impairment in graphophonemic conversion abilities, one has the impression that translexical-meaning attribution is a mandatory (although sometimes not sufficient) condition to spoken verbal output. Of course, it is easier for the listener to decide if meaning attribution is being made in line with convention in the case of reading than in that of spontaneous speech (one who reads *bird* instead of *sparrow* makes an error, whereas the lexical choice of one saying *bird* when one means *sparrow* can easily be perceived as normal in a conversational exchange).

The Non-Word Characteristic

It is legitimate to assert that, consistent with current teachings, Dr. François was "unable to make non lexical derivation of phonology from print" (Coltheart, 1980a). He was unable to read non-words. This being said, his case brings to light a number of points concerning the non-word characteristic of deep dyslexia. Indeed, there are circumstances in which, but for the problem in naming letters, the behaviour of a deep dyslexic hardly differs from that one would expect from a normal reader. Another is that non-words are often recognized as such by deep dyslexics. Irrespective of the above, a third point is that, provided a patient with a rich background of reading habits and an experimental situation which does not induce guardedness, the most likely behaviour to be expected in response to non-word stimuli is paralexia rather than absence of response. Clearly, Dr. François' own behaviour in this respect is best characterized by stating that non-word stimuli led him to formal paralexia whenever such stimuli were visually close enough to a verbal unit with an entry in his logographic input lexicon, which would be consistent with observations reported by Patterson (1978), by Coltheart (1980b), and by Saffran and Marin (1977). As shown in (63) below, it also led him to semic extraction behaviour in some instances:

(63) nipitir ⇒ ...
    Dr. François: Ah! Come now! What's that?
    Not to read. Don't know. Ah! Yes.
    Nif...
    Antique Egypt.
    Ni-fre...
    Ah! Dash! Can't!
    ARL: *Néfertiti?*
    Dr. François: Yes, yes, yes. *Néfertiti.* Good!

At that point, Dr. François remained unaware that the suggested response was wrong. His sublexical pathway was broken but the testing situation allowed him to go into his logographic input lexicon and from there into his semantic knowledge.

A Model

The clinical observation of acquired reading disorders has allowed systematic documentation of a number of facts from which one can infer more or less complex metaphoric representations of the psychological operations behind reading skills (in the present context, reading single words and non-words aloud). The following are examples of such behaviours: as the result of a cerebral disease, (A) certain readers of an alphabetic code can no longer read phonologically legal non-words although their capacity to read familiar words remains intact or nearly so, a nosological entity now labeled as *phonological dyslexia* (Beauvois & Derouesné, 1979; Job & Sartori,

Figure 1.

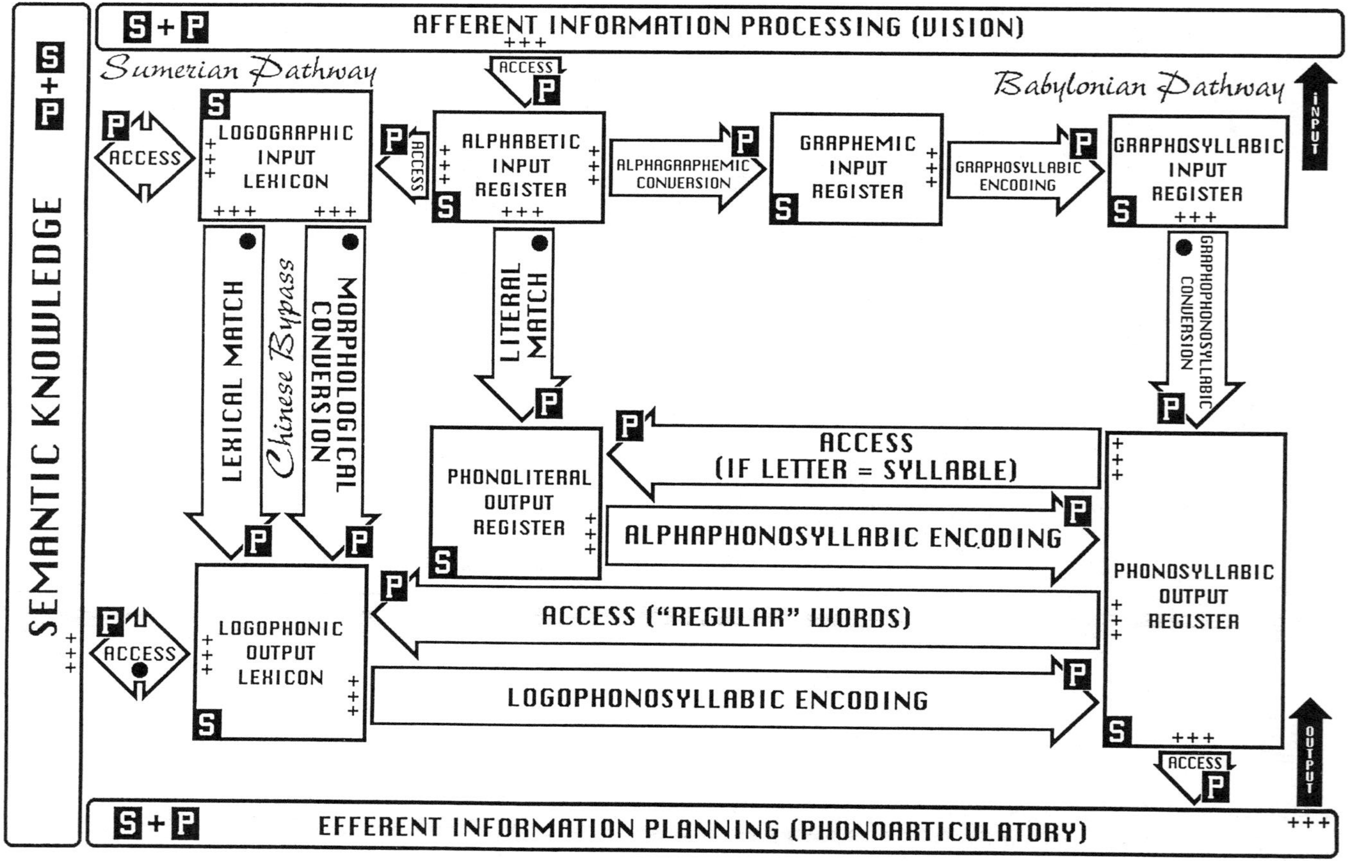

1984); (B) other readers of certain alphabetic codes can no longer conventionally read "irregular" words although their capacity to read "regular" ones remains intact, another exceptional nosological entity now labeled as *surface dyslexia* (Marshall & Newcombe, 1973; Patterson, Coltheart, & Marshall, 1985); and (C) certain brain-damaged readers of a logographic code remain capable of reading isolated words although they no longer access their semantic counterparts (Huang, 1987), a condition we suggest labeling *asemantic reading*.

As to the metaphors, they take the form of *models* usually represented by sets of boxes and arrows as in Figure 1. In this model (Lecours, 1996a), the boxes labeled as *registers* and *lexicons* represent specialized stock memories, whereas all of the arrows represent procedural memories (authorizing interactions between stocks). The boxes labeled as *afferent information processing, efferent information programming,* and *semantic knowledge* include both (unspecified) stock and procedural memories dedicated to particular sets of information (Lecours, 1996a; Lecours & Belleville, 1989). It should be noted at this point that the neural autonomy of all the boxes and of some of the arrows in Figure 1 is demonstrated by clinical observation of various forms of reading disorders resulting from brain lesions, and also by normative experiments (Bub & Lecours, 1987; Joubert & Lecours, in preparation; Lecours, 1996a; Lecours & Tainturier, 1990).

Concerning Figure 1, let us specify (A) that a white *S* within a black square identifies a "stock," (B) that a white *P* within a black square identifies a "procedure," (C) that the hardly specified *S* and *P* within three of the boxes should both be perceived as being more than one, (D) that the "input registers" and the "input lexicon" are postulated to gather abstract entities of exteroceptive origin (visual in the present case) whereas the "output registers" and the "output lexicon" are postulated to gather abstract entities which are at least in part of proprioceptive origin (phonoarticulatory in the present case); (E) that if the components of the "pathways" in this model are assumed to activate themselves sequentially, nothing in it excludes that more than one "pathway" can be working at the same time; (F) that the sets of "+++" within boxes represents the "activation" of sublexical or lexical entities within a stock (another manner of representing "buffers"); and (G) that the five black circles within Figure 1 are there to identify the components which are, in our opinion, dysfunctional in deep dyslexia (we will suggest at a later point that four of the five black circles are compatible with human brain anatomy).

With regard to "pathways," all of them depend at the begining with on afferent (visual) information processing and, for reading aloud, they all depend at the end on efferent (phonoarticulatory) information planning. Two of them are translexical. They rely on direct access to the *logographic input lexicon*; from there, one goes to semantic knowledge and the other to the *logophonic output lexicon*[5]. The other two are sublexical. One transforms letters or groups of letters into graphemes, then into syllables of eye origin; from there, conversion is made into syllables of ear-mouth origin and access to semantic knowledge is eventually possible through the

---

[5] According to Hillis and Caramazza (1991), no scientifically documented evidence has so far been published as to the psychological reality of the interlexical pathway; nonetheless, we consider the anecdotal evidence mentioned above (reading logograms aloud without access to semantic knowledge) as acceptable evidence.

logophonic output lexicon. The other one authorizes arbitrary matching of one's memory of letters sent to eyes into that of letters linked to sound and articulation (Lecours, 1996a).

Our cognitivist interpretation (for alphabetic writing systems) of Dr. François' semiology includes five paper lesions. Two of them impair the sublexical pathways: the patient can neither read phonologically legitimate non-words nor name the letters of a word read conventionally (although the allographic forms of a letter can be identified, orthographic errors can be detected, and recitation of the alphabet is possible). The other two paper lesions disrupt the direct interactions between lexicons, that is *lexical match* and *morphological conversion* (Figure 1). If Dr. François made a number of paralexias facing closed-class words of very high frequency presented in isolation, other patients remain mute when presented such words. On the other hand, Dr. François' morphological paralexias were the most frequent ones and it is known that closed-class bound morphemes can be lexicalized (Tainturier, 1986). As to the 5th paper lesion, if it is indeed a "lesion," it impairs the interactions between semantic knowledge and the logophonic output lexicon.

It has been suggested that the interactions between the logographic input lexicon and semantic knowledge and/or the latter itself can be impaired in deep dyslexia (Bub & Lecours, 1987). Given some of his reading behaviors, our impression is that it was not so in the case of Dr. François. Unless we have misunderstood, it has also been suggested that there is a possibility of direct access to the logographic input lexicon from *afferent information processing* and that this procedure is damaged in deep dyslexia (Coltheart, Patterson, & Marshall, 1987; Gordon, Goodman, & Caramazza, 1986). In our opinion, the existence of this procedure is unlikely if one considers cases of deep dyslexia where the patient can identify the allographic forms of letters he cannot name.

Given that Dr. François either did not read phonologically legitimate non-words or else hesitantly transformed them into an open-class lexical entity, it is clear that the sublexical pathway authorizing access to semantic knowledge for regular words was not functional, in our opinion, at the level of *graphophonosyllabic conversion* (Figure 1), because he could detect faulty graphemes. On the other hand, although the patient could often name letters presented in isolation at the time when he was given the François Reading Test, he nearly always could not name the letters of words he had read correctly even if the stimulus was still in front of his eyes, which no doubt testifies to the fact that his "literal match" procedure (Figure 1) was still dysfunctional at this point. Finally, because Dr. François could not read words – correctly or producing paralexias – without attributing meaning to them, and given his frequent production of morphological paralexias, we postulate that his lexical match and his morphological conversion procedures were also impaired (Figure 1).

As far as we can see, it is a necessity inherent in our "model" that access from written information to the *alphabetic input register* and thereafter to the logographic input lexicon and to semantic knowledge took place normally when Dr. François produced semantic paralexias or semic extraction behaviour. In our opinion, errors were then generated further in the information processing chain. On the other hand, we remain perplexed with regard to the production of formal verbal paralexias. If one does not agree with the possibility of parallel working of more than one pathway, one would then have to postulate that these are the result of mismatches between alphabetic information and logographic entries, which would lead to the addition of a sixth paper lesion.

Now, we remain under the impression that the constitution of a logographic input lexicon among fluent readers (for instance of a highly irregular alphabetic writing system) represents a long-lasting process, the diachrony of which might extend as long as a given individual keeps being exposed to written materials comprising words that he or she has so far not met. Moreover, it seems likely to us that a number of exposures to any given word or morpheme are necessary before stable entries are set in one's lexical memories, and that a stable entry might have better chances to remain so if reinforced once in a while. In other words, it is likely that, at any one time in the life of a given person, a number of entries remain in an unstable state and can only be decoded, in the normal, through several pathways at the same time. Maybe isolation of the first lexical pathway defined above (without damage to it) could be at the origin of deep dyslexia in cases such as that of Dr. François. Perhaps the term *isolation of direct lexicosemantic reading* (the result of an interaction between a morbid biological parameter and a premorbid sociocultural parameter) would befit such a reading disorder.

It might be that the label *isolation of direct lexicosemantic reading* is original but the idea it is meant to convey is not, because the *cas princeps* (seminal case) of deep dyslexia was interpreted in the very same manner by Marshall and Newcombe in 1966 and 1973 and by Newcombe and Marshall in 1980. Various reasons have later led to the rejection of this interpretation (Coltheart, 1980b; Coltheart, Patterson, & Marshall, 1987; Ellis, 1984; Rapp & Caramazza, 1991; Shallice, 1988) including (A) the description of phonological dyslexia by Beauvois and Derouesné (1979), and (B) the fact that normal subjects have been proven capable of lexical reading without resorting to extralexical phonology (Carr & Pollatsek, 1985; Humphreys & Evett, 1985). The latter two motives might be acceptable if it were reasonable – and we do not believe it is – to assert that logographic stock memories are identical from one individual to another within a given cultural community.

Be this as it may, and within the isolation conceptual framework, the production of formal verbal paralexias would be expected, in case of isolation of direct lexicosemantic reading, whenever a less familiar piece of written information (a less stable entry within one's logographic input lexicon) would be in competition with a formally related word having a more stable entry. The quantitative importance of production of visual errors would be linked to the stability and size of the individual's logographic lexical memory (frequency effects and length effects). The production of semantic paralexias, on the other hand, would not only depend on the size and stability of one's semantic knowledge but also on the lesser or greater impact of contextless presentation on the potential meaning(s) of a given stimulus.

This being said, and although we see no reason to postulate the existence of damage to the interacting device between the logographic input lexicon and semantic knowledge in cases such as that of Dr. François, we observe that some of his behaviours might be taken to indicate that, in the normal, the device between semantic knowledge and the logophonic output lexicon (Figure 1) might not be sufficient to insure access to the phonological representations of certain entities, in particular to those of lexicalized closed-class bound morphemes. In this respect, the examples of Dr. François' behaviors are, it seems to us, particularly convincing: indeed, he proved able to access the visual representations of closed-class bound morphemes and to show evidence of an exhaustive knowledge of their semic attribute while their phonoarticulatory representations remained inaccessible. In other words, if one were to insist on the necessity of a functional lesion between semantics and lexicons, one might find reasons to point at the gadget between semantics and logophonic output (Lecours, Lupien, & Bub, 1990).

Given the model presented in Figure 1, a legitimate question might be formulated concerning the effect of brain lesions impairing the direct interactions between lexicons (Figure 1) among readers of a logographic writing system such as that used in China. Before tackling this question, one would probably do well first to find out about the reading behaviors of neurologically healthy logographic readers with a relatively limited level of school education. The reason for this preliminary study would of course be to find out whether or not healthy individuals with a limited knowledge of a writing system of this sort might, in certain circumstances, display a reading behavior somewhat akin to that identified in the present context as deep dyslexia. On the other hand, we know nothing about the clinical manifestations of deep dyslexia among speakers/writers of polysynthetic languages (Hjelmslev, 1966; Lecours, in press), that is of languages with an astounding number of prefixes and suffixes attuning roots. Clearly, agrammatism and deep dyslexia must be quite different in such cases.

In conclusion, it is clear that in order to become a spectacular deep dyslexic, as Dr. François did following his surgical misfortune, one must have a rich premorbid reading background. There are cases in which brain damage of comparable location leads to total alexia or nearly so. As a matter of fact, if Broca's aphasia with agrammatism is sometimes associated with deep dyslexia, it also happens that a patient with Broca's aphasia and agrammatism – presumably resulting from comparable brain lesions – cannot read at all. In our opinion, it is likely that the latter clinical picture occurs either in patients whose reading activities, for some reason or another, have always depended on graphophonemic conversion, or else in patients with a social history characterized by a relatively short period of school education followed by limited and sparse reading-writing activities past this period. Aphasic alexia no doubt varies with site of brain lesions, with writing systems, with level of school education, and with reading and writing habits.

REFERENCES

Adams, R. D. & Victor, M. (1985). *Principles of neurology*. New York: McGraw-Hill.
Alajouanine, T., L'hermitte, F., & de Ribaucourt-Ducarne, B. (1960). Les alexies agnosiques et aphasiques. In T. Alajouanine (Ed.), *Les grandes activités du lobe occipital* (pp. 235-260). Paris: Masson.
Ardila, A. (1989). Personal communication to ARL, Buenos Aires, Argentina.
Badecker, W. & Caramazza, A. (1987). The analysis of morphological errors in a case of acquired dyslexia. *Brain and Language, 32*, 278-305.
Beauvois, M. F & Derouesné, J. (1979). Phonological alexia: Three dissociations. *Journal of Neurology, Neurosurgery and Psychiatry, 42*, 1115-1124.

Bub, D. & Lecours, A. R. (1987). Les troubles acquis de la lecture et de l'écriture des mots: L'approche cognitiviste. In M. I. Botez (Ed.), *Neuropsychologie clinique et neurologie du comportement* (pp. 325-336). Montréal: PUM; Paris: Masson.
Bunge, M. (1980). *The mind-body problem.* Oxford: Pergamon.
Caramazza, A. & Hillls, A. E. (1990). Where do semantic errors come from? *Cortex, 26,* 95-122.
Carr, T. & Pollatsek, A. (1985). Recognizing printed words: A look at current models. In D. Besner, T. G. Walker, & G. E. MacKinnon (Ed.), *Reading research: Advances in theory and practice* (Vol. 5). Orlando: Academic Press.
Célérier, P. (1991). Personal communication to ARL, Bordeaux, France.
Coltheart, M. (1980a). Deep dyslexia: A review of the syndrome. In M. Coltheart, K. Patterson, & J. C. Marshall (Eds.), *Deep dyslexia.* London: Routledge & Kegan Paul.
Coltheart, M. (1980b). Reading, phonological recoding and deep dyslexia. In M. Coltheart, K. Patterson, & J. C. Marshall (Eds.), *Deep dyslexia.* London: Routledge & Kegan Paul.
Coltheart, M. (1980c). Deep dyslexia: A right hemisphere hypothesis. In M. Coltheart, K. Patterson, & J. C. Marshall (Eds.), *Deep dyslexia.* London: Routledge & Kegan Paul.
Coltheart, M. (1983). The right hemisphere and disorders of reading. In A. W. Young (Ed.), *Functions of the right hemisphere* (pp. 172-201). New York: Academic Press.
Coltheart, M., Patterson, K., & Marshall, J. C. (Eds.). (1980). *Deep dyslexia.* London: Routledge & Kegan Paul.
Coltheart, M., Patterson, K., & Marshall, J. C. (1987). Deep dyslexia since 1980. In M. Coltheart, K. Patterson, & J. C. Marshall (Eds.), *Deep dyslexia* (2nd ed.). London: Routledge & Kegan Paul.
Ducarne, B. (1964). *Test pour l'examen de l'aphasie.* Paris: Éditions du Centre de psychologie appliquée.
Ducarne, B. (1966). Personal communication to ARL, Paris.
Ellis, A. W. (1984). *Reading, writing and dyslexia: A cognitive analysis.* Hillsdale, NJ: Lawrence Earlbaum.
Friedrich, F. J., Walker, J. A., & Posner, M. I. (1985). Effects of parietal lesions on visual matching: Implications for reading errors. *Cognitive Neuropsycholoy, 2,* 253-264.
Funnel, E. (1987). Morphological errors in acquired dyslexia: A case of mistaken identity. *Quarterly Journal of Experimental Psychology, 39,* 497-539.
Gordon, B., Goodman, R., & Caramazza, A. (1986). Separating the stages of reading errors. *The Johns Hopkins Cognitive Neuropsychology Laboratory* (Report #28).
Gougenheim, G. (1958). *Dictionnaire fondamental de la langue française.* Paris: Didier.
Hécaen, H. (1972). L'alexie littérale. In H. Hécaen (Ed.), *Introduction à la neuropsychologie* (pp. 45-46). Paris: Larousse.
Hillis, A. E. & Caramazza, A. (1991). Mechanisms for accessing lexical representations for output: Evidence from a case with category-specific semantic deficit. *Brain and Cognition, 40,* 106-144.
Hillis, A. E., Rapp, B., Romani, C., & Caramazza, A. (1990). Selective impairments of semantics in lexical processing. *Cognitive Neuropsychology, 7,* 191-243.
Hinton, G. E. & Shallice, T. (1991). Lesioning an attractor network: Investigations of acquired dyslexia. *Psychologia Review, 98,* 74-95.
Hjelmslev, L. (1966). *Le langage.* Paris: Minuit.
Huang, S. Y. (1987). Personal communication to ARL.
Humphreys, G. W. & Evett, L. J. (1985). Are there independent lexical and nonlexical routes in word processing? An evaluation of the dual-route theory of reading. *The Behavioral and Brain Sciences, 8,* 689-739.
Joanette, Y., Goulet, P., & Hannequin, D. (1990). *Right hemisphere and verbal communication.* New York: Springer-Verlag.
Job, R. & Sartori, G. (1984). Morphological decomposition: Evidence from crossed phonological dyslexia. *Journal of Experimental Psychology, 36,* 435-458.
Joubert, S. & Lecours, A. R. (in preparation). The effect of graphemic parsing in non-word reading.
Joubert, S. & Lecours, A. R. (in preparation). Lettres jouant un rôle diacritique en lecture française.
Joubert, S. & Lecours, A. R. (in preparation). Sublexical frequency effect in non-word reading.
Kaplan, E. & Goodglass, H. (1981). Aphasia-related disorders. In M. Taylor Sarno (Ed.), *Acquired aphasia* (pp. 303-325). New York: Academic Press.
Lecours, A. R. (1996a). *Langage écrit: Histoire, théorie et maladie.* Molinghem: Ortho.
Lecours, A. R. (1996b). Le duel. *Neuropsychologia Latina, 2,* 15-25.

Lecours, A. R. (in press). Language contrivance on consciousness (and vice versa). In H. Jasper, L. Descarries, V. Castelluci, & S. Rossignol (Ed.), *Consciousness: At the frontiers of neurosciences*. New York: Lippincott-Raven.
Lecours, A. R. & Belleville, S. (1989). Structures mutuelles du lexique et de la mémoire. *Rééducation Orthophonique, 27*, 267-302.
Lecours, A. R., Chain, F., Poncet, M., Nespoulous, J. L., & Joanette, Y. (1992). Paris 1908: "The hot summer of aphasiology" or "A season in the life of a chair." *Brain and Language, 42*, 105-152.
Lecours, A. R. & L'hermitte, F. (1970). Recherches sur le langage des aphasiques: 2. Mesure des relations de similarité entre unités linguistiques et modèle de référence pour la description des transformations aphasiques. *Encéphale, 59*, 547-574.
Lecours, A. R., L'hermitte, F., & Bryans, B. (1983). *Aphasiology*. London: Baillière Tindall.
Lecours, A. R., Lupien, S., & Bub, D. (1990). Semic extraction behaviour in deep dyslexia: Morphological errors. In J. L. Nespoulous & P. Villiard (Eds.), *Morphology, phonology, and aphasia* (pp. 60-71). New York: Springer-Verlag.
Lecours, A. R., Lupien, S., & Parente, M. A. (1989). Visual attention in left Sylvian strokes. *Journal of Neurolinguistics, 4*, 255-271.
Lecours, A. R., Mehler, J., Parente, M. A., & collaborators. (1987). Illiteracy and brain damage: 2. Manifestations of unilateral neglect in testing "auditory comprehension" with iconographic materials. *Brain and Cognition, 6*, 243-265.
Lecours, A. R. & Tainturier, M. J. (1990). Perturbations reconnues et perturbations pensables du lexique mental. In P. Morin, F. Viader, F. Eustache, & J. Lambert (Eds.), *Les agraphies* (pp. 243-275). Paris: Masson.
Lordat, J. (1843). Leçons tirées du cours de physiologie de l'année scolaire 1842-1843: Analyse de la parole pour servir à la théorie de divers cas d'alalie et de paralalie que les nosologistes ont mal connus (publiées, avec l'autorisation de Lordat, par son élève Kuhnholtz). *Journal de la Société de Médecine Pratique de Monpellier, 7*, 333-353, 417-433; *8*, 1-17.
Marshall, J. C. & Newcombe, F. (1966). Syntactic and semantic errors in paralexia. *Neuropsychologia, 4*, 169-176.
Marshall, J. C. & Newcombe, F. (1973). Patterns of paralexia. *Journal of Psycholinguistic Research, 2*, 175-199.
Marshall, J. C. & Newcombe, F. (1980). The conceptual status of deep dyslexia: An historical perspective. In M. Colthart, K. Patterson, & J. C. Marshall (Eds.), *Deep dyslexia* (pp. 1-21). London: Routledge & Kegan Paul.
Martinet, A. (1970). *Éléments de linguistique générale*. Paris: Armand Colin.
Morton, J. & Patterson, K. (1980). A new attempt at an interpretation or an attempt at a new interpretation. In M. Coltheart, K. Patterson, & J. C. Marshall (Eds.), *Deep dyslexia* (pp. 22-47). London: Routledge & Kegan Paul.
Patterson, K. E. (1978). Phonemic dyslexia: Errors of meaning or the meaning of errors. *Quarterly Journal of Experimental Psychology, 30*, 587-608.
Patterson, K. E., Coltheart, M., & Marshall, J. C (Eds.). (1985). *Surface dyslexia*. London: Erlbaum.
Patterson, K. E. & Marcel, A. J. (1977). Aphasia, dyslexia and phonological coding of written words. *Quarterly Journal of Experimental Psychology, 29*, 307-318.
Potier, B. (1968). *Introduction à l'étude des structures grammaticales fontamentales*. Université de Nancy.
Rapp, B. C. & Caramazza, A. (1991). Lexical deficits. In M. Taylor Sarno (Ed.), *Acquired aphasia*. Orlando: Academic Press.
Richardson, J. T. E. (1975). The effect of word imageability in acquired dyslexia. *Neuropsychologia, 13*, 281-288.
Ruiz, A., Ansaldo, A. I., & Lecours, A. R. (1994). Two cases of deep dyslexia in unilingual hispanophone aphasics. *Brain and Language, 46*, 245-256.
Saffran, E. M. & Marin, O. S. M. (1977). Reading without phonology: Evidence from aphasia. *Quarterly Journal of Experimental Psychology, 29*, 515-525.
Seindeberg, M. S. & McClelland, J. L. (1989). A distributed, developmental model of word recognition and naming. *Psychological Review, 96*, 523-568.
Shallice, T. (1988). *From neuropsychology to mental structure*. Cambridge, MA: Cambridge University Press.
Shallice, T. & McGill, J. (1978). The origins of mixed errors. In J. Requin (Ed.), *Attention performance*. Hillsdale, NJ: Erlbaum.

Shallice, T. & Warrington, E. K. (1975). Word recognition in a phonemic dyslexic patient. *Quarterly Journal of Experimental Psychology, 27*, 187-199.

Shallice, T. & Warrington, E. K. (1980). Single and multiple components of central dyslexic syndromes. In M. Coltheart, K. Patterson, & J. C. Marshall (Ed.), *Deep dyslexia*. London: Routledge & Kegan Paul.

Taft, M. (1990). Lexical processing of functionally constrained words. *Journal of Memory and Language, 29, 245-25*.

Tainturier, M. J. (1986). *Accès au lexique chez le sujet normal et chez l'aphasique de Broca, mémoire de maîtrise*. Département de psychologie, Université de Montréal, Montréal.

Tyler, H. R. (1969). Defective stimulus exploration in aphasic patients. *Neurology, 19*, 106-11.

DISSOCIATING SPEED FROM AUTOMATICITY IN THE STROOP TASK: EVIDENCE FROM A CASE OF PROGRESSIVE POSTERIOR CORTICAL ATROPHY

Kimberly C. Lindfield,
Harold Goodglass,
and Arthur Wingfield

INTRODUCTION

There have been clinical reports within the last decade (Benson, Davis, & Snyder, 1988; Victoroff, Ross, Benson, Verity, & Vinters, 1994) of a progressive dementia arising from atrophy of the posterior regions of the cerebral cortex. These patients often show an early development of visual agnosia, alexia, anomia, and difficulties in controlling visual gaze. Problems in memory are mild or absent in the early stages, but become severe with the later stages of the illness. Insight is also preserved. According to the Victoroff et al. (1994) report, the three patients who shared this early onset pattern progressed to three different forms of dementia: subcortical gliosis, Alzheimer's disease, and Creutzfeldt-Jakob disease. The implication of this finding is that this form of posterior cortical atrophy is not a disease entity in itself, but, rather, represents an occasional onset pattern of a number of different dementias.

In this paper we describe the clinical course of a patient (J.D.) with a very similar progression of posterior cortical atrophy. He presented initially with focal symptoms of hemianopia and alexia, secondary to parietal lobe atrophy, without a focal lesion. In addition to some unusual clinical observations during the course of his disease, this patient is of interest because of experimental studies carried out on his reading processing, which have theoretical implications for contributions of speed and automaticity during reading.

CASE DESCRIPTION AND EVOLUTION OF THE DISEASE

Initial Presentation

On initial admission to the Aphasia/Neurobehavior Service of the Boston Department of Veterans Affairs Medical Center in February, 1995, J.D. was a 64 year-old right-handed retired salesman with two years of college education. He complained of a three-year history of deteriorating reading and word-finding in addition to increased clumsiness. J.D. was alert and oriented on neurological examination, with normally fluent speech that was marked by occasional word-finding pauses. His auditory comprehension was intact and he followed multiple commands well. His mother had had Alzheimer's disease and died at age 91, two weeks prior to his admission.

J.D.'s ability to read was extremely limited, with difficulty in matching letters and poor matching of easy words to pictures. He could write simple sentences, albeit with spelling errors, but he could not read back what he had written. He had occasional misperceptions of simple line drawings but disproportionately more difficulty in identifying objects in complex scenes, showing a tendency to confabulate for parts of pictures that he could not recognize. He also had difficulty in locating particular objects on a page and in the testing room. He was not prosopagnosic. However, he was apraxic, with very poor imitation of the examiner's movements, albeit with some fluctuation in performance. In addition, J.D. had a right homonymous hemianopia.

Magnetic Resonance Imaging (MRI) revealed severe central and cortical atrophy. No focal abnormalities were seen. The left occipital horn was slightly more enlarged than the right occipital horn, however, suggesting somewhat greater atrophy on the left than on the right. Single Photon Emission Computerized Tomography (SPECT) imaging revealed bilateral posterior temporoparietal hypoperfusion, somewhat more severe on the left than on the right. J.D.'s clinical picture was almost identical to that of Case 1 in the series of cases with posterior cortical atrophy described by Benson et al. (1988).

Because of the absence of a focal lesion, a concerted effort was made to determine whether J.D.'s hemianopia was due to neglect of the right visual field. Both words and pictures were shown to him tachistoscopically on a computer screen, crossing the midline, in such a way that the left portion of the display could be seen as a complete word or picture if the patient did not complete the percept across the midline. In no case did J.D.'s report suggest that he was using information from the right side of the display. It was concluded that he probably had a hemianopia, although the possibility of profound neglect of the right visual field could not be excluded.

Neuropsychological examination estimated J.D.'s Wechsler Adult Intelligence Scale-Revised (WAIS-R) (Wechsler, 1981) Verbal IQ score as 103, with superior scores on Vocabulary, Similarities, and Comprehension subtests, but depressed scores on Digit Span and on Arithmetic subtests. He was virtually unable to do the Performance subtests of the WAIS-R, earning scaled scores of 1 on Picture Completion and Block Design. J.D. attained a Verbal Memory Index of 100 on the Revised Wechsler Memory Scale (WMS-R) (Wechsler, 1988); he was able to learn both easy and hard paired associates by the third trial, and he showed a clear learning curve on the California Verbal Learning Test (Delis, Kramer, Kaplan, & Ober, 1987), with some spontaneous semantic clustering in recall. Although his verbal memory was good, his visual memory was extremely poor, with a Visual Memory index of only 51. His General Memory index was 79.

J.D. was generally very poor in visual perceptual tasks. He performed randomly in matching simple designs to a multiple choice array and solved only 20% of the fragmented objects in the Hooper Visual Organization test (Hooper, 1982). He performed particularly poorly on the Figural Memory subtest of the WMS-R. Tests of executive function revealed difficulty in getting into and maintaining set, and he showed some occurrences of perseveration.

Language examination with the Boston Diagnostic Aphasia Examination (BDAE) (Goodglass & Kaplan, 1983) revealed normally fluent speech output with good articulation and normal sentence construction. His auditory comprehension was in the 70th percentile. His score on the Boston Naming Test (BNT) (Kaplan, Goodglass, & Weintraub, 1983) was in the impaired range, with 33 of 60 pictures correctly named, failures being due to both misperceptions and word retrieval difficulty.

Examination of August 1995

J.D. was reexamined with the reading and writing portions of the BDAE approximately six months after his initial examination. At this time he showed significant deterioration in both modalities. His identification of individual letters was extremely slow and accuracy was undependable. Letter identification in words was dramatically worse than for letters in isolation. This made his ability to read words extremely difficult, both for words standing alone and in simple sentences. On rare occasions, J.D. was successful at reading short words. In contrast, when required to match a spoken stimulus word to a written word presented with foils, he made no errors and appeared to spot the desired word at a glance. Because two of the four foils were structurally similar to the target in this task, it was unlikely that he could have based his choice on the first letter. J.D. recognized eight of eight words spelled orally to him (W-H-I-S-K-E-Y being the most difficult), and he made no errors in spelling words aloud (the most difficult being *seven-twenty-one*).

At this time, J.D. was able to write most of the alphabet, to sign his name, and to write a few primer level words from dictation, but little else. He could not recall how to form an *L* or a *T* on dictation. In his attempt to describe the *Cookie Theft* picture from the BDAE, J.D. now displayed a severe simultanagnosia, focusing on small parts of larger objects without relating them to their wholes, unless asked. When asked what they were a part of, he had no difficulty shifting his gaze from one detail to another and in this way attempting to interpret the entire object.

In spite of these difficulties, J.D. was in excellent social contact, and found his way to the laboratory by himself from a remote suburb using public transportation.

Examination of October 1997

J.D. was admitted for a full work-up and disposition planning approximately two and a half years after his initial examination. His general cognitive status had deteriorated and he had gotten into difficulties by wandering off, which made it impossible to keep him in his custodial residence. At this time, he was no longer oriented to date or place. He believed that the year was 1970 and that the hospital was in Lynn, Massachusetts (the location of his custodial residence). Nevertheless, he remembered many of the details of his trips to the hospital of two years earlier. He was very much aware of the extent of his deterioration and exhibited appropriate affect.

J.D.'s conversation was still normally fluent, but with many more failures of word-finding than had been noted earlier. On formal testing of confrontation naming, his score had dropped to 3 items correct out of 60, without cues. He was now completely unable to name individual letters and he was no longer able to write his name correctly. Visuo-spatial testing revealed further decline since his last examination. He was unable to draw a circle or to copy even the simplest designs. Testing of his visual fields showed that he was no longer hemianopic, although he showed neglect on simultaneous visual stimulation.

Comment on Clinical Features

J.D.'s initial presentation was unusual because of the apparently focal neuropsychological deficits of alexia with partially preserved writing, and anomia, along with right hemianopia, in the absence of a focal lesion. Initially, J.D. had nearly normal memory performance and could give an accurate account of his difficulties. Although this pattern suggested an atypical onset of dementia, affecting some aspects of language, but not memory, his social contact was entirely preserved. Six months later, his written language had deteriorated further, but his memory was still relatively untouched.

On examination 24 months later, the dementing process had spread to include his memory, orientation, and executive functions. Nevertheless, there was a core of self-awareness and personality preservation that appeared to be disproportionate to his cognitive deficits. Remarkably, the apparent profound hemianopia that was initially observed had resolved to a relatively mild visual neglect that could be brought out only on simultaneous stimulation. Thus, the initial possibility that the apparent hemianopia was the result of severe visual neglect proved to be a more likely account. The change in the severity of the neglect might have been caused by changes in the visual attentional system during the progress of his illness.

Imaging Studies

MRI and SPECT studies were each conducted on two different occasions: February 1995 and October 1997.

MRI Results

Figure 1 shows eight MRI slices in axial view taken from each of the two occasions. The top panel shows images taken in February 1995, and the bottom panel presents the October 1997 examination. As can be seen, there is considerable cortical and central atrophy with no indication of localized destruction in either case. The degree of atrophy shown is out-of-proportion to the changes one may expect to see for J.D.'s age. Visual inspection discloses greater atrophy on the second occasion compared to the first. On this second occasion the degree of atrophy is greater within the left occipital region than the right occipital region.

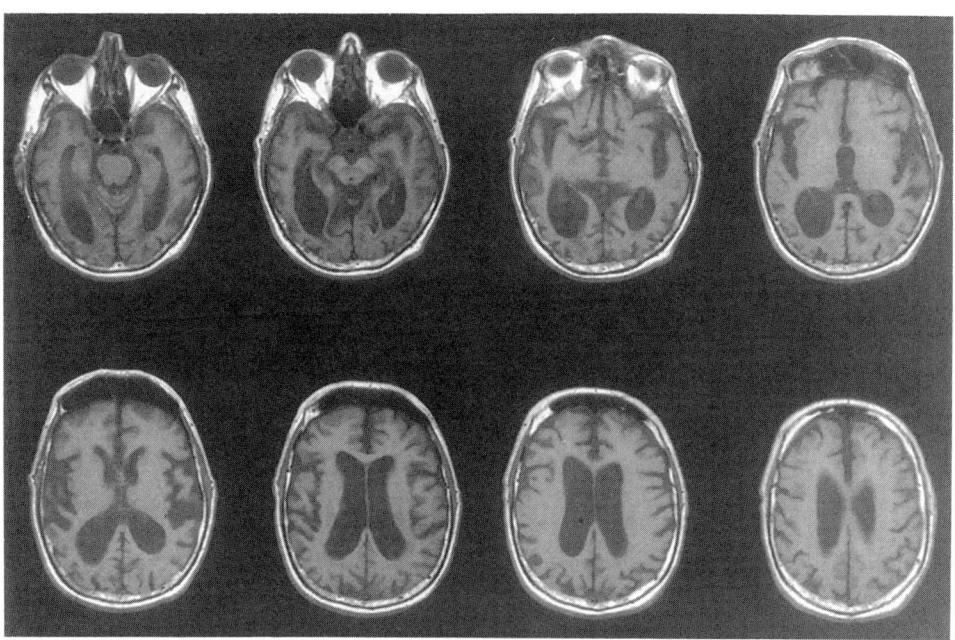

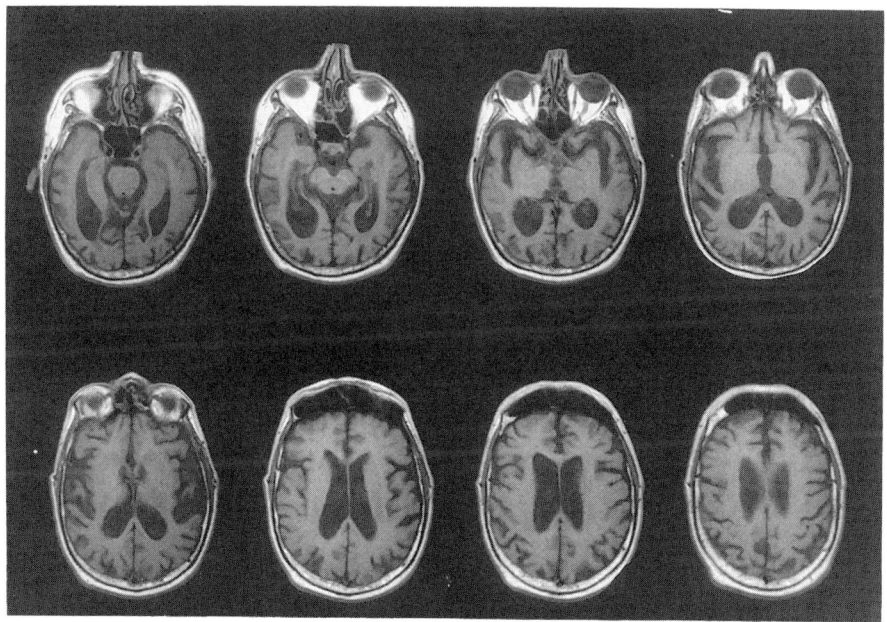

Figure 1. Eight MRI slices in axial view from February 1995 (top panel) and October 1997 (bottom panel) for patient J.D. showing progression of atrophy.

There is also a suggestion of greater atrophy within the occipital polar region as opposed to the frontal polar region, which is consistent with J.D.'s clinical picture.

In each case, the ventricles are enlarged to a degree constant with the level of atrophy. In order to get an estimate of the amount of brain volume loss that had occurred between the two imaging studies, volumetric measures of the ratio of ventricle size to brain size were calculated. This was done using the methods described by Albert, Naeser, Duffy, and McAnulty (1987) (Naeser, Palumbo, Prete, Fitzpatrick, Mimura, Samaraweera, & Albert, 1998). In this procedure, we first traced the borders of the ventricles for each MRI slice of interest. The areas in these tracings were then converted to volume by multiplying the areas on each tracing by the depth of the slice. These volumes were then summed across the eight slices of interest. A similar tracing procedure was used to determine the total volume of brain included in these eight slices. The ratio was determined by dividing the ventricle volume by the brain volume.

At the time of the first study (1995), ventricle volume was determined to be 13% of the total brain volume. This value had increased to 17% of brain volume in 1997, representing an approximate 31% increase in ventricle size over this two year period.

SPECT Results

The February 1995 and October 1997 SPECT studies revealed moderate to severe hypoperfusion bilaterally in the posterior temporoparietal cortex. On the October 1997 examination, greater hypoperfusion was evident in the posterior temporoparietal cortex in the left hemisphere. These findings were consistent with the atrophy noted on the MRI studies.

EXPERIMENTAL EXPLORATIONS

A task that has become automatic has undergone a qualitative change in the way it is carried out through practice (Raichle, Fiez, Videen, MacLeod, Pardo, Fox, & Petersen, 1994; Segalowitz & Segalowitz, 1993). Such tasks are ones that are involuntary and can be carried out with little or no attentional effort. Typically such tasks proceed very quickly and cannot be inhibited once they are initiated (LaBerge & Samuels, 1974; Logan, 1988; Posner & Snyder, 1975; Shiffrin & Schneider, 1977; Tzelgov, Yehene, & Naveh-Benjamin, in press).

Automaticity is essential for higher-order processes such as skilled reading (Logan, 1997; Naslund & Smolkin, 1997; Thurlow & VandenBrock, 1997). Indeed, it has been argued that the difficulty of dyslexic readers is due to an inability to automatize certain components of the reading task. Once the sub-skills of reading, such as phonemic decoding, are performed automatically, the higher-order aspects of the task, including comprehension and metacognitive functions, are performed effectively at the same time (Naslund & Smolkin, 1997; Samuels & Flor, 1997).

Probably the most striking experimental demonstration of reading as an automatic task is the Stroop effect. The Stroop effect is the dramatic difficulty skilled readers have when they are asked to name the ink color of a printed word that spells the name of a different color. The hallmark of this effect is that it is unidirectional. Namely, skilled readers show no difficulty reading color-words when they are presented in different color ink (Stroop, 1935; MacLeod, 1991).

We illustrate the traditional Stroop effect in Figure 2 with data from 16 healthy adults with no history of brain damage or other neuropathology. Their ages ranged from 61 to 70 years ($M = 65$ years), and they had completed an average of 16.7 years of education. The left panel of Figure 2 shows their mean speed of reading aloud color-words printed in black and white (baseline word reading) and their speed of reading color names printed in non-congruent colors (e.g., reading the word *blue* printed in red). In the left panel, we can see that reading the word printed in the non-congruent color did not differ appreciably from the baseline reading condition. The right panel shows the data for color naming. We can see that the time it takes to name a color in the baseline condition is longer than the time to read a word in the baseline condition as seen in the left panel. The final bar shows the critical Stroop interference condition in which subjects were asked to name the color in which words were printed when the word and the print color were non-congruent. We can see that this group of normal adults showed the traditional effect, taking significantly longer to name the print color when it spells the name of a different color-word.

In 1935, Stroop also demonstrated what has come to be known as the reverse Stroop effect. He showed that color naming could interfere with the ability to read color-words printed in different colored ink after giving subjects extensive practice with naming colors over an eight day period. This finding supported his view of the source of interference in these tasks. The extensive practice resulted in faster completion times for naming colors than for reading color-words. Interestingly, however, such interference was no longer apparent on a second testing occasion just a short time later. Reverse Stroop effects have also been demonstrated under conditions in which words were degraded, making them difficult to read (Gumenik & Glass, 1970; Dyer & Severance, 1972).

There are two major theoretical accounts of the Stroop effect (see MacLeod, 1991 for an exhaustive review of this literature). The first, that word reading is faster than color naming, is based on Stroop's original account and has to do with the relative differences in processing speed between the two competing responses. According to this view, the two potential responses, the name of the color ink and the color-word name, occur in parallel and compete with each other for a single output. If the faster of the two responses is not the required response, it would result in the observed interference. That is, the earlier response would interfere with, or block, the slower response. On the other hand, if the faster of the two responses is the required response, no interference would result. This model also nicely accounts for the reverse Stroop effect, since the direction of the interference effect depends on the time relations of the responses involved.

The relative speed of processing view is able to account for the vast majority of important empirical findings of the Stroop effect (MacLeod, 1991). Unfortunately, it fails on the most direct manipulation of its assumptions. Glaser and Glaser (1982) hypothesized that if interference in the Stroop task arises as a result of completion of the faster response before the required slower response, presenting subjects with the slower dimension ahead of time should reduce the amount of interference present in the task. Surprisingly, subjects always showed

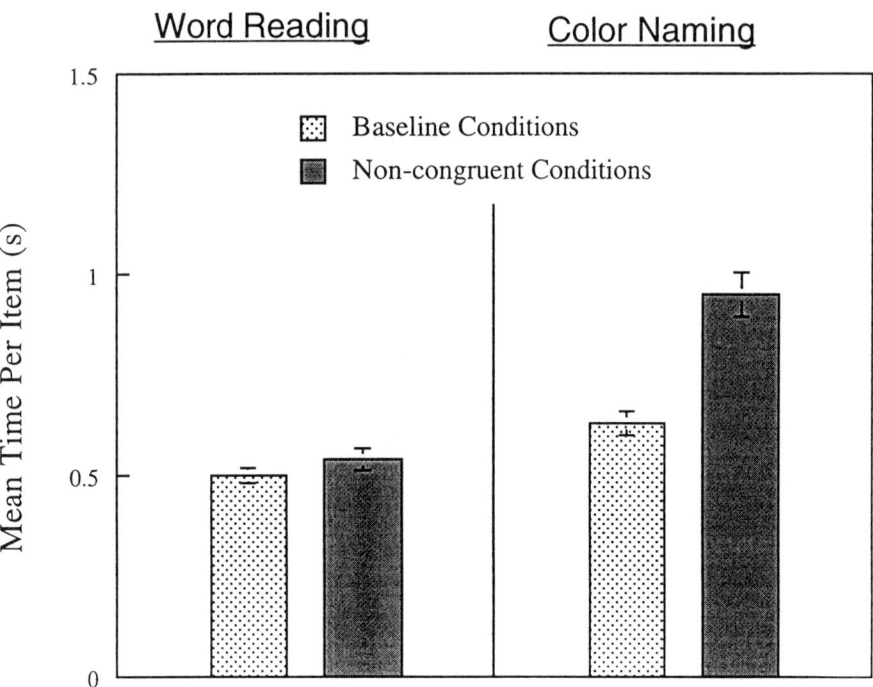

Figure 2. Mean response times per item for word reading (left panel) and color naming (right panel) in the baseline and non-congruent conditions for a group of normal adults.

difficulty in naming the color of the ink (the traditional Stroop effect), even in the condition where the competing color-word was shown 100 milliseconds after the ink color, giving the ink color response a head start. Furthermore, the ability to read color-words was unaffected by manipulating the time intervals of the word and color.

In another study, Dunbar and MacLeod (1984) reported a traditional Stroop effect after altering the orientation of the words so that reading time was considerably slower than naming colors. If interference in this task were due simply to differences in the speed of responses that compete with each other for a single output, such conditions should have led to the observation of a reverse Stroop effect. Taken together with Glaser and Glaser's data, these findings question the idea that interference is due simply to words being processed faster than ink colors (MacLeod, 1991). Nevertheless, the relative speed of processing account is still a widely held view of the Stroop effect.

The second major theoretical account of the Stroop effect has to do with the automaticity of word reading in comparison to color naming. The automaticity of word reading relative to naming ability has been discussed since before the turn of the century (Cattell, 1886). As previously indicated, criteria of automaticity are that the process requires minimal attentional resources, is obligatory, and cannot be interrupted once engaged (LaBerge & Samuels, 1974; Logan, 1988; Posner & Snyder, 1975). Thus, in principle, an automatic but slow response could interfere with a less well-learned but faster response.

Because speed and automaticity are usually inextricably bound in normal behavior, the opportunities in which one can observe the effects of automaticity independent of the effects of speed are quite rare. Our patient J.D. allowed us this rare opportunity. J.D. was tested with the Stroop paradigm on two separate occasions during the course of his progressive dementia. On the first occasion, his reading ability had deteriorated considerably, resulting in his speed of naming colors to be faster than his ability to read color names, the opposite of what is observed in normal behavior.

On the second occasion (approximately six months later), in addition to further decline in his reading ability, J.D. complained of increased difficulty in his ability to name colors. At this time, J.D.'s abilities had deteriorated to a point where there was no difference in his response times for reading color-words and naming colors. Thus, we were given the unique opportunity to examine the effect of automaticity on performance, independent of the advantage of speed.

A description of J.D.'s performance when he was first tested on the Stroop task was reported by Goodglass, Wingfield, Shonewill, and Howerton (1995), and his performance on the second testing session was reported by Wingfield, Goodglass, and Lindfield (1997). In this present paper we place these observations within a more complete context of the clinical course of his illness, and we draw several theoretical inferences concerning the significance of the change in his performance pattern between these two occasions.

Time 1 Testing on the Stroop Task

J.D. was presented with a series of displays on a computer screen consisting of 20 items presented in two parallel columns of 10 items each. Each display required J.D. to either name colors or read color-words presented under the following four conditions.

(1) *Reading Baseline Condition*: In this condition, J.D. was presented with 20 words representing the names of four different colors (red, yellow, green, and blue) printed in black ink. These color names were arranged in random order with each appearing five times. J.D. read the words as rapidly and accurately as he could.

(2) *Color Naming Baseline Condition*: In this condition, each stimulus consisted of a row of four *x's* (*XXXX*) printed in one of the four colors corresponding to the color names (red, yellow, green, and blue). In this case, J.D.'s task was to name the color of each stimulus in succession as quickly and accurately as he could. Each of the four colors appeared five times in random order.

(3) *Reading Color Names Printed in Conflicting Colors*: In this condition, each of the 20 color-words was printed in a color that was different from the name of the printed word (e.g., the word *red* printed in blue, *yellow* printed in green, and so forth). J.D.'s task was to read the printed color names in succession as rapidly and accurately as he could, ignoring the difference in their ink color.

(4) *Naming Colors on Conflicting Words*: In this condition, J.D. saw the same 20 color-words printed in colors different from the color names spelled out by the printed words. This time J.D. was required to report the print color of the words while ignoring the names that they spelled.

Scoring was based on the total time taken from presentation of the set of 20 stimulus items in a particular condition to J.D.'s completing his reading or naming for all of the 20 items. J.D. made very few errors on either reading or color naming, with only one in each condition. He was thus successful in his reading for this small set of four color names, although his reading was slowed. J.D.'s latencies for all four experimental conditions are shown in Figure 3.

There are two key findings represented in this figure. The first is that J.D.'s baseline speed for color naming (right panel) is faster than his baseline speed for reading color-words (left panel). This is the opposite of what one would observe in normal behavior, as typified in Figure 2, where word reading would be faster than color naming. This is presumably a result of the change in J.D.'s reading ability. The second key finding is that J.D.'s reading of words in the non-congruent color condition was very much slower than his baseline reading condition (left panel). That is, opposite to the standard Stroop result, the color of the print interfered with J.D.'s reading of the words. Conversely, in contrast to the normal Stroop results, naming the print colors of non-congruent words was not appreciably slower than the baseline color naming condition (right panel). This constitutes a reverse Stroop effect.

Time 2 Testing on the Stroop Task

On this second testing session, held approximately six months later, J.D. complained of increased reading difficulty as well as further deterioration in his

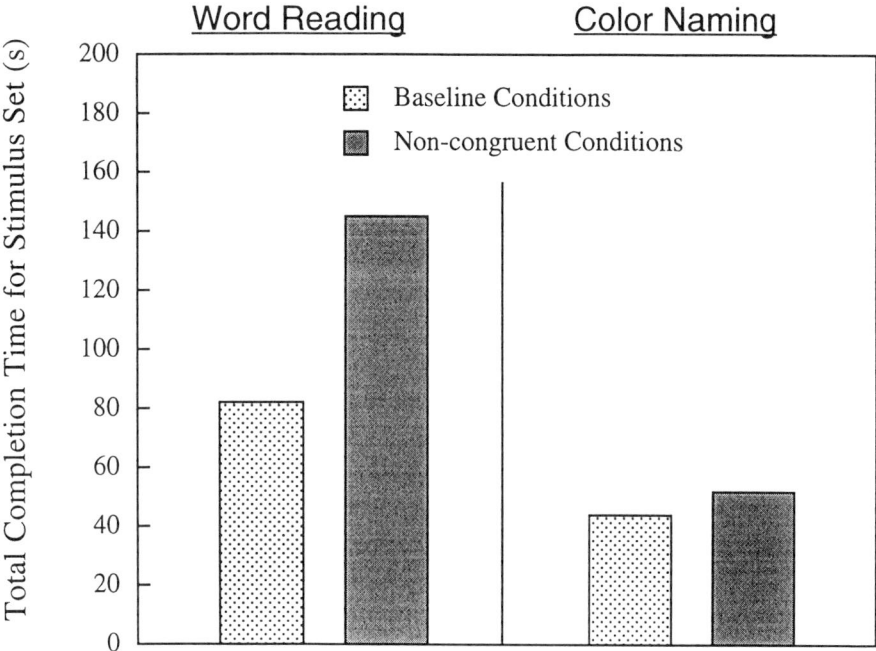

Figure 3. Total times to complete stimulus sets for word reading (left panel) and color naming (right panel) in the baseline and non-congruent conditions for J.D. (first testing session).

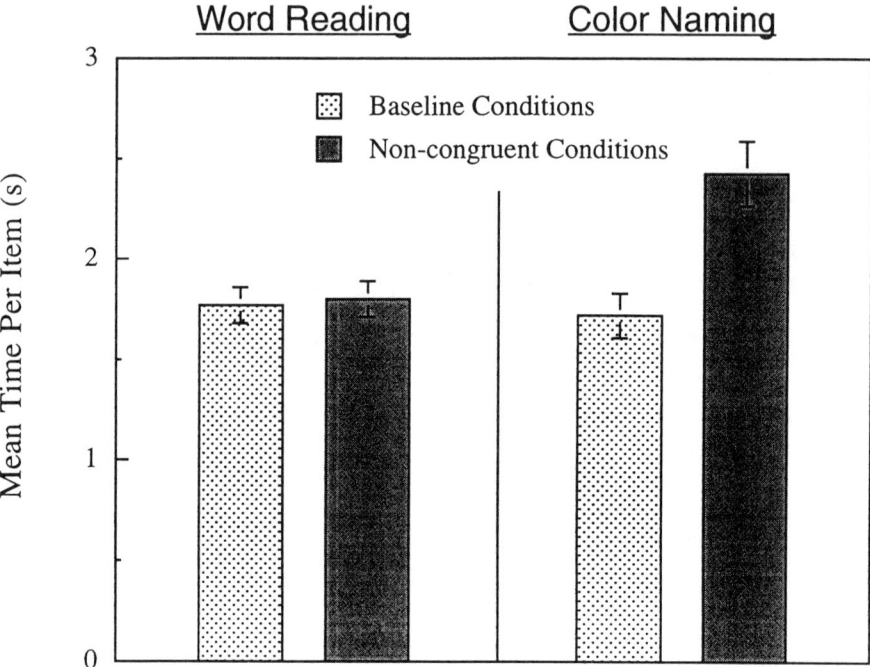

Figure 4. Mean response times per item for word reading (left panel) and color naming (right panel) in the baseline and non-congruent conditions for J.D. (second testing session).

word retrieval, including color naming. J.D. was tested on the Stroop task with the same four conditions. On this occasion, however, the stimuli for each condition were shown one at a time on a computer screen. As each item appeared, J.D. was instructed to respond as quickly as possible into a desk-mounted microphone. Response latencies to his spoken responses were measured via a voice-operated relay with latency measurements made from the moment the stimulus appeared on the computer screen to the onset of his verbal response. This procedure allowed us to obtain individual latencies for each response that was produced.

The mean response latencies per item for this second testing are shown in Figure 4. This time, the latencies for the baseline color naming and word reading conditions did not differ. This finding reflects a greater decline in J.D.'s color naming ability as compared to his reading ability relative to the first testing occasion. As shown in the left panel of Figure 4, J.D.'s speed of reading color-words in the non-congruent color did not differ from his baseline reading condition in this case. Thus, as in the normal subjects, J.D.'s ability to read color names was no longer affected by the presence of a conflicting print color. His speed of naming colors in the non-congruent condition, however, was very much slower than the baseline naming condition, shown in the right panel. That is, on this occasion he showed the traditional Stroop effect as one would expect to see it in normal behavior as illustrated with our normal subject group in Figure 2 (MacLeod, 1991; Stroop, 1935).

Discussion

We have reported on a patient with a progressive reading disorder (J.D.) in whom we have examined performance in the Stroop paradigm on two different occasions during the course of his illness. On the first testing occasion, J.D. presented with a decreased reading ability and a relative preservation in his ability to name colors. This was reflected in his performance in the two Stroop test baseline conditions in which the response times to reading color-words were much longer than his response times to naming colors. On this first occasion, J.D. also showed a reverse Stroop effect. Namely, he required more time to read color-words when they were presented in a non-congruent color in comparison to the baseline condition. J.D.'s ability to name colors, however, was unaffected by the appearance of an interfering color-word.

On the second testing occasion, conducted approximately six months later, J.D. complained of difficulty in his ability to read and name colors. This time, the mean time required to read a color-word was identical to the mean time required to name a color. In addition, J.D.'s ability to read color-words did not differ in the two reading conditions. However, J.D. required more time to name colors when they appeared in the context of non-congruent color-words than when they appeared in the baseline condition. Thus, in this case, J.D. showed the traditional Stroop effect.

This demonstration of Stroop interference in the absence of an advantage in reading speed is consistent with the data reported by Glaser and Glaser (1982) and by Dunbar and MacLeod (1984) that challenge the speed of reading account of the Stroop effect. Under the relative speed of processing view, no interference effects should have been observed in this instance since there is no advantage of processing speed. Our finding of a Stroop effect in the absence of an advantage in reading speed is consistent, however, with the automaticity account of the Stroop effect (Cohen, Dunbar, & McClelland, 1990) (see MacLeod's 1991 review). According to this view, the obligatory nature of word reading would result in interference in color naming when one is asked to name the ink color of a word that spells the name of a different color.

We attribute the finding of a reverse Stroop effect on the first testing occasion to the observation that the response times for the word reading baseline condition were very much longer than those required for the color naming baseline condition, the reverse of the normal relationship (Cattell, 1886). This great disparity in response time for retrieving the color name versus the phonology of the printed word resulted in prior activation of the name of the print color in the non-congruent reading condition, and, hence, the observed difficulty in reading the color-word. Thus, we would like to argue that a large advantage in processing speed of the non-automatic task (e.g., color naming) can result in interference on the automatic task (e.g., word reading) to result in a reverse Stroop effect. In other words, a sufficiently great disparity in processing speed can have the effect of masking or blocking the effects of automaticity.

In the present study, the different combinations of J.D.'s reading and naming ability allowed us to observe performance patterns that could be duplicated in normals only through manipulation of the task stimuli (e.g., Dunbar & MacLeod, 1984) or by presenting the word and the color at different time intervals (e.g., Glaser & Glaser, 1982). That is, in the study of the factors contributing to the Stroop effect in normals, one cannot escape from artificial manipulations of stimulus variables which result in changing the nature of the task. The Stroop effect, however, depends on certain relationships both between subject variables and stimulus characteristics. In J.D., nature has produced changes in his capacities that allowed us to look at the modification of the relationship between subject variables and stimulus variables under standard Stroop administration conditions. This case illustrates the value of unique cases of brain injury in the study of psychological processes such as the Stroop effect.

ACKNOWLEDGMENTS

The research reported here was supported by NIH grant P50 DC00081. The first author acknowledges support from training grant T32 DC00017 to the Boston University School of Medicine. We thank Dr. Margaret Naeser, Dr. Carole Palumbo, and Steven Hodge for their assistance with the imaging studies.

REFERENCES

Albert, M. S., Naeser, M. A., Duffy, F. H., & McAnulty, G. (1987). CT and EEG validators for Alzheimer's disease. In L. W. Poon (Ed.), *Handbook of memory assessment of older adults* (pp. 383-392). Washington, DC: American Psychological Association.
Benson, D. F., Davis, H. J., & Snyder, B. D. (1988). Posterior cortical atrophy. *Archives of Neurology*, *45*, 789-793.
Cattell, J. M. (1886). The time it takes to see and name objects. *Mind*, *11*, 63-65.
Cohen, J. D., Dunbar, K., & McClelland, J. L. (1990). On the control of automatic processes: A parallel distributed processing account of the Stroop effect. *Psychological Review*, *97*, 332-361.

Delis, D. C., Kramer, J. H., Kaplan, E., & Ober, B. A. (1987). *The California verbal learning test-research edition*. New York: Psychological Corporation.

Dunbar, K. & MacLeod, C. M. (1984). A horse race of a different color: Stroop interference patterns with transformed words. *Journal of Experimental Psychology: Human Perception and Performance, 10*, 622-639.

Dyer, F. N. & Severance, L. G. (1972). Effects of irrelevant colors on reading of color names: A controlled replication of the "reverse Stroop" effect. *Psychonomic Science, 28*, 336-338.

Glaser, M. O. & Glaser, W. R. (1982). Time course analysis of the Stroop phenomenon. *Journal of Experimental Psychology: Human Perception and Performance, 8*, 875-894.

Goodglass, H. & Kaplan, E. (1983). *The assessment of aphasia and related disorders* (2nd ed.). Philadelphia: Lea and Febiger.

Goodglass, H., Wingfield, A., Schonewill, W., & Howerton, B. (1995). Alexia and a reverse Stroop effect in a case of posterior cerebral atrophy without focal lesion. *Brain and Language, 51*, 173-176.

Gumenik, W. E. & Glass, R. (1970). Effects of reducing the readability of the words in the Stroop Color-Word Test. *Psychonomic Science, 20*, 247-248.

Hooper, H. E. (1982). *The Hooper visual organization test*. Concordville, PA: Brandywine Associates.

Kaplan, E., Goodglass, H., & Weintraub, S. (1983). *Boston naming test*. Philadelphia: Lea and Febiger.

LaBerge, D. & Samuels, S. J. (1974). Toward a theory of automatic information processing in reading. *Cognitive Psychology, 6*, 293-323.

Logan, G. D. (1988). Toward an instance theory of automatization. *Psychological Review, 95*, 492-527.

Logan, G. D. (1997). Automaticity and reading: Perspectives from the instance theory of automatization. *Reading and Writing Quarterly, 13*, 123-146.

MacLeod, C. M. (1991). Half a century of research on the Stroop effect: An integrative review. *Psychological Bulletin, 109*, 163-203.

Naeser, M. A., Palumbo, C. L., Prete, M. N., Fitzpatrick, P. N., Mimura, M., Samaraweera, R., & Albert, M. L. (1998). Visible changes in lesion borders on CT scan after five years poststroke, and long-term recovery in aphasia. *Brain and Language, 62*, 1-28.

Naslund, J. C. & Smolkin, S. B. (1997). Automaticity and phonemic representations: Perceptual and cognitive building blocks for reading. *Reading and Writing Quarterly, 13*, 147-154.

Posner, M. I. & Snyder, C. R. R. (1975). Attention and cognitive control. In R. L. Solso (Ed.), *Information processing and cognition: The Loyola symposium* (pp. 55-85). Hillsdale, NJ: Erlbaum.

Raichle, M. E., Fiez, J. A., Videen, T. O., MacLeod, A. K., Pardo, J. V., Fox, P. T., & Petersen, S. E. (1994). Practice-related changes in human brain functional anatomy during nonmotor learning. *Cerebral Cortex, 4*, 8-26.

Samuels, S. J. & Flor, R. F. (1997). The importance of automaticity for developing expertise in reading. *Reading and Writing Quarterly, 13*, 107-121.

Segalowitz, N. S. & Segalowitz, S. J. (1993). Skilled performance, practice, and the differentiation of speed-up from automatization effects: Evidence from second language word recognition. *Applied Psycholinguistics, 14*, 369-385.

Shiffrin, R. M. & Schneider, W. (1977). Controlled and automatic human information processing: II. Perceptual learning, automatic attending and a general theory. *Psychological Review, 84*, 127-190.

Stroop, J. R. (1935). Studies of interference in serial verbal reactions. *Journal of Experimental Psychology, 47*, 499-504.

Thurlow, R. & VandenBrock, P. (1997). Automaticity and inference generation during reading comprehension. *Reading and Writing Quarterly, 13*, 165-181.

Tzelgov, J., Yehene, V., & Naveh-Benjamin, M. (1997). From automaticity to memory and vice versa: On the relations between automaticity and memory. In J. Brezinski, B. Krause, & T. Maryszewski (Eds.), *Idealization in psychology: Poznan studies of the sciences and humanities* (pp. 239-261). Amsterdam-Atlanta: Rodopi.

Wechsler, D. (1981). *Wechsler adult intelligence scale* (Rev. ed.). New York: The Psychological Corporation.

Wechsler, D. (1988). *Wechsler memory scale* (Rev. ed.). New York: Psychological Corporation.

Victoroff, J., Ross, G. W., Benson, F., Verity, M. A., & Vinters, H. V. (1994). Posterior cortical atrophy. *Archives of Neurology, 51*, 269-274.

Wingfield, A., Goodglass, H., & Lindfield, K. C. (1997). Separating speed from automaticity in a patient with focal brain atrophy. *Psychological Science, 8*, 247-249.

THE ROLE OF MEMORY IN ESTIMATING TIME: A NEUROPSYCHOLOGICAL ANALYSIS

Marcel Kinsbourne

I am soft sift in an hourglass.
  -Gerard Manley Hopkins, The Wreck of the Deutschland

The yardsticks for the fourth dimension are the hourglass, the sundial, and the clock. But when people remember how long ago a remote event occurred, no clocks are still running, and their estimates are based on inferences from episodic memory. But is that also true for intervals of time measured in seconds rather than years?

In this discussion, I consider evidence about how people go about estimating the duration of intervals of time (of intermediate length, more than a second or two, but not much in excess of a minute). I characterize difficulties that patients with Korsakoff's syndrome and patients with frontal lobe damage experience with time estimation and use these findings to choose between competing models of the underlying brain mechanism. The studies further clarify both the nature of the patients' cognitive difficulties and the nature of the mental operations that normal people deploy when they judge how long a sequence of events has lasted.

Aristotle (reprinted in McKeon, 1941) was of the opinion that "the organ whereby [animals] perceive time is also that whereby they remember." Current opinion is at odds with Aristotle's claim and adopts a less parsimonious position: that a "biological clock" underlies the ability to estimate past time. The functioning of this hypothetical facility does not implicate memory. I shall review neuropsychological evidence that weakens the case for a clock and supports Aristotle's unitary point of view with respect to the critical role of memory in estimating past time.

The ability to estimate the duration of intervals of time is paralleled by a subjective sense of time passing. Does this subjective awareness of time passing imply that the passing of time is directly perceived – a sixth sense for the fourth dimension, as it were – or does the brain preconsciously infer time by attending to cues that arise during intervals, regardless of modalities involved? Contrary to Bergson (1896), who championed a "pure time sense," no amodal sensors for time have been discovered, and estimates of past time are subject to a number of well documented biases related to what people are doing during the interval and to what their expectations are. Time is inferred rather than directly experienced. By what mechanism, where represented in the brain, is this accomplished?

In uncontrolled naturalistic settings there are numerous, qualitatively different, routes to estimating distance in time (analogous to the several ways of visually estimating distance in space). Duration may be inferred based on expectancy (how long it *should* take), experience (how long it *usually* takes), task difficulty (how long it *could* take), and, for longer intervals, on factors such as fatigue, impatience, and boredom. We look for a mechanism that estimates duration when such factors are irrelevant or held constant. To quantitate estimates of the duration of past time, the following controlled paradigms are used: (1) Time production: The subject is told how long (in seconds or minutes) the desired interval should be. He indicates the point in time after the trial has begun at which he feels the specified duration has been reached. (2) Time reproduction: The subject attends to a duration demarcated by the investigator and reproduces it. (3) Time estimation: A specified period of time elapses, at the end of which the subject offers a duration estimate (in seconds or minutes). In each case, the interval is either left empty – that is, void of task requirements – or is filled by a uniform succession of displays and uniform requirements for performance by the subject.

Present time is estimated by a production method. For instance, the subject advances a counter at what she takes to be a one-per-second rate. The actual rate of advance, as a function of clock rate, represents the individual's subjective rate of present time passing, or cognitive tempo, moment by moment. Theoretically, one could also have a counter automatically advanced at a given rate and have the subject estimate that rate in units of time per count. In contrast, reproduction inevitably implicates past time and therefore cannot be used to evaluate present time.

For past time estimation, time reproduction is also not the optimal procedure, because it is confounded by a memory requirement. In addition, time production and reproduction are subject to confounding by individual variation in the ability to inhibit responding. An impulsive individual may prematurely terminate the production or reproduction. If this happens, then the estimate of duration that results does not reflect time past but the impairment in impulse control. Individuals with attention deficit hyperactivity disorder and with prefrontal damage are particularly apt to terminate actions prematurely for lack of impulse control. Production is therefore not a straightforward measure of time past in patients like those that are pertinent for the present discussion, namely patients with frontal lobe damage and also those with Korsakoff's syndrome, some of whom are thought to exhibit symptoms of frontal lobe dysfunction as well.

The method of time estimation, when corrected for rate of present time passing (Frankenhauser, 1959) is not subject to confounding by impulsivity or by the need to hold the standard in memory and is preferable for studying the sense of time passing. It does utilize an intervening variable, the semantic memory of the length of time units (seconds or minutes) and would not be suitable for those in whom that knowledge is in question. Time estimation is performed under either of two conditions: retrospective and prospective.

The retrospective paradigm has the subject engage in an activity without being forewarned that duration will be an issue. Only when he is done, or when he is interrupted by the experimenter, is he told to estimate how long he was engaged in the activity. To do this he has to think back over what he has done, and infer, as best he can from what he can remember, how long it took. This is a single trial method. After one trial the subject is alerted to the fact that duration may be an issue, and subsequent trials necessarily incorporate a prospective element.

The prospective paradigm has the subject alerted at the start of the first trial to the fact that she will be asked to estimate the time the trial took when it is over. She is therefore at liberty to engage in whatever maneuvers she believes might assist time estimation during the period to be timed.

Holding intervening activity constant normal, subjects make shorter estimates under retrospective than prospective conditions (Hicks, Miller, & Kinsbourne, 1976; Kinsbourne & Hicks, 1990). Retrospectively, the subject has to rely on memory to recapture what happened and base his estimate on as many events as he can recall (*storage-size hypothesis* of Ornstein, 1969). Assuming some loss from perception to memory, this will be less than what actually happened, and the retrospective judgments are indeed typically underestimates. Prospectively, the subject is able to combine his ongoing activity with any mental operation that might help him come closer to correct (clock) answer than he can in retrospect. What does he do to bring this about? Explanations fall into two classes. One proposes two quite different mechanisms for the two types of time estimation, and one proposes similar mechanisms. The first assumes a metric of duration that does not involve memory; the second supposes that, as in the retrospective paradigm, memory is crucially involved. In this analysis, I use the findings from patients with memory impairments to determine whether prospective time judgments depend on accurate remembering or not.

The prevalent view, invoked among others by Hicks, Miller, and Kinsbourne (1976) is that, forewarned about the relevance of time, the subject foregoes memory-related strategies and instead activates a clock or counter that is represented in some form in her brain (Thomas & Weaver, 1975). At the end of the interval the amount of time past can be read from the "clock face," or its equivalent. The existence of such a counter has been proposed by many theorists after it was first broached by Hoagland (1935). It is widely applied to issues of temporal sequencing of responses as well as timing per se, in animals and man. This hypothetical counter is either started when the trial begins, or its then current reading is noted (unconsciously). It is cumulatively incremented as time passes, and at the end of the trial the brain "reads off" the sum total time, and the subject responds accordingly. According to scalar timing theory (Church, 1984), the following components exist: a pacemaker, an accumulator that tallies the count, and a switch between them that opens when the subject attends to time.

If patients with brain lesions render flawed estimates of duration, this could manifest in either or both of two ways: They are randomly more variable than normal, or they systematically deviate from clock time (over- or under-estimating). In terms of scalar timing theory, excess variability could reflect a damaged counter which has become unstable, or a switch that sticks at some times and swings loose at others. Underestimates could be due to one of two reasons: the counter runs too slowly, or the counter's capacity is pathologically restricted (the switch sticks?). In overestimates the counter runs too fast.

The clock metaphor at the neurological level bears a one-to-one relationship with the ability to estimate past time at the level of behavior. Whenever a theoretical model, which is attributed to a lower level of organization, is in one-to-one relationship to the higher level phenomenon to be explained, it should be questioned as lacking in explanatory value. In neuropsychology one is not content to assume complete transparency of the underlying brain, and for instance ascribe a reading deficit to damage in the reading center, a writing deficit to an impaired writing center, and so forth. The cognitive neuropsychologist searches for underlying component processes or primitives on which the performance is based. Ascribing prospective timing to a timing device in the brain, and a timing deficit to damage of such a device, is similarly uninformative. Certainly, because people can estimate time, something in the brain enables them to do so. But simply switching a clock on and off seems to be a simplistic construct. Could time instead be transduced from other already known sources of information?

I suggest an alternative view for consideration in light of the neuropsychological evidence. This view does not require the assumption of a counter. Instead, time past is inferred from the number of transitions in the situation or task that can be ascribed to the target interval (cf. Fraisse, 1963), similar to the cues that Block (1978) hypothesized to underlie time estimations performed retrospectively. According to this view, which I shall call *encoding for timing theory*, subjects use their memory ability in prospective time estimation, just as they do in the retrospective condition. But when they know ahead of time that time is an issue, then they can enhance their prospects for subsequent accurate time estimation by encoding events during the interval in such a way as to render them easier to retrieve at judgment time. During the test interval, they specifically attend to cues for transitions between events, as it were to fixate them for subsequent retrieval. The more cues they retrieve, the longer the duration estimates at which they arrive, and the closer they are to actual clock time.

A transition can occur in the display, or in the mind of the observer. It is change in the contents of experience from moment to moment, or a change in a subjective state that is sensitive to, anticipates, or longs for, such transitions. The sense of a transition happening would then depend, at least, on the display, the activity required, the extent to which the activity leaves attention available for registering transitions in the circumstances or the subjective state (Hicks, Miller, & Kinsbourne, 1976), the amount of information that can be maintained in parallel in the present or working memory, and the subjects' expectation of (Jones & Boltz, 1989) and desire for (Curton & Lordahl, 1974; Cahoon & Edmonds, 1985) changes.

Given an interval during which the task the individual performs and his mental set do not change, a strong prediction of the counter mechanism is that the ratio of estimated time to clock time should be roughly constant across duration, as should be the associated Weber fraction (either indefinitely, or until the counter grinds to a halt). This predicted linear relationship between the two variables is indeed found in normal subjects across the time intervals of current interest. The ratio of estimated time to clock time is typically 0.9 (Eisler, 1976).

If the counter is lesioned, how might this affect time judgments? Total inactivation would render every duration judgment retrospective, and the difference in estimates that the two paradigms yield would disappear. If the pacemaker slows down or speeds up, present time judgments will correspondingly deviate. If the accumulator becomes limited in its capacity, duration judgments would be veridical up to a limit, beyond which they would progress no further. If the switch becomes sticky, then the tally from which duration is inferred would lag, and time past would be underestimated. Note that in all these hypothetical situations, though the ratio of estimated to clock time would change, the linear relationship between the two variables is preserved (over the range across which they vary). Does this invariance over time of the ratio also obtain in people with brain injury? I first address the experience of time of patients with alcoholic Korsakoff's syndrome (Butter & Cermak, 1980).

The literature that implicates subjective time sense in Korsakoff's syndrome originated in Korsakoff's own pioneering (1890) report, and extends through multiple publications to the present time. Case descriptions of temporal disorientation abound (e.g., Williams & Zangwill, 1950), and these difficulties with past time have even been considered to be the root cause of the Korsakoff amnesia (van der Horst, 1932). Events in the public domain are frequently misdated by many years, and their sequence in time is often reversed. Specifically, underestimation of time (for instance, after admission to the hospital) is very commonly noted, for instance by Talland (1965). He writes of

> the collapse of the amnesic patients' time scale, their tendency to telescope oft-repeated occurrences into one or a few occasions, and their frequent confusion of the order of events.

There has been speculation about an absence of normally available time markers for events. Lacking these, forgetting of events is thought to be inevitable and perhaps also of the duration that the forgotten events occupied. However, what exactly a time marker is supposed to be is not clear. If it is the clarity of the event memory that indicates how recent the corresponding event is, then the unclear event memories of Korsakoff patients should lead them to overestimate the intervening interval. Overestimation of time is not the predominant tendency in Korsakoff's syndrome. However, if Korsakoff patients are simply unable to estimate time past beyond very short intervals, then the distinction between different time intervals collapses, and it becomes understandable why they are so confused about when things happened.

Talland (1965), Richards (1973), Oscar-Berman, Zola-Morgan, and Oberg (1982), and Shaw and Aggleton (1994) all reported impaired, specifically curtailed, time judgments in Korsakoff's syndrome. But because of the time judgment paradigms they used, all three studies were confounded by a failure to rule out diminished response inhibition, as discussed above. Using an experimental design adapted from Frankenhauser (1959) that had subjects read digits presented singly at a one-per-second rate, Kinsbourne and Hicks (1990) reported on time estimations of Korsakoff's syndrome patients, with chronic alcoholic and normal contrast groups. They found the following: a normal rate of present time (inferred from the rate at which they advanced a memory drum at a requested one per second rate); normal or near normal prospective time estimates for intervals up to 30 seconds; and grossly curtailed estimates for longer intervals, in proportion to their length. At each interval, including the briefest, the estimates of the Korsakoff patients were much more variable than those of the contrast groups.

Because the Korsakoff group's rate of present time passing was normal, the impaired time estimates cannot be attributed to a slowed cognitive tempo. The apparent discontinuity between estimates below and above 30 seconds fits poorly with clock theory; one would not expect a change in the rate of increment of a counter, holding constant the task, as intervals increase. Nor, if one were to fit a single exponential curve to the data, would one expect so dramatic a departure from linearity. The discontinuity/nonlinearity does fit, however, with a noncounter theory that invokes both selective attention and episodic remembering, as invoked above.

According to this account, subjects who are forewarned about an impending requirement to estimate duration still have to remember relevant aspects of the contents of the test interval, like they do when estimating purely retrospectively when the time for the judgment arrives. But for the duration of the trial, and to the extent they are not preoccupied with the task at hand, they can selectively attend so as to fixate interval-related cues for easier subsequent retrieval. These cues are perhaps transitions between external features and/or internal states, as suggested above. If the task is difficult and attention-consuming, they have less opportunity for temporally-related selective attending, and their estimates are correspondingly shorter (*shared attention model* of Hicks, Miller, & Kinsbourne, 1976). When the task is easy and routine, as it was in the Kinsbourne and Hicks study, there is ample opportunity for selective attention followed by attempted retrieval. But, in the case of Korsakoff's syndrome, the hallmark impairment of episodic memory (Kinsbourne & Wood, 1975; 1982) intervenes. Even though the subjects presumably attend with the set to remember, their episodic memory system is so compromised that they can retrieve hardly any event that is not extremely recent.

Korsakoff patients can hold information in mind for an appreciable period of time, as attested by their normal memory spans (Talland, 1965). But the least interference or change in mental set results in strikingly rapid forgetting (Kinsbourne & Wood, 1975). So, in the Kinsbourne and Hicks experimental situation, the patient can recover contents accumulated up to one internal wavering of mental set, which leaves him virtually unable further to increase his estimate. So a group of Korsakoff patients can on average, to some diminishing extent, recover contents accumulated during the previous 10 to 30 seconds, and extract appropriate cues on which to base a judgment which is only a modest underestimate. But for longer durations, the patient could only increment his estimate if he could recover, in addition to recent cues, ones that are one-half or one minute old and have slipped from immediate awareness, a challenge his impaired episodic retrieval ability cannot meet. The Korsakoff patient therefore increments his estimate only minimally with respect to the cues on which normal subjects base their estimates in excess of about half a minute.

The Korsakoff group mean estimates are close to normal below one-half a minute, and the widening shortfall thereafter is paralleled in part by a similar discrepancy between prospective and retrospective time estimates in normal subjects. For durations up to about one-half minute, they are nearly the same. For longer durations, the retrospective performance falls off (Kinsbourne & Hicks, 1990; Predebon, 1995) – though by no means as steeply as in the amnesics.

The variability of estimates at all tested durations further documents the negative effect of the memory deficit on the subjective sense of time past. Talland (1965) remarked on Korsakoff amnesic patients' very general propensity to close their search for the correct response prematurely, leaving their estimates of time (and other variables) rough and approximate. Properly executed episodic remembering is an indispensable component of time estimation, prospective as well as retrospective. The metaphor of a clock/counter does not accommodate this memory constraint. Can the clock model be salvaged nonetheless?

In proposing a mechanism for any neuropsychological deficit, two options are available. One can attribute the defective performance to an impairment of functioning of the processor that performs the mental operation in question in the intact brain. The form that this impairment assumes can be used as evidence about the manner in which the mental operation is normally executed in the brain. Or one can suppose that this processor was completely inactivated by the lesion and has relinquished control over the task. One then attributes the residual performance to an effort at compensation by residual undamaged but less appropriately specialized brain. In the latter case, one can maintain that the strategy the patient uses is not representative of the way the mental operation in question is normally performed. The findings are then not relevant for normal functioning. In the first case, the nature of the deficit can cast light on the nature of the corresponding intact performance, whereas in the second case it cannot.

According to the second, less parsimonious but nonetheless viable option, one could argue that, in addition to the episodic memory system, the time counter is lesioned in Korsakoff's syndrome, as a second independent deficit. In the absence of an available clock the patients are thrown back upon a memory strategy, as in retrospective judgments, which, however, given their memory problem, serves them poorly. More specifically, it cannot be the counter element that becomes unavailable to Korsakoff patient, because his subjective rate of present time passing is normal. It would have to be the accumulator element of the scalar timing model that is limited in capacity (or the switch that sticks in the closed position). Such an explanation is not ruled out, but its tortured post-hoc character counts against it. It would be premature to assume it, and to abdicate responsibility for using the findings to contribute to the main goal of cognitive neuropsychology: to discover how the brain normally works.

Our findings also address van der Horst's time deficit theory of the mechanism of Korsakoff amnesia. Because these patients are virtually unable to experience durations longer than a minute or so, they are understandably at a loss when they search their memory for the time that has elapsed after some personally important or publicly notable event has occurred. They search their preserved knowledge base, and come up with estimates that are little more than guesses. They cannot critically monitor against their subjective sense of time past, because that sense fails them. In sum, their problem with timing is fully explained by their memory deficit, and need not be considered primary or independently present.

Our recent findings with frontally lesioned patients complement this account. Using a similar paradigm to that of Kinsbourne and Hicks (1990), Mimura,

Kinsbourne and O'Connor (in press) found estimates that for short (less than 30 seconds) durations were pathologically increased. As the interval extended from ten through 20 to 30 seconds, the relative excess over normal duration judgment decreased, and ultimately reversed to a mild shortfall. This effect was found in proportion to defective performance on the Wisconsin Card Sorting Test, a test that is sensitive to prefrontal functioning (Greve, Williams, Haas, Littell, & Reinoso, 1996), both in the frontal group and in a Korsakoff contrast group. The relationship was contributed by Greve et al.'s factor 1 of the test, representing perseveration of mental set.

Frontally lesioned patients are well known to find it difficult to hold multiple items of information concurrently in awareness; their episodic memory may be intact or mildly impaired. I propose that the subjective sense of time passing within the short (less than 30 seconds) memory range is based on the extent to which items have turned over (faded from awareness and been replaced) after the duration began. The rapid fading and replacement of contents from short term store suggests to the frontal patient that more time has elapsed than is actually the case. (That is, it offers more than the expected number of transitions.) Correspondingly, their duration estimates are excessively long. In the Mimura et al. (in press) data, this effect is greatest for the shortest interval tested, 10 seconds, and declines as the interval grows longer, to reverse beyond 30 seconds. I propose that as durations become longer, the inflationary tendency due to over-rapid turnover in awareness is increasingly counteracted by a degree of episodic memory weakness, so that the resultant estimates become progressively more attenuated.

Though it is different from that found in Korsakoff's syndrome, the function that describes the relationship of frontal patients' time estimates relative to the duration of the interval similarly fits poorly with the assumptions of clock/counter theory. Again one could salvage the model by invoking an inactivated clock, and the use of a memory strategy of limited efficacy in its place. Again, the post hoc nature of the assumption weakens the clock/counter theory.

It is no more mandatory to infer a clock for estimates within the short term range than it is beyond that range. The clock metaphor is an instance of a type of model that shifts level of analysis without gaining generality. The logic is as follows: The person can estimate time without explicitly counting. Therefore, there is a clock in his brain that implicitly counts for him. To date, no such clock has been discovered in the brain. Such one-to-one correspondences between the question and the answer may truly exist, but before making the shift from behavior to brain, it is appropriate to attempt a solution at the behavioral level. The behavior-brain correspondence that then becomes apparent may be closer to the truth.

In summary, the dominant clock/counter metaphor predicts an invariant ratio of estimated time to clock time across durations during which subjects are uniformly engaged. This linearity has often been confirmed for normal subjects. But a linear model fails to describe the performance of certain patients whose neural equipment for antecedents of the subjective time sense has been fractionated by focal injury. The neuropsychological evidence enables us to approximate more closely the mechanism of this very general and widely available ability to estimate past time, without the ad hoc assumption of a counter instantiated in the neural network. With respect to the role of memory in time estimation, Aristotle's claim is supported.

REFERENCES

Bergson, H. (1896). *Matière et mémoire*. Paris: Alcan.
Block, R. A. (1978). Remembered duration: Effects of event and sequence complexity. *Memory and Cognition*, 6, 320-326.
Butters, N. & Cermak, L. S. (1980). *Alcoholic Korsakoff syndrome: An information processing approach to amnesia*. New York: Academic Press.
Cahoon, D. & Edmonds, E. M. (1985). The watched pot still won't boil: Expectancy as a variable in estimating the passage of time. *Bulletin of the Psychonomic Society*, 16, 115-116.
Church, R. M. (1984). Properties of the internal clock. *Annals of the New York Academy of Sciences*, 423, 566-584.
Curton, E. D. & Lordahl, D. S. (1974). Effects of attentional focus and arousal on time estimation. *Journal of Experimental Psychology*, 103, 861-867.
Eisler, H. (1976). Experiments on subjective duration 1868-1975: A collection of power function exponents. *Psychological Bulletin*, 83, 1154-1171.
Fraisse, P. (1963). *The psychology of time*. New York: Harper and Row.
Frankenhauser, M. (1959). *Estimation of time*. Stockholm: Alquist and Wiskell.
Greve, K. W., Williams, M. C., Haas, W. G., Littell, R. R., & Reinoso, C. (1996). The role of attention in Wisconsin Card Sorting performance. *Archives of Clinical Neuropsychology*, 11, 215-222.
Hicks, R. E., Miller, G. W., & Kinsbourne, M. (1976). Prospective and retrospective judgment of time as a function of the information processed. *American Journal of Psychology*, 89, 719-730.
Hoagland, H. (1935). *Pacemakers in relation to aspects of behavior*. New York: Macmillan.
Jones, M. R. & Boltz, M. (1989). Dynamic attending and responses to time. *Psychological Review*, 96, 459-491.
Kinsbourne, M & Hicks, R. E. (1990). The extended present: Evidence from time estimation by amnesics and normals. In G. Vallar & T. Shallice (Eds.), *Neuropsychological impairments of short-term memory* (pp. 319-330). London: Cambridge University Press.
Kinsbourne, M. & Wood, F. (1975). Short-term memory processes and the amnesic syndrome. In J. A. Deutsch (Ed.), *Short-term memory* (pp. 258-291). New York: Academic Press.
Kinsbourne, M. & Wood, F. (1982). Theoretical considerations regarding the episodic-semantic distinction. In L. Cermak (Ed.), *Human memory and amnesia* (pp. 195-218). Hillsdale, NJ: Erlbaum.
Korsakoff, S. S. (1890). Eine Psychische Störung Combiniert mit Multipler Neuritis (Psychosis polyneuritica seu cerebropathia psychica toxaemica). *Allgemeine Zeitschrift für Psychiatrie*, 46, 475-485.
McKeon, R. P. (Ed.) (1941). *The basic works of Aristotle*. New York: Random House.
Mimura, M., Kinsbourne, M., & O'Connor, M. (in press). Time estimation by patients with frontal lesions and by Korsakoff amnesics. *Journal of the International Neuropsychological Society*.
Ornstein, R. E. (1969). *On the experience of time*. Baltimore: Penguin.
Oscar-Berman, M. Zola-Morgan, S. M., Oberg, R. G. E., & Bonner, R. T. (1982). Comparative neuropsychology and Korsakoff's syndrome. Ill-Delayed response, delayed alternation and DRL performance. *Neuropsychologia*, 20, 187-202.
Predebon, J. (1995). Prospective and retrospective time estimates as a function of clock duration. *Perceptual and Motor Skills*, 80, 941-942.
Richards, W. (1973). Time reproductions by H. M. *Acta Psychologica*, 37, 279-282.
Shaw, C. & Aggleton, J. P. (1994). The ability of amnesic subjects to estimate time intervals. *Neuropsychologia*, 32, 857-873.
Talland, G. A. (1965). *Deranged memory*. New York: Academic Press.
Thomas, E. A. & Weaver, W. B. (1975). Cognitive processing and time perception. *Perception and Psychophysics*, 17, 363-367.
van der Horst, L. (1932). Über die Psychologie des Korsakows Syndrom. *Monatschrift der Psychiatrie und Neurologie*, 83, 65-84.
Williams, M. & Zangwill, O. L. (1950). Disorders of temporal judgment associated with amnesic states. *Journal of Mental Science*, 96, 484-493.

NEUROBEHAVIORAL ASSESSMENT

NEUROPSYCHIATRIC SYMPTOMS IN ALZHEIMER'S DISEASE: ASSESSMENT AND MANAGEMENT

Susan McPherson and Jeffrey Cummings

INTRODUCTION

Dementia is a multi-faceted clinical disorder characterized by impairment of memory with disturbances of language, executive functions, and visuospatial skills and is often accompanied by neuropsychiatric and emotional disturbances. It can be differentiated from other disorders by decline from a previous level of intellectual function, persistence of symptoms, and the presence of deficits in multiple cognitive domains (Cummings & Benson, 1992). Impairment in the ability to perform tasks of daily living such as using the telephone, check writing, and driving can be present in mildly-affected patients with more advanced patients exhibiting difficulties in toileting, feeding, and dressing themselves.

Dementia is primarily a problem of old age and the number of cases of dementia increase as the population ages, thereby making it a significant and expanding public health problem. The frequency of dementia in the population doubles every five years, affecting 1 percent of 60 to 64 year-olds and increasing to affect 30 to 40 percent of 85 year-olds (Jorm, Korten, & Henderson, 1987). In the United States, the total direct and indirect cost of caring for patients with dementia is estimated at $113 billion annually (National Foundation for Brain Research, 1992). The majority of care for dementia patients is provided by family members, often referred to as the "hidden victims" of dementia. Studies have found an increase in the rates of depression, psychotropic medication use, and stress-related illnesses among caregivers (Morris, Morris, & Briton, 1988). The Council on Scientific Affairs (1993) recommends that the caregiver be evaluated and referred for appropriate services as part of the assessment and on-going care of a dementia patient.

ALZHEIMER'S DISEASE

The most common cause of dementia is Alzheimer's disease (AD), a progressive degenerative disorder accounting for 60 to 70 percent of the dementias of old age. Alzheimer's disease is manifested by insidious onset, gradual decline with death approximately ten years after onset. One of the earliest neuropsychological deficits in AD is the inability to learn new information. This memory deficit is the cardinal feature of AD and is accompanied by impaired language skills, including naming and comprehension, impaired construction abilities, poor environmental orientation, and deficits in calculation, abstraction, and judgment. Ultimately, almost all cognitive capacities are lost. Several risk factors have been identified for AD, including advanced age, family history of AD, apolipoprotein E-4 genotype, prior head trauma, Down's syndrome, and low level of education.

Although the pathogenesis of AD is not completely known, aggregation of amyloid, protein in a distinctive beta-pleated configuration, appears to be one of the central pathologic events (Selkoe, 1993). The histologic changes of AD, neuritic plaques and neurofibrillary tangles, are most marked in the medial temporal lobe regions and the neocortex of the temporo-parietal-occipital junction; they are least abundant in the primary motor and sensory regions of the brain. Neurochemical changes characteristic of AD include a marked deficiency of choline acetyltransferase (ChAT), the enzyme that catalyzes the synthesis of acetylcholine (Koo & Price, 1993), as well as reductions in norepinephrine, serotonin, gamma-aminobutyric acid, glutamate, and somatostatin.

Neuropsychiatric abnormalities are common in AD and manifest early in the course of the disease with disengagement, indifference, and diminished affection. Agitation, anxiety, aggression, depression, personality changes, paranoia with persecutory delusions, and psychomotor activity disturbances also are common (Cummings & Victoroff, 1990; Reisberg, Franssen, Sclan, Kluger, & Ferris, 1989). Neuropsychiatric symptoms may lead to a more rapid decline in cognitive function (Chui, Lyness, Sobel, & Schneider, 1994; Mortimer, Ebbitt, Jun, & Finch, 1992; Stern et al., 1994). The neuropsychiatric manifestations of AD are frequently cited as the most distressing aspects of the disease, both from the perspective of the patient and caregiver. Studies have suggested that neuropsychiatric alterations are ultimately responsible for the decision to institutionalize the patient (O'Donnell et al., 1992). Recent studies have found similar rates and similar types of neuropsychiatric disturbances in AD across cultural settings (Cummings, Diaz, Levy, Binetti, & Litvan, 1996).

This chapter will focus on the assessment and management of the neuropsychiatric symptoms associated with AD, including: (1) the behavioral disturbances common to AD; (2) common rating scales used to assess the disturbances; (3) treatment of behavioral manifestations and (4) the importance of using changes in behavioral disturbances as outcome measures in clinical trials.

THE SPECTRUM OF BEHAVIORAL DISTURBANCES IN ALZHEIMER'S DISEASE

Alzheimer's disease manifests in a wide range of neuropsychiatric disturbances (see Table 1). The most common alterations in behavior include mood changes, psychosis, personality alterations, anxiety, agitation, aberrant motor behavior, and neurovegetative disturbances including alterations in sleep patterns

Table 1. Common Behavioral Disturbances in Alzheimer's Disease

Behavior	Percentage of Patients Reported
Aggression	18-65%
Aberrant Motor Behaviors	
Restlessness	21-60%
Wandering	10-61%
Alterations of Mood	
Anxiety	24-65%
Depression	0-50%
Elevated Mood	4-17%
Irritability/Labile Mood	30-45%
Psychosis	
Delusions	10-73%
Hallucinations	3-49%

and appetite (Cummings & Victoroff, 1990; Mega, Cummings, Fiorello, & Gornbein, 1996; Wragg & Jeste, 1989).

Alterations of Mood

Alterations of mood are common in AD and are usually evident as minor depressive symptoms such as sadness, hopelessness, and tearfulness, with severe depression relatively uncommon (Mega et al., 1996; Weiner, Edland, & Luszcynska, 1994). Studies have varied in reported rate of depressive symptoms among AD patients, possibly as a result of differing criteria, the population studied, and the approach used to identify depression and AD. Studies report rates of major depression between zero to ten percent (Burns, Folstein, Brandt, & Folstein, 1990; Cummings, Ross, Absher, Gornbein, & Hadjiaghai, 1995; Weiner et al., 1994); other studies find rates of depressive symptoms (less severe than major depression) between 25 and 50 percent (Burns et al., 1990; Mega et al., 1996; Migliorelli et al., 1995). An emerging consensus points to findings which suggest that major depressive episodes are infrequent once the cognitive impairment of AD is evident.

Disorders of elevated mood are less common in AD with reported frequencies varying between four and eight percent (Burns et al., 1990; Mega et al., 1996). Irritability and labile mood are present in approximately 40 percent of AD patients and are characterized by rapid shifting from one mood state to another (Mega et al., 1996).

Psychosis

Psychosis has been reported in 30 to 60 percent of patients, making it one of the more common neuropsychiatric disturbances in AD (Mega et al., 1996; Reisberg et al., 1987; Wragg & Jeste, 1989). The hallmark of psychosis is the presence of either hallucinations or delusions or both. Delusions are more common than hallucinations in AD. Delusions are fixed, false beliefs not commonly held by the patient's culture that are firmly held despite evidence to the contrary. Reports of delusions of theft, infidelity, or beliefs that the patients fear they will be harmed are frequent. Other manifestations of psychosis include the false beliefs that their spouses are not who they claim to be (misidentification or Capgrass syndrome), a stranger is living in the home (phantom boarder), individuals seen on television are present in the home (picture sign) (Flynn, Cummings, & Gornbein, 1991; Reisberg et al., 1987), and that their residences are not really their homes (Cummings & Victoroff, 1990).

Hallucinations are sensory perceptions that occur in the absence of external stimuli (e.g., hearing voices, seeing visions). Auditory, tactile, visual, and olfactory hallucinations can be present in AD. Patients may hear voices arguing about them or commanding them. Visual hallucinations are most common, including seeing animals, people, and complex scenes (Cummings & Victoroff, 1990; Mendez, Martin, Smyth, & Whitehouse, 1990).

Personality Alterations

Alterations in personality are frequently reported in AD and are among the more subtle of the behavioral changes (Mega et al., 1996; Petry, Cummings, Hill, & Shapira, 1988; 1989; Rubin & Kinscherf, 1989). Patients are often described by family members as apathetic, indifferent, less interested in family affairs, and less affectionate. There is a loss of interest and enthusiasm for previous hobbies and diminished initiative in conversation and social interaction. Reduced motivation permeates every aspect of the patient's life. Approximately one-third of patients manifest disinhibited behaviors (Mega et al., 1996), and, although more characteristic in the frontotemporal degenerations, mild disinhibition with tactlessness and impulsivity is not uncommon in AD (Levy, Miller, Cummings, Fairbanks, & Craig, 1996).

Anxiety

Anxiety is common in AD and occurs throughout most of the course of the illness. Reisberg and colleagues (1989) divided 120 patients with AD into stages based on the Global Deterioration Scale (GDS) (Reisberg, Ferris, de Leon, & Crook, 1982) and rated the patients' anxiety about upcoming events. Anxiety was most frequently reported at GDS 5 (46.4%), with moderate amounts reported at GDS 3 (42.9%); GDS 6 (31.7%) and GDS 4 (22.7%). When the frequency of any anxiety symptom was recorded, percentages in each stage rose dramatically for all stages except for GDS 7 (GDS 2: 42%; GDS 3: 68%; GDS 4: 45%; GDS 5: 80%; GDS 6: 66%; and GDS 7: 0%). In a similar approach, Mega and colleagues (1996) used the Mini-Mental State Examination (MMSE) (Folstein, Folstein, & McHugh, 1975) to compare anxiety among patients with differing severities of cognitive disturbance. Results of this study found symptoms of anxiety present in 24% of patients with mild cognitive impairment (MMSE 30-21), 65% with moderate dementia (MMSE 20-11), and 54% of those with severe intellectual compromise (MMSE 10-0).

Agitation

Agitation is among the most disabling symptoms of AD. Agitation is an extremely diverse phenomenon manifested by severe distress in the patient marked by emotional upset with inappropriate vocal or motor activity which cannot be explained by cognitive impairment or by identifiable needs of the patient. It not only affects the patient but also causes marked emotional distress in the caregiver. Specific examples of agitated behavior include cursing, screaming, oppositional behavior, and active resistance to care (Cohen-Mansfield & Billig, 1986). Relatively little is known about the pathophysiologic basis of agitation in AD. Agitation varies among patients and in different phases of the illness. Mega et al. (1996) found correlations between agitation and anxiety, disinhibition and irritability in patients with mild cognitive impairment, and correlations between agitation and delusions and hallucinations in patients with moderate cognitive impairment. In patients with severe impairment, no correlations of agitation with other neuropsychiatric symptoms were identified.

Catastrophic reactions are extreme emotional outbursts that include behaviors such as shouting, cursing, and striking out. They are at the interface between mood changes and agitation, are usually associated with frustration over failures or confrontations with family members, and are generally short-lived. They are very distressing to the family members of the AD patient (Rabins, Mace, & Lucas, 1982).

Aberrant Motor Behavior

Patients with AD engage in a variety of purposeless aberrant motor behaviors, such as pacing, rummaging through drawers and closets, packing, unpacking, and endless rearranging. In the later stages of the illness, stereotypic behaviors such as tying and untying knots, unraveling thread, or repetitively picking at clothes (carphologia) are common.

Neurovegetative Disturbances

Neurovegetative disturbances, including changes in sleep, appetite, and libido, are particularly common in advanced patients. Sleep architecture is abnormal in AD and is marked by increased arousals and awakenings. Patients may awaken in the middle of the night and dress or prepare to go out. Patients often exhibit decreased total sleep time, decreased slow wave and rapid-eye-movement sleep, and reduced sleep efficiency (Bliwise, 1994; Swearer, Drachman, O'Donnell, & Mitchell, 1988). The neurobiological changes in AD contribute importantly to anorexia and weight loss, and most patients in the advanced phases of the disease experience weight loss (Burns et al., 1990; Morris, Hope, & Fairburn, 1989; Tariot et al., 1995). Abnormal eating behaviors such as periods of increased appetite or putting too much food in the mouth at once can occur (Morris et al., 1989). A marked reduction in interest in sexual activity is evident from the initial phases of the illness. A few patients may exhibit periods of increased sexual interest that recede as the disease progresses (Burns et al., 1990; Shapira & Cummings, 1989). Kluver-Bucy syndrome, marked by increased sexual behavior, hyperorality, and hypermetamorphosis (compulsive attraction to high stimulus items in the environment), has been observed in some patients (Lilly, Cummings, Benson, & Frankel, 1983).

ASSESSMENT OF BEHAVIORAL DISTURBANCES IN AD

Several behavioral rating scales have been developed to assess the behavior of dementia patients. The scales vary according to whether the source of information is patient-based versus caregiver-based, the anticipated use of the tool (e.g., behavioral characterization, longitudinal follow-up, differential diagnosis), and the type of behavior assessed (e.g. mood, agitation, anxiety). Scales also differ according to the origin of the scale and whether it has been adapted from another scale or developed specifically for dementia. The commonly used scales are listed in Table 2. Although the theoretical frameworks on which the scales were based are rarely articulated, they can often be inferred from the structure of the scale.

SOURCE OF INFORMATION

Four sources of information have been used to gather behavioral ratings on patients; (1) family caregivers, (2) professional caregivers, (3) patient observation by physicians, and (4) patient self-report. The advantages to family caregivers as raters include the fact that they are intimately familiar with the behavior of the patient and are able to report changes in daily behavior patterns. Family caregiver rating scales are generally used for outpatients. Unfortunately, caregiver report formats may be biased by the mood state, education, and sophistication of the caregiver as an observer. The BEHAVE-AD (Reisberg et al., 1987) and Neuropsychiatric Inventory (NPI) (Cummings et al., 1994) are two examples of caregiver-based rating scales.

Professional caregiver scales are generally used in institutional settings such as hospitals, nursing homes, or other residential care facilities. Because they are usually completed by nursing staff, they have the advantage of being based on information from individuals more experienced in behavioral observation. They have the disadvantage of being based on data derived from individuals who observed the patient during only one shift of work; and some institutional caregivers receive relatively little specialized training. The Nurses' Observation Scale for Inpatient Evaluation (NOSIE) (Honigfeld & Klett, 1965), the Ward Daily Behaviour Scale (Blunden, Hodgkiss, Klemperer, McCarthy, & Watson, 1994), and the Multidimensional Observation Scale for Elderly Subjects (MOSES) (Helmes, Csapo, & Short, 1987) are examples of professional caregiver rating scales.

Another source of behavioral information is the direct observation of patients by physicians. This evaluation is usually conducted in a clinic. The

Table 2. Behavior Rating Scales

Patient-based Rating Scales
Geriatric Depression Scale
Patient-based/Caregiver-based Rating Scales
Alzheimer's Disease Assessment Scale (ADAS)
Cornell Scale for Depression in Dementia (CSDD)
Hamilton Depression Inventory
Professional Caregiver Rating Scales (Physicians/Nurses)
Gottfries, Brane, Steen (GBS)
Neurobehavior Rating Scale (NRS)
Nurses' Observation Scale for Inpatient Evaluation (NOSIE)
Ward Daily Behaviour Scale
Multidimensional Observation Scale for Elderly Subjects (MOSESE)
Caregiver-Based Rating Scales
Behavioral Pathology in Alzheimer's Disease Rating Scale (BEHAVE-AD)
Caregiver Obstreperous-Behavior Rating Assessment (COBRA)
Cohen-Mansfield Agitation Inventory (CMAI)
Columbia University Score for Psychopathology in Alzheimer's Disease (CUSPAD)
Neuropsychiatric Inventory (NPI) (Cummings et al., 1994)

advantages of this method include the use of highly skilled observers and assurances of validity. The major disadvantage to this method is that only those behaviors observed during a very limited observation period are captured. The Neurobehavior Rating Scale (NRS) (Levin et al., 1987) is an example of a tool of this type.

A final source of behavior rating is patient self-report. This form is reliable only in the early phases of a dementing illness, and validity is also difficult to assess except in the earliest phases. The Geriatric Depression Scale (GDS) (Yesavage, Brink, Rose, & Lum, 1983), which is a self-rating instrument, is often used in studies as a rating of mood changes.

CONTENT OF BEHAVIORAL SCALES

Differing approaches to assessing behavior in dementia are reflected in the content of the behavior rating scale. Traditional psychopathologic disorders such as depression or psychosis are reflected in scales such as the Cornell Scale for

Depression in Dementia (Alexopoulos, Abrams, Young, & Shimoian, 1988) and the Columbia University Scale for Psychopathology in Alzheimer's Disease (Devanand et al., 1992). An example of a scale that assesses behavioral changes that are common in dementia but rare in other disorders is the Cohen-Mansfield Agitation Inventory (Cohen-Mansfield, Marx, & Rosenthal, 1989).

Some scales, such as the BEHAVE-AD, NPI, Hamilton Depression Rating Scale (Hamilton, 1967), Cornell Scale for Depression in Dementia, and Columbia University Scale for Psychopathology in Alzheimer's Disease, rate psychopathology only. Other scales rate both psychopathology and other abnormalities. For example, the NRS and Gottfries, Brane, and Steen Scale (GBS) (Gottfries, Brane, Guilberg, & Steen, 1982) include both behavior and cognitive changes, and scale scores of individual component behaviors can be obtained. Aggression, personality, mechanical skills, and vegetative functions are all evaluated by the Caretaker Obstreperous-Behavior Rating Assessment (COBRA) (Drachman, Swearer, O'Donnell, Mitchell, & Maloon, 1992). The Memory and Behavior Checklist (Teri et al., 1992) includes both cognitive and behavioral items and the non-cognitive portion of the Alzheimer's Disease Assessment Scale (ADAS-noncog) sums behavior changes, weight alterations, and tremor.

Several measures have been developed to provide information on individual behaviors, global behavioral scores, or both. The BEHAVE-AD, NPI, and Behavior Rating Scale for Dementia (BRSD) (Tariot et al., 1995) score both individual behaviors as well as providing global or summary ratings (BEHAVE-AD and NPI) or factor scores (BRSD).

The selection of a rating instrument should be made on the basis of the behaviors to be evaluated and the characteristics of the tool. Scales which provide overall summary scores may give a global impression of the patient in a single score but may be insensitive to individual behaviors. Conversely, highly focused tools provide precise information on one specific behavioral attribute but do not reflect the entire spectrum of behaviors exhibited by a patient.

SOURCE OF INSTRUMENTS

Behavioral rating scales for dementia have been imported from a variety of sources. In some cases, scales have been imported directly from psychiatry or neurology, and adapted for use with the dementia population; in others they were developed specifically for use with dementia patients.

The Hamilton Depression Rating Scale (Hamilton, 1967) was imported from psychiatry for use with dementia patients from psychiatric investigations of depressed patients. This scale allows for direct comparison of depression in patients with and without dementia. Unfortunately, it has the disadvantage of scoring symptoms common in dementia, such as weight loss and agitation, as aspects of depression. Other instruments imported directly from psychiatry include the Brief Psychiatric Rating Scale and the Geriatric Depression Scale.

Scales which have been modified for use with the dementia population include the Cornell Scale for Depression in Dementia, with items adapted from the approach of the Hamilton Depression Rating Scale for application in dementia. The

NRS was adapted from the Brief Psychiatric Rating Scale for use with patients with head trauma before being used in dementia research. The BRSD has items from the Hamilton Depression Rating Scale and the BEHAVE-AD. Examples of tools originally developed for use with dementia patients include the BEHAVE-AD, Cohen-Mansfield Agitation Inventory, and NPI.

PROPERTIES OF RATING SCALES

The underlying theory of how best to capture behavioral data is reflected in the structure and properties of behavioral rating scales. In some cases, behaviors are rated as merely present or absent using a checklist approach. In other cases, behaviors are rated using a fixed interval scale (e.g., mild-1, moderate-2, severe-3) as is done with the Revised Memory and Behavior Problem Checklist and the NPI. Other instruments rely on an analog scale with the patient or caregiver choosing a point between two polar extremes that best characterizes the patient's behavior (e.g., between happy and sad). In addition, scales may rate the frequency of behaviors (e.g., the BRSD), severity of behaviors (as in the BEHAVE-AD), or both (NPI and COBRA).

Behavioral rating scales vary from relatively brief, with only a few questions in each behavioral domain (ADAS-noncog) to comprehensive (e.g., BRSD). The NPI uses a somewhat novel approach in which screening questions are asked for each domain. If the screen is answered positively, more extended questioning is pursued; if the screen is negative, the domain is not explored in depth.

OUTCOME OF ASSESSMENT

Behavioral rating scales have been used primarily in cross-sectional research studies. There is little information available regarding their usefulness for tracking behaviors over time or their sensitivity to behavioral changes produced by specific interventions. The available research suggests, however, that tools that accurately rate behaviors will be sensitive in monitoring either spontaneous or treatment-induced behavioral changes. Substantial literature exists on the use of the Hamilton Depression Rating Scale in monitoring the response to antidepressant therapy, and the ADAS (including the noncognitive portion) has been used extensively in clinical trials of antidementia drugs (Farlow et al., 1992; Knapp et al., 1994; Rogers & Friedhoff, 1996). The NPI was found to be sensitive to behavioral changes associated with the use of tacrine and of metrifonate in the treatment of AD (Kaufer, Cummings, & Christine, 1996; 1998; Morris et al., 1998). Additional longitudinal studies are needed to ascertain the usefulness of these scales for defining whether behaviors characterize a subgroup of patients in whom the behaviors occur continuously, or if the behaviors are more indicative of transient phenomena that occur less regularly in different individuals during the course of a dementing disease.

TREATMENT OF BEHAVIORAL DISTURBANCES IN AD

Two major approaches exist for the treatment of behavioral disturbances in AD: non-pharmacologic and pharmacologic. Nonpharmacologic management is generally the first line of treatment with the dementia patient, given that these patients are often sensitive to medication side effects and considering that behaviors such as repetitive questions, verbal outbursts and wandering are not remediated by medication (Sultzer & Cummings, 1993). Environmental adjustments such as adequate lighting, reducing distractions, and using objects that help with orientation (clocks and calendars) can also be useful (Alessi, 1991). The environment should be simplified and patients given the opportunity to participate in planning the daily routine (Deutsch & Rovner, 1991). Communication should be simplified through use of yes/no questions and single step instructions. Soothing music, reassurance, and redirection can be used to avoid minor agitation episodes (Sultzer & Cummings, 1993; Cohen-Mansfield, Marx, & Rosenthal, 1989). Caregivers need to learn to be aware of how nonverbal cues, such as frowning, can be threatening to a demented patient (Alessi, 1991).

Treatment with medication becomes necessary when nonpharmacologic management approaches do not control the target behavior. Psychotropic agents are generally the first line of pharmacologic treatment in the management of agitation, anxiety, psychoses, and depression. More recently, it has been observed that the currently approved cholinergic agents may be useful in treating some behavioral symptoms in AD. These agents generally have fewer side effects than conventional psychotropic agents and may add to the armamentarium of drugs available to the practicing clinician to improve the behavior of AD patients.

PSYCHOTROPIC AGENTS

Antipsychotics

Antipsychotics are the most commonly prescribed medication for the treatment of agitation and psychosis in dementia. The efficacy of antipsychotic agents for the treatment of agitation is modest, with some authors suggesting that the benefit of antipsychotic medication is only 18% greater than the response from placebo (Schneider, Pollock, & Lyness, 1990). The low efficacy rate coupled with the potential side effects of the drugs warrant the use of antipsychotics only when agitation is clearly secondary to psychosis or when patients do not respond to other medications (Kunik, Yudofsky, Silver, & Hales, 1994). A variety of antipsychotics may be used and specific agents should be selected on the basis of the side-effect profile. Initial dosages should be small and should be increased slowly.

There are a number of adverse reactions associated with the use of antipsychotics (Baldessarini, 1985; Jenicke, 1989). Patients may become overly sedated, leading to confusion, or develop orthostatic hypotension, leading to falls and fractures (Ray, Griffen, Schaffner, Baugh, & Melton, 1987). Confusion, constipation, and urinary retention can result from use of agents with anticholinergic side effects. Other potential complications include cardiac conduction delays, cholestatic jaundice, agranulocytosis, and worsening of pre-existing epilepsy with specific agents. Use of higher potency antipsychotics can lead to motor restlessness (akathisia) and parkinsonism, or worsen the patient's cognitive condition (Devanand, Sackeim, Brown, & Mayeux, 1989).

In terms of psychosis, patients with systematized delusions are probably most helped by antipsychotic medications. Medication is not as effective for patients with delusions of theft and vague episodic fears (Morris, Rovner, Folstein, & German, 1990). Atypical antipsychotics such as clozapine, olanzapine, and risperidone can be used to control agitation and psychosis. These agents are particularly useful for patients with dementia with Lewy bodies, parkinsonism, or antipsychotic sensitivity (Factor, Brown, Molho, & Podskalny, 1994; McKeith, Fairbairn, Perry, Thompson, & Perry, 1992; Chacko, Hurley, & Jankovic, 1993). Use of clozapine necessitates weekly white blood cell counts because of the risk of agranulocytosis. Olanzapine and risperdone are effective in controlling agitation and do not carry the risk of agranulocytosis. The atypical agents are sedating, and risperdone carries a potential risk of parkinsonism at higher doses (Wright & Cummings, 1996).

Nonantipsychotic Medications

Several nonantipsychotic medications have been used to treat agitation in dementia, including benzodiazepines, antiepileptic drugs, antidepressants, buspirone, and trozodone. Benzodiazepines may be useful for agitation related to anxiety and control occasional episodes of nonpsychotic agitation but have a potential for disinhibition, delirium, sedation, falls, and dependency. Propranolol or other beta-blockers have been used to treat agitation in patients with a wide variety of brain insults (Schneider & Sobin, 1992), but their use is limited in patients with cardiac disease, chronic obstructive pulmonary disease, and diabetes. Agents such as buspirone and carbamazepine reduce agitation, but have a delayed onset of action (Schneider & Sobin, 1992). Trazodone has been found to be most effective in patients with repetitive utterances and mannerisms, verbal aggression, and oppositional behavior (Sultzer, Gray, Gunay, Berisford, & Mahler, 1995). Potential side effects for carbamazepine and trazodone include sedation, and use of trazodone can lead to priapism in younger patients.

Anxiolytics

The prevalence of anxiety in AD ranges between 7 and 30 percent (Reisberg et al., 1987; Deutsch & Rovner, 1991). However, pharmacologic treatment with traditional benzodiazepines can lead to several side effects, as noted above. Nonbenzodiazepine anxiolytics such as buspirone can be used to effectively treat anxiety and have fewer physical, cognitive, and behavioral side effects.

Antidepressants

Tricyclic antidepressants (TCA's) and selective serotonergic reuptake inhibitors (SSRI's) are useful when anxiety is thought to be secondary to depression and panic attacks, or when long-term treatment is necessary (Jenicke, 1989; Rosenbaum & Pollack, 1991; Schneider, 1993). Wright and Cummings (1996) suggest that antidepressant medications should be given in dosages one third to one half of the initial dose recommended for young, healthy adults and should be increased slowly. Other important recommendations include giving more sedating medications at bedtime and activating medications during the daytime.

Medications that cause sedation, orthostatic hypotension, and anticholinergic side effects, such as the TCA's amitriptyline and imipramine, should generally not be prescribed for demented elderly patients. Secondary amine TCA's (nortriptyline, desipramine) have fewer side effects and can be used safely provided the patient receives a pretreatment electrocardiogram and is watched closely for adverse effects. Monamine oxidase (MAO) inhibitors require strict dietary and medication restrictions and often cause orthostasis and should not be used with demented patients (Baldessarini, 1985). SSRI's cause less sedation, fewer antichonlingeric side effects, and less orthostasis and are better tolerated by dementia patients. Possible side effects include the onset or exacerbation of apathy (Hoehn-Saric, Lipsey, & McLeod, 1990), agitation, gastrointestinal distress, and interaction with other medications via the altering of hepatic metabolism. Patients on selegiline cannot take SSRI's given the risk of a serotonin syndrome (Bodner, Lynch, Lewis, & Kahn, 1995).

Cholinergic Therapy

The neurochemical changes associated with AD include deficiencies of acetylcholine, norepinephrine, and serotonin, with severe cholinergic deficiencies in the paralimbic and heteromodal association cortex. The neuroanatomical source of choline acetyltransferase (CAT), the enzyme necessary for the synthesis of cortical acetylcholine, is the nucleus basalis of Meynert (NBM). Atrophy of the NBM occurs early in the course of AD, resulting in a deficiency of cortical acetylcholine (Whitehouse, Price, Clark, Coyle, & DeLong, 1981). The cholinergic deficiency of AD has been hypothesized as a major contributing factor to the cognitive abnormalities of the dementia syndrome (Coyle, Price, & DeLong, 1983).

Cholinergic deficiency also has been implicated as playing an important role in causing the behavioral disturbances that commonly accompany AD (Cummings & Kaufer, 1996). The relationship between behavioral changes and cholinergic deficiency is based on the following evidence: 1) the limbic system provides the principal afferents to the NBM, suggesting a role for NBM processing of emotional information and predicting emotional disturbances with NBM dysfunction; 2) depletion of acetylcholine occurs in frontal and temporal brain areas involved in the production of neuropsychiatric symptoms in AD; 3) use of anticholinergic agents produces behavioral disturbances similar to AD, including delusions, hallucinations, and agitation; 4) use of cholinergic substances ameliorates the neuropsychiatric symptoms of AD.

At present, several cholinesterase inhibitors are available for the treatment of AD and other disorders, including intravenous physostigmine for the treatment of acute anticholinergic delirium, and tacrine (Cognex) and donepezil (Aricept) for treatment of AD. Drugs currently under review by the FDA for treatment of AD include: rivastigmine (Exelon), metrifonate (Pro-Mem), and long-acting oral physostigmine (Synapton). These agents have similar efficacy and adverse event profiles including gastrointestinal effects such as cramping, diarrhea, anorexia, nausea, and vomiting.

The cholinesterase inhibitor physostigmine has been reported to improve psychosis and worsen depression, (Molchan, Vitiello, Minichiello, & Sunderland, 1991) and to reduce delusions (Cummings, Gorman, & Shapira, 1993) in patients with AD. Gorman and colleagues conducted a double-blind crossover trial comparing physostigmine and haloperidol, and found that BEHAVE-AD scores were reduced to an equal extent by both agents, with an increase in parkinsonism in patients treated with haloperidol and a decrease in parkinsonian features in patients treated with physostigmine (Gorman, Read, & Cummings, 1993).

Tacrine also has been investigated as a possible treatment intervention for the behavioral manifestations of AD. Results of studies on tacrine have demonstrated declines in symptoms of anxiety, disinhibition, and aberrant motor behavior such as pacing and rummaging, as measured by the NPI (Kaufer et al., 1996), with significant reductions in apathy and disinhibition in a follow-up study with a larger sample size (Kaufer et al., 1998). Raskind and colleagues reanalyzed data on patients using tacrine and found a statistically significant reduction in the number of patients experiencing delusions (Raskind, Sadowsky, Signund, Beitler, & Auster, 1997). Similar effects have been found with metrifonate with reduction in NPI scores for hallucinations, apathy, and depression (Cummings et al., 1998).

Although few studies are available, cholinergic receptor agonists also have been investigated as possibly efficacious in moderating the behavioral disturbances of AD. A dose-dependent reduction in vocal outbursts, suspiciousness, delusions, agitation, and hallucinations has been found in one study using xanomeline, a selective muscarinic cholinergic receptor agonist (Bodick et al., 1997). As compared with patients on placebo, there was suppression of other behavioral manifestations including the emergence of delusions, suspiciousness, wandering, vocal outbursts, hallucinations, dangerous driving, fearfulness, agitation, and threatening behavior.

Cummings and Back (1998) developed a cholinergic hypothesis for the neuropsychiatric symptoms of AD based upon the available evidence. The postulate holds that cholinergic agents are psychotropic drugs that are mechanism-based and disease-specific in that the psychotropic benefit is based on the cholinergic actions of the drugs (i.e. "mechanism based") and they are likely to be beneficial only in patients who have a cholinergic deficiency (i.e. "disease specific"). They further hypothesized that the beneficial effect of cholinergic enhancement is mediated in frontal, temporal, and paralimbic structures, all of which are affected in AD. Although sparse, the available research supports the use of cholinergic agents in the treatment of the behavioral disturbances associated with AD.

INCLUSION OF BEHAVIORAL DISTURBANCES AS OUTCOME MEASURES IN CLINICAL TRIALS

Outcome measures of clinical trials for drugs used to treat AD have been carefully considered by the International Harmonization Work Group and a consensus has been achieved that measures of cognition and function as well as global measures are necessary in all studies of AD-related drugs. Controversy exists regarding the role of neuropsychiatric measures in anti-AD drug trials. Nonetheless, the available research supports the inclusion of neuropsychiatric assessments as outcomes in all trials and the role of neuropsychiatric symptom assessment as primary outcome measures in specific types of anti-AD drug trials.

As detailed above, behavioral symptoms are common in AD, affecting nearly all patients (Mega et al., 1996; Reisberg et al., 1987). Behavioral symptoms are neither necessary nor sufficient to define AD, but, like the motor manifestations that emerge in the late stages of AD, they are integral parts of the illness and define much of the associated disability (Rabins et al., 1982; Steele, Rovner, Chase, & Folstein, 1990). There is increasing evidence from neuroimaging, neurochemical, and neuropathologic studies that the neuropsychiatric symptoms of AD reflect underlying causative neurobiological alterations (Kotrla, Chacko, Harper, Jhingran, & Doody, 1995; Sultzer et al., 1995; Zubenko, Mossy, & Kopp, 1990; Zubenko et al., 1991). The cholinergic deficiency of AD contributes to the neuropsychiatric symptoms of the disorder. Behaviors that may be related to the cholinergic deficit include apathy, agitation, psychosis, anxiety, disinhibition, and purposeless behaviors (Cummings & Kaufer, 1996). Preliminary evidence cited above suggests that these behaviors can be ameliorated with cholinesterase inhibitors and muscarinic receptor agonists (Bodick et al., 1997; Cummings et al., 1993; Gorman et al., 1993; Kaufer et al., 1996). Patients who exhibit cognitive improvement with cholinergic treatment are most likely to have a concomitant decrease in behavioral symptoms, but the two types of response are not linked in all cases. Patients may manifest behavioral improvements and no cognitive change, particularly when in advanced phases of AD (Kaufer et al., 1996). This group of patients is an example of a population in whom changes in neuropsychiatric symptoms could appropriately be the primary outcome measures of a trial of anti-AD agents including cholinergic compounds.

Global measures are used as outcomes in all clinical trials of anti-AD drugs. These measures reflect a clinician's overall assessment of changes that have occurred since the patient entered into a clinical trial (Knopman, Knapp, Gracon, & Davis, 1994). Global assessments reflect cognitive alterations, functional changes, and variations in behavior. Without separate measures of neuropsychiatric symptoms, it is impossible to conduct analyses that provide insight into the contribution of behavioral changes to global alterations. Global changes due in part to behavioral improvement may be inappropriately attributed to cognitive responses. Thus, behavioral evaluations are necessary to adequately interpret the results of all clinical trials in which a global assessment is a primary outcome measure of anti-AD therapy.

Issues specific to assessment of neuropsychiatric symptoms in clinical trials and important in the deliberations of the harmonization effort include:
(1) Cholinergic therapy and other biologic interventions may exert beneficial behavioral effects by reducing existing symptoms or by suppressing the emergence of new symptoms; different populations and different strategies will be necessary to study these two pharmacologic effects. Likewise, neuropsychiatric symptoms may

spontaneously remit, and symptom reductions in treated populations must be compared to spontaneous remission rates in control populations.

(2) The psychotropic effects of anti-AD drugs may simultaneously exert influences on several symptoms or symptom complexes, and monitoring of several dimensions of behavior in clinical trials will be necessary. Multidimensional instruments such as the NPI, BEHAVE-AD, and BRSD are appropriate to this type of assessment.

(3) Recruitment of patient populations with behavioral symptoms may result in greater diagnostic heterogeneity than is present in conventional anti-AD clinical trials since more patients with frontotemporal dementias and Lewy body dementia – conditions with more neuropsychiatric abnormalities than typical AD (Levy et al., 1996; Perry, Kerwin, Perry, Blessed, & Fairburn, 1990) – may be identified. Diagnostic approaches sensitive to the neuropsychiatric symptoms characteristic of different disorders will be required to assure diagnostic specificity.

(4) Biologic markers specific to AD patients with neuropsychiatric disorders must be sought and monitored in the course of treatment. EEG (Lopez et al., 1991) and imaging (Kotrla et al., 1995; Sultzer et al., 1995) correlates of behavioral disorders have been suggested and require further investigation.

(5) Contributions of improved behavior to changes in other measures commonly used in clinical trials such as global assessments, caregiver distress, delayed nursing home placement, and performance of instrumental activities of daily living must be monitored.

(6) The relationship of neuropsychiatric symptoms to caregiver burden, caregiver behavior, and environmental stimuli requires study, and their effects must be accounted for in the course of anti-AD drug trials that include changes in behavior as outcomes.

(7) Patients usually are not insightful reporters of their own neuropsychiatric symptoms and surrogate information sources will be necessary to monitor changes in symptoms as a result of treatment. Instruments appropriate to different patient circumstances – family caregiver, professional caregiver, home environment, and institutional environment – are needed.

SUMMARY

Neuropsychiatric disorders are common in AD and other dementias and reflect changes in brain function. Regional pathological and neurochemical alterations determine the profile of neuropsychiatric symptoms observed in different disorders and among different patients with the same disorder. Clinical trials of agents intended to improve cognition in AD should include behavioral assessment. Behavioral changes may influence cognition, activities of daily living, caregiver burden, and quality of life; neuropsychiatric assessments are needed to understand changes in these domains. The psychotropic effects of anti-AD drugs may be of benefit to AD patients who have no cognitive response to the agents, and behavioral changes may be the primary outcome measures of some trials of anti-AD therapies. Conventional psychotropic agents may benefit patients unresponsive to cholinergic compounds.

ACKNOWLEDGMENTS

This project was supported by a National Institute on Aging Alzheimer's Disease Core Center grant (AG 10123), an Alzheimer's Disease Research Center of California grant, and the Sidell-Kagan Foundation.

REFERENCES

Alessi, C. A. (1991). Managing the behavioral problems of dementia in the home. *Clinics in Geriatric Medicine, 7,* 787-801.

Alexopoulos, G. S., Abrams, R. C., Young, R. C., & Shamoian, C. A. (1988). Cornell scale for depression in dementia. *Biological Psychiatry, 23,* 271-284.

Baldessarini, R. J. (1985). *Chemotherapy in psychiatry. Principles and practice* (Rev. ed.). Cambridge, MA: Harvard University Press.

Bliwise, D. L. (1994). Dementia. In M. H. Kryger, T. Roth, & W. C. Dement (Eds.), *Principles and practice of sleep medicine* (2nd ed., pp. 790-800). Philadelphia: W. B. Saunders Company.

Blunden, J., Hodgkiss, A., Klemperer, F., McCarthy, A., & Watson, J. P. (1994). The ward daily behaviour scale. *British Journal of Psychiatry, 165,* 87-93.

Bodick, N. C., Offen, W. W., Levey, A. I., Cutler, N. R., Gauthier, S. G., Satlin, A., Shannon, H. E., Tollefson, G. D., Rasmussen, K., Bymaster, F. P. Hurley, D. J., Potter, W. Z., & Paul, S. M. (1997). Effects of xanomeline, a selective muscarinic receptor agonist, on cognitive function and behavioral symptoms in Alzheimer disease. *Archives of Neurology, 54,* 465-473.

Bodner, R. A., Lynch, R., Lewis, L., & Kahn, D. (1995). Serotonin syndrome. Neurology, 45, 219-223.

Burns, A., Folstein, S., Brandt, J., & Folstein, M. (1990). Clinical assessment of irritability, aggression, and apathy in Huntington and Alzheimer disease. *Journal of Nervous and Mental Disorders, 178,* 20-26.

Chacko, R. C., Hurley, R. A., & Jankovic, J. (1993). Clozapine use in diffuse Lewy body disease. *Journal of Neuropsychiatry and Clinical Neuroscience, 5,* 206-208.

Chui, H. C., Lyness, S. A., Sobel, E., & Schneider, L.S. (1994). Extrapyramidal signs and psychiatric symptoms predict faster cognitive decline in Alzheimer's disease. *Archives of Neurology, 51,* 676-681.

Cohen-Mansfield, J. & Billig, N. (1986). Agitated behaviors in the elderly, I: a conceptual overview. *Journal of the American Geriatric Society, 34,* 711-721.

Cohen-Mansfield, J., Marx, M. S., & Rosenthal, A. S. (1989). A description of agitation in a nursing home. *Journal of Gerontology, 44,* M77-84.

Council on Scientific Affairs, American Medical Association. (1993). Physicians and family caregivers: a model for partnership. *Journal of the American Medical Association, 269,* 1282-1284.

Coyle, J. T., Price, D. L., & DeLong, M. R. (1983). Alzheimer's disease: A disorder of cortical cholinergic innervation. *Science, 219,* 1184-1190.

Cummings, J. L. & Back, C. (1998). The cholinergic hypothesis of neuropsychiatric symptoms in Alzheimer's disease. *American Journal of Geriatric Psychiatry, 6,* 564-578.

Cummings, J. L. & Benson, D. F. (1992). *Dementia: A clinical approach.* Butterworth-Heinemann, Boston.

Cummings, J. L., Cyrus, P., Bieber, F., Orazem, J., Mas, J., & Gulanski, B. (March, 1998). *The effect of metrifonate on the cognitive, functonal, and behavioral symptoms of Alzheimer's disease.* Abstract presented at the American Association for Geriatric Psychiatry, San Diego, CA.

Cummings, J. L., Diaz, C., Levy, M., Binetti, G., & Litvan, I. (1996). Neuropsychiatric syndromes in neurodegenerative diseases: frequency and significance. *Seminars in Clinical Neuropsychiatry, 1,* 241-247.

Cummings, J. L., Gorman, D. G., & Shapira, J. (1993). Physostigmine ameliorates the delusions of Alzheimer's disease. *Biological Psychiatry, 33,* 536-541.

Cummings, J. L. & Kaufer, D. I. (1996). Neuropsychiatric aspects of Alzheimer's disease: the cholinergic hypothesis revisited. *Neurology, 47,* 876-883.

Cummings, J. L., Mega, M., Gray, K., Rosenberg-Thompson, S., Carusi, D. A., & Gornbein, J. (1994). The Neuropsychiatric Inventory: comprehensive assessment of psychopathology in dementia. *Neurology, 44,* 2308-2314.

Cummings, J. L., Ross, W., Absher, J., Gornbein, J., & Hadjiaghai, L. (1995). Depressive symptoms in Alzheimer's disease: assessment and determinants. *Alzheimer's Disease and Associated Disorders, 9*, 87-93.

Cummings, J. L. & Victoroff, J. I. (1990). Noncognitive neuropsychiatric syndromes in Alzheimer's disease. *Neuropsychiatry, Neuropsychology, and Behavioral Neurology, 3*, 140-158.

Deutsch, L. H. & Rovner, B. W. (1991). Agitation and other non-cognitive abnormalities in Alzheimer's disease. *Psychiatric Clinics of North America, 14*, 341-351.

Devanand, D. P., Miller, L., Richards, M., Marder, K., Bell, K., Mayeux, R., & Stern, Y. (1992). The Columbia University Scale for Psychopathology in Alzheimer's Disease. *Archives of Neurology, 49*, 371-376.

Devanand, D. P., Sackheim, H. A., Brown, R. P., & Mayeux, R. (1989). A pilot study of haloperidol treatment of psychosis and behavioral disturbance in Alzheimer's disease. *Archives of Neurology, 46*, 854-857.

Drachman, D. S., Swearer, J. M., O'Donnell, B. F., Mitchell, A. L., & Maloon, A. (1992). The Caretaker Obstreperous Behavior Rating Assessment (COBRA) scale. *Journal of the American Geriatric Society, 40*, 463-480.

Factor, S. A., Brown, D., Molho, E. S., & Podansky, G. D. (1994). Clozapine: A 2-year open trial in Parkinson's disease patients with psychosis. *Neurology, 44*, 544-546.

Farlow, M., Gracon, S. I., Hershey, L. A., Lewis, K. W., Sadowsky, C. H., & Dolan-Ureno, J. (1992). A controlled trial of tacrine in Alzhiemer's disease. The Tacrine Study. *Journal of the American Medical Association, 268*, 2523-2529.

Flynn, F. G., Cummings, J. L, & Gornbein, J. (1991). Delusions in dementia syndromes: Investigation of behavioral and neuropsychological correlates. *Journal of Neuropsychiatry and Clinical Neuroscience, 3*, 364-370.

Folstein, M. F., Folstein, S. E., & McHugh, P. R. (1975). Mini-Mental State. A practical method for grading the cognitive state of patients for the clinician. *Journal of Psychiatric Research, 12*, 189-198.

Gorman, D. G., Read, S., & Cummings, J. L. (1993). Cholinergic therapy of behavioral disturbances in Alzheimer's disease. *Neuropsychiatry, Neuropsychology, and Behavioral Neurology, 6*, 229-234.

Gottfries, C-G., Brane, G., Guilberg, B., & Steen, G. (1982). A new rating scale for dementia symptoms. *Archives of Gerontology and Geriatrics, 1*, 311-330.

Hamilton, M. (1967). Development of a rating scale for primary depressive illness. *British Journal of Social and Clinical Psychology, 6*, 278-296.

Helmes, E., Csapo, K., & Short, J. A. (1987). Standardization and validation of the Multidimensional Observation Scale for Elderly Subjects (MOSES). *Journal of Gerontology, 42*, 395-405.

Hoehn-Saric, R., Lipsey, J. R., & McLeod, D. R. (1990). Apathy and indifference in patients on fluvoxamine and fluoxetine. *Journal of Clinical Psychopharmacology, 10*, 343-345.

Honigfeld, G. & Klett, C. J. (1965). The Nurses' Observation Scale for Inpatient Evaluation. *Journal of Clinical Psychology, 21*, 65-71.

Jenike, M. A. (1989). *Geriatric psychiatry and pharmacology: A clinical approach*. Chicago: Year Book Medical Publishers.

Jorm, A. F., Korten, A. E., & Henderson, A. S. (1987). The prevalence of dementia: A quantitative integration of the literature. *Acta Psychiatrica Scandinavica, 76*, 464-479.

Kaufer, D. I., Cummings, J. L., & Christine, D. (1996). Effect of tacrine on behavioral symptoms in Alzheimer's disease: an open label study. *Journal of Geriatric Psychiatry and Neurology, 9*, 1-6.

Kaufer, D. I., Cummings, J. L., & Christine, D. (1998). Differential neuropsychiatric symptom responses to tacrine in Alzheimer's disease: relationship to dementia severity. *Journal of Neuropsychiatry and Clinical Neuroscience, 10*, 55-63.

Knapp, M. J., Knopman, D. S., Soloman, P. R., Pendlebury, W. W., Davis, C. S., & Gracon, S. I. (1994). A 30-week randomized controlled trial of high-dose tacrine in patients with Alzheimer's disease. *Journal of the American Medical Association, 271*, 985-991.

Koo, E. H. & Price, D. L. (1993). The neurobiology of dementia. In P. J. Whitehouse (Ed.). *Dementia* (pp. 55-91). F.A. Davis Company, Philadelphia.

Kotrla, K. J., Chacko, R. C., Harper, R. G., Jhingran, S., & Doody, R. (1995). SPECT findings on psychosis in Alzheimer's disease. *American Journal of Psychiatry, 152*, 1470-1475.

Knopman, D. S, Knapp, M. J., Gracon, S. I., & Davis, C. S. (1994). The Clinician Interview-Based Impression (CIBI): A clinician's global change rating scale in Alzheimer's disease. *Neurology, 44*, 2315-2321.

Kunik, M. E., Yudofsky, S. C., Silver, J. M., & Hales, R. E. (1994). Pharmacologic approach to management of agitation associated with dementia. *Journal of Clinical Psychiatry, 55,* (2), 13-17.

Levin, H. S., High, W. M., Goethe, K. E., Sisson, R. A., Overall, J. E., Rhoades, H. M., Eisenberg, H. M., Kalisky, Z., & Gary, H. E. (1987). The Neurobehavior Rating Scale: Assessment of the sequelae of head injury by the clinician. *Journal of Neurology, Neurosurgery and Psychiatry, 50,* 183-193.

Levy, M. L., Miller, B. L., Cummings, J. L., Fairbanks, L. A., & Craig, A. (1996). Alzheimer's disease and frontotemporal dementias: Behavioral distinctions. *Archives of Neurology, 53,* 687-90.

Lilly, R., Cummings, J. L., Benson, D. F., & Frankel, M. (1983). Clinical features of the human Kluver-Bucy syndrome. *Neurology, 33,* 1141-1145.

Lopez, O. L., Becker, J. T., Brenner, R. P., Rosen, J., Bajulaiye, O. I., & Reynolds, C. F. III. (1991). Alzheimer's disease with delusions and hallucinations: Neuropsychological and electroencephalographic correlates. *Neurology, 41,* 906-912.

McKeith, I., Fairbairn, A., Perry, R., Thompson, P., & Perry, E. (1992). Neuroleptic sensitivity with senile dementia of the Lewy body type. *BMJ, 305,* 673-678.

Mega, M., Cummings, J. L., Fiorello, T., & Gornbein, J. (1996). The spectrum of behavioral changes in Alzheimer's disease. *Neurology, 46,* 130-135.

Mendez, M. F., Martin, R. J., Smyth, K. A., & Whitehouse, P. J. (1990). Psychiatric symptoms associated with Alzheimer's disease. *Journal of Neuropsychiatry and Clinical Neuroscience, 2,* 28-33.

Migliorelli, R., Teson, A., Sabe, L., Petracchi, M., Leiguarda, R., & Starkstein, S. E. (1995). Prevalence and correlates of dysthymia and major depression among patients with Alzheimer's disease. *American Journal of Psychiatry, 152,* 37-44.

Molchan, S. E., Vitiello, B., Minichiello, M., & Sunderland, T. (1991). Reciprocal changes in psychosis and mood after physostigmine in a patient with Alzheimer's disease. *Archives of General Psychiatry, 48,* 1113.

Morris, J. C., Cyrus, P. A., Orazem, J., Mas, J., Bieber, F., Ruzicka, B. B., Gulanski, B. (1998). Metrifonate benefits cognitive, behavioral, and global function in patients with Alzheimer's disease. *Neurology, 50,* 1222-1230.

Morris, C. H., Hope, R. A., & Fairburn, C. G. (1989). Eating habits in dementia. *British Journal of Psychiatry, 154,* 801-806.

Morris, R. G., Morris, L. W., & Britton, P. G. (1988). Factors affecting the emotional well-being of the caregivers of dementia sufferers. *British Journal of Psychiatry, 153,* 147-156.

Morris, R. K., Rovner, B. W., Folstein, M. F., & German, P. S. (1990). Delusions in newly admitted residents of nursing homes. *American Journal of Psychiatry, 147,* 299-302.

Mortimer, J. A., Ebbitt, B., Jun S-P., & Finch, M. D. (1992). Predictors of cognitive and functional progression in patients with probable Alzheimer's disease. *Neurology, 42,* 1689-1696.

National Foundation for Brain Research Archives. (1992). *The cost of disorders of the brain.* National foundation for Brain Research Archives, Washington, D.C.

O'Donnell, B. F., Drachman, D. A., Barnes, H. J., Peterson, K. E., Swearer, J. M., & Lew, R. A. (1992). Incontinence and troublesome behaviors predict institutionalization in dementia. *Journal of Geriatric Psychiatry and Neurology, 5,* 45-52.

Perry, E. K., Kerwin, J., Perry, R. H., Blessed, G, Fairbairn, A. F. (1990). Visual hallucinations and the cholinergic system in dementia [letter]. *Journal of Neurology, Neurosurgery and Psychiatry, 53,* 88.

Petry, S., Cummings, J. L, Hill, M. A., & Shapira, J. (1988). Personality alterations in dementia of the Alzheimer type. *Archives of Neurology, 45,* 1187-1190.

Petry, S., Cummings, J. L., Hill, M. A., & Shapira, J. (1989). Personality alterations in dementia of the Alzheimer type: A three-year follow-up study. *Journal of Geriatric Psychiatry and Neurology, 2,* 203-207.

Rabins, P. V., Mace, N. L, & Lucas, M. J. (1982). The impact of dementia on the family. *Journal of the American Medical Association, 248,* 333-335.

Raskind, M. A., Sadowsky, C. H., Sigmund, W. R., Beitler, P. J., & Auster, S. B. (1997). Effect of tacrine on language, praxis, and noncognitive behavioral problems in Alzheimer's disease. *Archives of Neurology, 54,* 836-840.

Ray, W. A., Griffen, M. R., Schaffner, W., Baugh, D. K., & Melton, L. J. (1987). Psychotropic drug use and the risk of hip fracture. *New England Journal of Medicine, 316,* 363-369.

Reisberg, B., Borenstein, J., Salob, S. P., Ferris, S. H., Franssen, E., & Georgotas, A. (1987). Behavioral symptoms in Alzheimer's disease: Phenomenology and treatment. *Journal of Clinical Psychiatry*, *48*, (5), 9-15.

Reisberg, B., Ferris, S. H., de Leon, M. J., & Crook, T. (1982). The Global Deterioration Scale for assessment of primary degenerative dementia. *American Journal of Psychiatry*, *139*, 1136-1139.

Reisberg, B., Franssen, E., Sclan, S. G., Kluger, A., & Ferris, S. H. (1989). Stage specific incidence of potentially remediable behavioral symptoms in aging and Alzheimer disease. *Bulletin of Clinical Neuroscience*, *54*, 95-112.

Rogers, S. L. & Friedhoff, L. T. (1996). The efficacy and safety of donepezil in patients with Alzheimer's disease: results of a US Muticentre, Randomized, Double-blind, Placebo-controlled Trial: The Donepezil Study Group. *Dementia*, *7*, 293-303.

Rosenbaum, J. F. & Pollack, M. H. (1991). Anxiety. In N. H. Cassem, (Ed.), *Massachusetts General Hospital handbook of general hospital psychiatry* (3rd ed., pp. 159-190). St. Louis, MO: Mosby-Year Book.

Rubin, E. H. & Kinscherf, D. A. (1988). Psychopathology of very mild dementia of the Alzheimer type. *American Journal of Psychiatry*, *146*, 1017-1021.

Schneider, L. S. (1993). Efficacy of treatment for geropsychiatric patients with severe mental illness. *Psychopharmacology Bulletin*, *29*, 501-524.

Schneider, L. S., Pollock, V. E., Lyness, S. A. (1990). A meta-analysis of controlled trials of neuroleptic treatment in dementia. *Journal of the American Geriatrics Society*, *38* (5), 553-563.

Schneider, L. S. & Sobin, P. B. (1992). Non-Neuroleptic treatment of behavioral symptoms and agitation in Alzheimer's disease and other dementias. *Psychopharmacology Bulletin*, *28*, 71-79.

Selkoe, D. J. (1993) Physiological production of the ß-amyloid protein and the mechanism of Alzheimer's disease. *Trends in Neuroscience*, *16*, 403-409.

Shapira, J. & Cummings, J. L. (1989). Alzheimer's disease: Changes in sexual behavior. *Medical Aspects of Human Sexuality*, *23*, 32-35.

Sival, R. C., Haffmans, P. M. J., van Gent, P. P., van Nieuwkerk, J. F., & Jansen, P. A. F. (1994). The effects of sodium valproate on disturbed behavior in dementia [letter]. *Journal of the American Geriatric Society*, *42*, 906-907.

Sobin, P., Schneider, L., & McDermott, H. (1989). Fluoxetine in the treatment of agitated dementia [letter]. *American Journal of Psychiatry*, *146*, 1636.

Steele, C., Rovner, B., Chase, G. A., & Folstein, M. (1990). Psychiatric symptoms and nursing home placement of patients with Alzheimer's disease. *American Journal of Psychiatry*, *147*, 1049-51

Stern, Y., Brandt, J., Jacobs, D. M., Marder, K., Bell, K., Sano, M., Devanand, D. P., Bylsma, R., & Laffeche G. (1994). Utility of extrapyramidal signs and psychosis as predictors of cognitive and functional decline, nursing home admission, and death in Alzheimer's disease: prospective analyses from the Predictors Study. *Neurology*, *44*, 2300-2307.

Sultzer, D. L. & Cummings, J. L. (1993). Alzheimer's disease. In R. E. Rakel (Ed.), *Conn's current therapy* (pp. 838-840). Philadelphia: WB Saunders.

Sultzer, D. L., Gray, K. F., Gunay, I., Berisford, M. A., & Mahler, M. E. (1995, May). *A comparison of trazodone and haloperidol for treatment of agitation in dementia.* Paper presented at the annual meeting of the American Psychiatric Association, Miami, FL.

Swearer, J. M., Drachman, D. A., O'Donnell, B. F., & Mitchell, A. L. (1988). Troublesome and disruptive behaviors in dementia. *Journal of the American Geriatric Society*, *36*, 784-790.

Tariot, P. N., Mack, J. L., Patterson, M. B., Edland, S. D., Weiner, M. F., Fillenbaum, G., Blazina, L., Teri, L., Rubin, E., Mortimer, J. A., Stern, Y., & the Behavioral Pathology Committee of the Consortium to Establish a Registry for Alzheimer's Disease. (1995). The Behavior Rating Scale for dementia of the Consortium to Establish a Registry for Alzheimer's Disease. *American Journal of Psychiatry*, *152*, 1349-1357.

Teri, L., Truax, P., Logsdon, R., Uomoto, J., Zarit, S., & Vitaliano, P. P. (1992). Assessment of behavioral problems in dementia: The Revised Memory and Behavior Problems Checklist. *Psychology and Aging*, *7*, 627-631.

Weiner, M. F., Edland, S. D., & Luszczynska, H. (1994). Prevalence and incidence of major depression in Alzheimer's disease. *American Journal of Psychiatry*, *151*, 1006-1009.

Whitehouse, P. J., Price, D. L., Clark, A. W., Coyle, J. T., & DeLong, M. R. (1981). Alzheimer disease: evidence for selective loss of cholinergic neurons in the nucleus basalis. *Annals of Neurology*, *10*, 122-126.

Wragg, R. E. & Jeste, D. V. (1989). Overview of depression and psychosis in Alzheimer's disease. *American Journal of Psychiatry, 146*, 577-587.

Wright, M. T. & Cummings, J. L. (1996). Neuropsychiatric disturbances in Alzheimer's disease and other dementias: Recognition and management. *The Neurologist, 2*, 207-218.

Yesavage, J. A., Brink, T. L., Rose, T. L., & Lum, O. (1983). Development and validation of a geriatric depression screening scale: a preliminary report. *Journal of Psychiatric Research, 17*, 37-49.

Zubenko, G. S., Moossy, J., & Kopp, U. (1990). Neurochemical correlates of major depression in primary dementia. *Archives of Neurology, 47*, 209-214.

Zubenko, G. S., Moossy, J., Martinez, J., Rao, G., Claassen, D., Rosen, J., & Kopp, U. (1991). Neuropathologic and neurochemical correlates of psychosis in primary dementia. *Archives of Neurology, 48*, 619-624.

CROSS-CULTURAL NEUROPSYCHOLOGY OF AGING AND DEMENTIA: AN UPDATE

Nicola Wolfe

INTRODUCTION

As the population of the United States ages and regional demographics change, neuropsychologists have been challenged to adapt to a range of clinical populations. Cross-cultural approaches to the neuropsychology of aging are in increasing demand for two major applications. First, the ethnic, racial, linguistic, and cultural diversity within the United States has called for tools of assessment and research that are appropriate for each of these groups with differing backgrounds. Second, research on aging and dementia has increasingly moved toward epidemiological studies that compare rate s and expression of illness across nations or between ethnic groups with different linguistic, racial, or socio-cultural identities.

A RECENT HISTORICAL PERSPECTIVE

The need for a cross-cultural approach to neuropsychology has been increasingly recognized over the past few years. In 1992, Matthews' presidential address to the International Neuropsychological Society (INS) called for increasing the *international* role of the INS (Matthews, 1992). In 1993, the first INS symposium on *Cross-cultural Neuropsychology* was held at the annual INS meeting in Galveston, Texas. Interest among professionals was growing, and several instruments were already developed specifically designed for cross-cultural use. By 1995, Ardila pointed to the need for a new field called *cross-cultural neuropsychology*. He described this as a "critical new direction of research" for the 21st century (Ardila, 1995). There has been a surge in interest in comparative rate s of dementing illnesses, for example, between the U.S. and Asia (White, Petrovitch, Ross, Masaki, Abbott, Wergowske, Chiu, Foley, Murdaugh, & Curb, 1996; Graves, Larsen, White, Teng, & Homma, 1996), and between the U.S. and East African populations (Friedland & Kalaria, 1998). Key in this process is the development of standardized diagnostic methods.

Historically, neuropsychologists have generally relied on standard normative data obtained from a cross-section of the American population and extrapolated to the individual, knowing only limited information about a client's culture and language. With non-English speakers, neuropsychologists relied on simple translation of items, assuming that the test instruments administered in an individual's own language would still yield valid information in spite of the lack of norms based on that client's cultural or linguistic group.

LIMITATIONS OF EXISTING INSTRUMENTS

However, in neuropsychological assessment, as has occurred in educational assessment, many of the existing neuropsychological instruments used to evaluate neuropsychological functioning in the elderly have been demonstrated to have limitations in cross-cultural use. For example, the Mini Mental State Exam (MMSE), a standard instrument for screening for cognitive decline and dementia, has been reported to be biased by education level (Escobar, Burnam, Karno, Forsythe, Landsverk, & Golding, 1986; Anthony, Le Resche, Niaz, et al., 1982) and culture (Katzman, Zhang, Orang-Ya-Qu, Wang, Liu, Wong, Salmon, & Grant, 1988). Gurland, Wilder, Cross, Teresi, and Barrett (1992) applied a compendium of five widely used screening scales in cross-cultural application. The five scales examined were the CARE Diagnostic (Golden, Teresi, & Gurland, 1983), the Kahn-Goldfarb Mental Status Questionnaire (Kahn, Goldfarb, Pollack, & Peck, 1960), the Short Portable Mental Status Questionnaire (Pfeiffer, 1975), the Blessed Memory Information Concentration (Blessed, Tomlinson, & Roth, 1968), and the MMSE (Folstein, Folstein, & McHugh, 1975). In application with Black, Hispanic, and White groups, Gurland et al. found drastically conflicting results for absolute and culturally relative rates of cognitive impairment. They concluded that differences between the scales were mostly due to their varying sensitivities, but that socio-cultural bias also played a role. Education bias also has been reported on many other neuropsychological instruments such as the Wisconsin Card Sort Test (WCST) (Rosselli & Ardila, 1993).

Advances in the cross-cultural neuropsychology of aging can be grouped into three general areas: (1) Modification of existing tests – translation and adaptation of existing instruments for different linguistic and socio-cultural groups; (2) *De novo* test construction – construction of completely new tests specifically designed for cross-cultural purposes (including item selection, item analysis, pilot studies, normative studies, validity, and reliability studies); (3) Norm development – developing norms for tests in a wide range of different populations (especially norms for age, education, and individual ethnic groups).

MODIFICATION OF EXISTING TESTS

In response to the need for cross-cultural neuropsychology, there has been a recent explosion of translations, modifications, and adaptations of existing instruments for a range of language and ethnic groups; these include Cree (Cree-speaking natives on reserves in Manitoba), Czech, Chamorro (Guam), Chinese (Shanghaiese, Cantonese, Mandarin, and Kinmen, a Chinese islet), Croatian, Danish, Dutch, Finnish, French, German, Spanish, Hindi (India, Pakistan, and

Bangladesh), Icelandic, Italian, Japanese, Malay (Singapore), South African, Vietnamese, and Yoruba (Yoruba-speaking population of Ibadan, Nigeria).

Increasingly, however, emphasis in cross-cultural neuropsychology has been shifting away from translation and adaptation (Brislin, Lanner, & Thorndike, 1973; Karno, Burman, Escobar, & Eaton, 1993) toward test development *de novo*, that is, new tests specifically designed for cross-cultural use (Wolfe, 1993).

THREE NEWER CROSS-CULTURAL DEMENTIA SCREENING INSTRUMENTS

In an attempt to assess elderly and demented persons with reduced cultural bias, there have been several excellent instruments developed over the past few years. Three of these instruments are briefly described below.

Cognitive Abilities Screening Instrument (CASI)

An excellent example of an instrument specifically designed for cross-cultural neuropsychology of the elderly is the Cognitive Abilities Screening Instrument (CASI) (Teng, 1996; Teng, Hasegawa, Homma, Imai, Larson, Graves, Sugimoto, Yamaguchi, Sasaki, Shui, & White, 1994). Evolving over years of research by Evelyn Teng and colleagues in the area of the epidemiology of dementia, the CASI offers tremendous advances in the field. The CASI has increasingly gained attention as a neuropsychological screening instrument for dementia that was designed for cross-cultural use. This instrument offers several advantages and has been applied especially in the international collaborative epidemiological research of dementia among Japan, the U.S., and China. White et al. (1996) used the CASI as the screening assessment instrument in a large scale epidemiological study of dementia called the Honolulu-Asia Aging Study. Briefly described,

> the CASI... provides quantitative assessment on attention, concentration, orientation, short-term memory, long-term memory, language abilities, visual construction, list-generating fluency, abstraction and judgement (Teng et al., 1994).

Scores on the MMSE, the Modified Mini-Mental State Test (3MS), and the Hasegawa Dementia Screening Scale can also be estimated from subsets of the CASI items. Pilot testing conducted in Japan and in the U.S. has demonstrated its cross-cultural applicability and its usefulness in screening for dementia, in monitoring disease progression, and in providing profiles of cognitive impairment. Typical administration time is 15 to 20 minutes. The CASI has a Short Form (4-item) which has been reported to perform comparably to the MMSE, the 3MS, and to the Hasegawa Dementia Scale in sensitivity and specificity for detecting dementia in individuals aged 51 to 93 in the U.S. and Japan (Teng et al., 1994). The CASI requires literacy, however, and thus may be less appropriate for populations with little or no formal education.

The Cross-Cultural Cognitive Examination (CCCE)

Filling a niche for use in non-literate populations, the Cross-Cultural Cognitive Examination (CCCE) (Glosser, Wolfe, Albert, et al., 1993) is an instrument similar to the CASI, designed for cross-cultural neuropsychological screening for dementia. The CCCE was also designed for epidemiological application, but specifically evolved out of demand for screening in *non-literate* populations. Originally constructed for an NIH neuroepidemiologic study of Guam-Parkinsonism-Dementia-Complex, the CCCE offers several unique advantages (Glosser, Wolfe, Albert, Lavine, Steele, Calne, & Schoenberg, 1993). The CCCE was designed to assess a range of basic cognitive functions over eight domains: attention, language, visuo-spatial, verbal memory, visual memory, recent memory, abstraction, and psychomotor speed. Incorporated in the CCCE, is the two-stage method of case identification used in population surveys. Thus, the test includes a five-minute brief screening procedure, designed to be highly sensitive, followed by a more extended 20 minute mental status examination, designed to be more specific for identifying dementia, intended for individuals who fail the screening portion. In several validation studies in mainland U.S. populations, Chamorro villagers in Guam, and in Japan, language, education, and social factors did not significantly compromise the high sensitivity and specificity of the CCCE for identifying cases of dementia (Wolfe, Imai, Otani, Nagatani, Hasegawa, Sugimoto, Tanaka, Kuroda, Glosser, & Albert, 1992; Tanaka, Miyazaki, Sugimoto, Yamaguchi, & Wolfe, 1992; Glosser et al., 1993). Criterion validity of the CCCE, with respect to other accepted dementia screening measures, was also demonstrated (Glosser et al., 1993). These findings support the usefulness of the CCCE in cross-cultural neuroepidemiological research.

Community Screening Instrument for Dementia (CSI'D)

The purpose of the Community Screening Instrument for Dementia (CSI'D) (Hall, Ogunniyi, Hendrie, Osuntokun, Hui, Musiek, Rodenberg, Unverzagt, Guerje, & Baiyewu, 1996) is, like the CCCE, to screen for dementia particularly in epidemiological studies. The CSI'D has a unique two-part design; one part includes cognitive and risk factors, the other an interview with a relative about daily functioning and general health of the subject. The inclusion of information on daily functioning has been recommended, for example, by Jorm and Jacomb (1989) as a way to avoid educational bias in cognitive testing. The CSI'D was developed and validated in a study comparing Cree Indians in Manitoba and Manitobans of European extraction (Hall, Hendrie, Rodgers, et al., 1993). It has been further applied to study incidence and prevalence of dementia in a cross-cultural study of elderly community-dwelling African Americans in Indianapolis and Yoruba in Ibadan, Nigeria. In each application, the instrument was adapted for the particular language and cultural setting. Although both the Cree language and Yoruba have written forms, they are predominantly spoken languages, and the subjects tested were largely unable to read or write.

In an interview of approximately 20 minutes, the cognitive items are designed to measure memory, abstract thinking, judgment, other disturbances of higher cortical function, personality changes, and functioning at work and in social relationships. Hall's careful development included item selection, adaptation, two independent translations, consensus translations, back-translation, two pilot tests and subsequent revisions, and determination of cut-off scores for screening (Hall et al., 1996).

In their study of the CSI'D (Hall et al., 1996) the screening stage was followed by a detailed diagnosis. Individuals identified as possibly demented based on performance on the CSI'D then completed a range of other evaluations (CERAD-NB, CAMCOG, CT scans, relative interview, neurological assessment, and laboratory tests). Results suggest that the sensitivity and specificity of the instrument in both sites combined was 87.0% (sensitivity) and 83.1% (specificity), respectively (Hall et al., 1996).

The three instruments above are among the best brief screening instruments for detecting possible dementia, but this list is not comprehensive. Tests of specific domains include the Taussig Cross-Cultural Memory Test (Taussig & Ponton, 1993), and instruments relying particularly on informant sources have also been developed for cross-cultural neuropsychological screening. One recent example of these is the Informant Questionnaire on Cognitive Decline in the Elderly (IQCODE) (Fuh, Teng, Lin, Larson, Wang, Lui, Chou, Kuo, & Lui, 1995). Valle (1994) has presented a so-called *culture-fair behavioral assessment and intervention model* for non-cognitive behaviors. For more in-depth clinical neuropsychological assessment there is the Spanish and English Neuropsychology Assessment Scale (SENAS) (Mungas, 1996). Still under development, the SENAS has been designed with 12 tests, 6 verbal and 6 non-verbal assessments of a range of cognitive domains. Ideally suited for assessment of elderly and demented subjects, it could have broader applications as well (Mungas, personal communication). This instrument should represent a substantial advance over available methods, as it is specifically designed *de novo* with cross-cultural application in mind, using rigorous psychometric methods including item-analysis.

SOME METHODS FOR CONSTRUCTING NEW CROSS-CULTURAL INSTRUMENTS (DE NOVO)

Some of the psychometric methods recommended by Mungas to reduce cultural bias are outlined in an excellent chapter in *Ethnicity and the dementias* (Mungas, 1996). Cultural sensitivity of the test developer may not be sufficient. Mungas suggests that one cannot always anticipate bias. Instead, he recommends specifically testing for bias. He emphasizes the importance of combining knowledge and experience with rigorous empirical methods (Mungas, 1996).

RECOMMENDATIONS

Define *Culturally Equivalent*

Ideally, a neuropsychological instrument or item used in cross-cultural application would be *culture-fair* or *culturally equivalent*. Cultural equivalence might be defined as equivalence of scores across national, cultural boundaries or ethnically non-discriminatory use within a society. Early attempts based on nonverbal and performance tests (Anastasi, 1988; Cattell, 1940) did not prove to be as culture-fair as hoped (Anastasi, 1988; Vernon, 1969). Unfortunately, non-verbal testing does not necessarily reduce cultural bias, and many non-verbal abilities, such as the ability to draw in three dimensions, are highly education-dependent (Cattell, 1979). Thus, it is probably more realistic to aim for *culturally-reduced tasks* rather than *culturally-loaded tasks*.

Documenting Population Demographics

In cross-cultural applications of neuropsychology it can be particularly helpful to start with a thorough delineation of population demographics; these include the more routinely obtained age, sex, and education information. In addition, to fully describe the sociocultural context, many other variables are relevant; these include race, socioeconomic status, occupation, religion, size of community (urban versus rural), and language preference. Demographic information is especially important when attempting to match samples and compare two cultural groups (Wolfe et al., 1992). Ardila has emphasized the importance of clearly distinguishing education and cultural variables. Differences resulting from education are sometimes attributed to cultural and even ethnic differences (Ardila, 1995). Ardila (1995) noted that less educated individuals sometimes perform on neuropsychological tests like some brain-injured subjects. This is called the *Ardila effect*. Thus, education should be coded and analyzed rigorously, including years of education and country of origin, to evaluate its contribution to a cohort effect (Taussig & Ponton, 1996).

Ethnicity can be difficult to define. Self-report is often relied upon. However, in ethnic minorities, variables such as the degree of acculturation and assimilation are difficult to quantify (Sue, 1996). In many cross-cultural applications, for example with immigrant populations, it helps to assess an individual's degree of acculturation and bilingualism. This can be accomplished with the aid of acculturation scales and by allowing for multiple responses in regional dialects. Multi-site studies help as well (Taussig & Ponton, 1996). Measures of acculturation generally include items such as age at immigration, educational history, social class, health care preferences, and beliefs.

Translation and Back Translation

Several useful translation methods outlined by Brislin (1980) include: back translation – a bilingual translator performs independent translation into the original language to ensure original meaning is preserved; bilingual technique – two groups of bilinguals compare items in each language, and items which yield discrepant responses can be identified; committee approach – translation by a committee of bilinguals; and pretest procedures – field testing to ensure items are well understood (Brislin, 1980).

Careful translation still does not necessarily solve all problems. Standard screening instruments such as the MMSE (Folstein et al., 1975) have been translated, but still require attention to individual items. For example, Katzman (1988) noted that the item that asks individuals to read *close your eyes* had a death connotation in Shanghai and was changed to the less offensive *raise your arms*.

Adaptation of individual test items must also preserve difficulty level. For example, for Digit Span tests repetition may be easier in languages where each digit is spoken in a single syllable, reducing the time and complexity of the task. Similarly, the task of naming the months of the year may be easier in Japan versus in the U.S. because names of the months are simply in numerical order (month one, month two, etc.).

Selection and Adaptation of Individual Item Selection

Jensen (1980) recommended several general methods in test construction that can help to reduce cultural loading. These include choosing the following: performance tests, oral instructions, pictorial responses, power tests (instead of speed tests), non-verbal content, abstract reasoning (instead of specific factual knowledge), non-scholastic tasks, and solving novel problems (instead of recall of past-learned information) (Jensen, 1980).

Several general principles for selecting items are suggested below: Items should (1) be understandable and meaningful to all subjects (i.e., items should have maximum ecological validity), (2) be interpretable by other neuropsychologists, and previously normed tests should be used when possible, (3) be able to be scored in an objective fashion, (4) be readily translatable, (5) not be obviously biased in one culture, (6) not require special training that some subjects do not have (e.g., literacy or mathematical ability), (7) be practical for administration, and (8) be as non-threatening as possible. In addition, Mungas (1996) suggests making more items than needed in order to have room to eliminate biased items during test development, and including a range of difficulties such that demented subjects are able to pass some items and healthy individuals may fail some items.

A key methodological consideration in new test construction is that two versions of an instrument must be matched for overall difficulty level. Chapman and Chapman (1973; 1988) note that scales must be matched according to their psychometric characteristics to reach valid conclusions about the presence of differential deficits in an ability.

DEFINING ITEM BIAS

An item can be defined as biased if "individuals with the same amount of an underlying trait, from different sub-populations, have different probabilities of responding to an item correctly" (Hulin, Drasgow, & Parsons, 1983). The use of item analysis is described well by Mungas (1996) in his development of SENAS. The item response approach is well suited to cross-cultural application because it uses non-linear regression of the probability of passing each item. An item is non-biased if the item curves are equal in two groups – that is, if two individuals of equal ability from different groups have the same expected outcome. The difficulty with using item response theory in the development of cross-cultural tests is the reliance on large normative sample sizes. While this has been somewhat easier to obtain with multiple choice tests used in educational assessment, the longer, more complex administration of the neuropsychological batteries makes large samples more difficult to obtain.

SPECIFIC ADAPTATIONS TO CONTROL FOR EDUCATION DIFFERENCES

Education clearly affects performance on neuropsychological tests and differs tremendously among sociocultural, racial, and ethnic groups. Two major methods for management of education effects have been proposed: A neuropsychological instrument could be statistically adjusted for education (Kittner, White, Farmer, Wolz, Kaplan, Moes, Brody, & Feinlieb, 1986) using a stratified regression or non-parametric method, or it could be designed to be less sensitive to education effects (Berkman, 1986). These two approaches, however, are not mutually exclusive. The best methods may be those that design instruments to be less sensitive to education effects and also adjust for education level. However, investigators differ in opinion on whether to develop items that are not education-biased. Some explain that because underlying abilities (cognitive processes) are education-biased, it is not appropriate to eliminate educational effects from instruments.

In order to reduce the cultural bias that is due to more than just educational differences, Mungas (1996) described psychometric methods (for example, the use of ANCOVA), which examine the relationship between scales or items, and variables such as age, education, and language.

VALIDITY AND RELIABILITY

The principles of test construction, including establishing validity and reliability, are particularly important in cross-cultural neuropsychology. New instruments require structured clinical validation protocols (LaRue & Markee, 1995). Studies of criterion validity, comparing the new instrument to some existing *gold standard*, are especially important to ensure interpretability of the new instrument in each culture. An example of the design of such a study can be found in Wolfe, Imai, Otani, Nagatani, Hasegawa, Sugimoto, Tanaka, Kuroda, Glosser, and Albert (1992). Excellent examples of test-retest and inter-rater reliability studies are also available (Hall et al., 1996).

TEST ADMINISTRATION/TRAINING GOALS

How does one adapt to *culture* that is not static? Training individuals for cross-cultural neuropsychology includes increasing awareness and knowledge of test items' relevance to different cultures, keeping abreast of research related to culturally diverse groups, and achieving some cultural competency greater than only written and spoken language (Hinkle, 1994). Researchers can familiarize themselves with those dimensions of culture most relevant to neuropsychological assessment such as language (dialects and idiom), religions, family structures, recent history, attitudes toward disclosure, non-verbal conventions (e.g., eye contact and interpersonal distance), and attitudes toward health and disability.

Some suggestions for the administration of cross-cultural instruments (Ardila, 1995) are that testers should speak the same language or dialect as the examinee. They should be familiar with principles of neuropsychological assessment such as maintaining a non-judgmental attitude, offering encouragement, confidentiality, and explaining the goals of the evaluation. Furthermore, test instructions should not be in a formal language that people do not use themselves and that could be misunderstood (Ardila, 1995). Testers should be well trained in the instruments to be administered.

An example of a sample tester training program is outlined below: (1) Select testers (bilingual, educated, and motivated); (2) Review goals of neuropsychological testing; (3) Provide detailed training with a written manual, video, and verbatim instructions; (4) Encourage testers to practice and provide detailed feedback; (5) Evaluate tester competency (e.g., quiz) to qualify the tester; and (6) Adapt the instrument and testing methods based on pilot results.

Implementation of some of the recommendations outlined above could help to reduce cultural bias, making neuropsychological assessment more cross-cultural.

FUTURE DIRECTIONS IN CROSS-CULTURAL NEUROPSYCHOLOGY

In some regions of the United States, ethnic minorities will soon be the majority of those over 65 years old. Thus, the demand for cross-cultural neuropsychology of aging is urgent. In response to immediate needs, investigators have been working to establish norms and to construct new cross-cultural neuropsychological instruments. The progress described in this chapter presents the first advances in this rapidly emerging field.

REFERENCES

Ardila, A. (1995). Directions of research in cross-cultural neuropsychology. *Journal of Clinical and Experimental Neuropsychology, 17*, 143-150.
Anastasi, A. (1988). *Psychological testing.* New York: Macmillan.
Anthony, J. S., Le Resche, L., Niaz, U., Vo-Korff, M. R., & Folstein, M. F. (1982). Limits of the "Mini-Mental State" as a screening test for dementia and delirium among hospital patients. *Psychological Medicine, 12*, 397-408.
Berkman, L. F. (1986). The association between educational attainment and mental status examinations, of etiologic significance for senile dementia or not? *Journal of Chronic Disease, 39*, 171-173.
Blessed, G., Tomlinson, B. E., & Roth, M. (1968). The association between qualitative measures of dementia and senile change with cerebral matter of elderly subjects. *British Journal of Psychiatry, 114*, 792-811.
Brislin, R. W. (1980). Translation and content analysis of oral and written materials. In H. C. Triandis & J. W. Berry (Eds.), *Handbook of cross-cultural psychology. Methodology* (Vol. 2, pp. 386-444). Boston: Allyn and Bacon, Inc.
Brislin, R. W., Lanner, W. J., & Thorndike, R. M. (1973). *Cross-cultural research methods.* New York: John Wiley.
Cattell, R. B. (1940). A culture free intelligence test. Part 1. *Journal of Educational Psychology, 31*, 161-179.
Cattell, R. B. (1979). Are culture fair intelligence tests possible and necessary? *Journal of Research and Development in Education, 12*, 3-13.
Chapman, L. S. & Chapman, J. D. (1973). *Disordered thought in schizophrenia.* New York: Appleton-Century-Crofts.
Chapman, L. C. & Chapman, J. C. (1988). Artifactual and genuine relationships of lateral difference scores to overall accuracy in studies of laterality. *Psychological Bulletin, 104*, 127-136.
Escobar, J. I., Burnam, A., Karno, M., Forsythe, A., Landsverk, J., & Golding, J. M. (1986). Use of the Mini-Mental State Examination (MMSE) in a community population of mixed ethnicity. Cultural and linguistic artifacts. *Journal of Nervous and Mental Disease, 174* (10), 607-614.

Foldi, N. S. (1988). Research in human neuropsychology: Issues of aging. In B. Kent & R. N Butler (Eds.), *Human aging research: Concepts and techniques* (pp. 285-297). New York: Raven Press.

Folstein, M. F., Folstein, S. E., & McHugh, P. R. (1975). The Mini-Mental State. A practical method of grading the cognitive state of patients for the clinician. *Journal of Psychiatric Research, 12*, 189-198.

Friedland, R. P. & Kalaria R. N. T (1998). The East African Dementia Project. Establishment of the Nyeri dementia study and training workshops in the clinical neurosciences. *IBRO News, 1*, 1.

Fuh, J. L., Teng, E. L., Lin, K. N., Larson, E. B., Wang, S. J., Lui, C. Y., Chou, P., Kuo, B. I., & Lui, H. C. (1995). The Informant Questionnaire on Cognitive Decline in the Elderly (IQCODE) as a screening tool for dementia for a predominantly illiterate Chinese population. *Neurology, 45*, 92-96.

Glosser, G., Wolfe, N., Albert, M. L., Lavine, L., Steele, J. C., Calne, D. B., & Schoenberg, B. S. (1993). Cross-cultural cognitive examination: Validation of a dementia screening instrument for neuroepidemiological research. *Journal of the American Geriatric Society, 41*, 931-939.

Golden, R. R., Teresi, J. A., & Gurland, B. J. (1983). Detection of dementia and depression cases with the Comprehensive Assessment and Referral Evaluation interview schedule. *International Journal of Aging and Human Development, 16*, 242-254.

Gurland, B. J., Wilder, D. E., Cross, T., Teresi, J., & Barrett V. W. (1992). Screening scales for dementia: Toward reconciliation of conflicting cross-cultural findings. *International Journal of Geriatric Psychiatry, 7*, 105-113.

Graves, A. B., Larsen, E. B., White, L. R., Teng, E. L., & Homma, A. (1994). Opportunities and challenges in international collaborative epidemiologic research of dementia and subtypes. Studies between Japan and the United States. *International Psychogeriatrics, 6* (2), 209-223.

Hall, K. S., Hendrie, H. C., & Rodgers, D. D. (1993). The development of a dementia screening interview in two distinct languages. *International Journal of Methods in Psychiatric Research, 3*, 1-28.

Hall, K. S., Ogunniyi, A. O., Hendrie, H. C., Osuntokun, B. O., Hui, S. L., Musick B. S., Rodenberg C. A., Unverzagt, F. W., Guerje, O., & Baiyewu, O. (1996). A cross-cultural community based study of dementias: Methods and performance of the survey instrument in Indianapolis, USA and Ibadan, Nigeria. *International Journal of Methods in Psychiatric Research, 6*, 129-142.

Hinkle, J. S. (1994). Practitioners of cross-cultural assessment: A practical guide to information and training. Special Issue: Multicultural assessment. *Measurement and Evaluation in Counseling and Development, 27*, 103-115.

Hulin, C. L., Drasgow, F., & Parsons, C. K. (1983). *Item response theory: Application to psychological measurement*. Homewood, IL: Dow Jones-Irwin.

Jensen, A. R. (1980). *Bias in mental testing*. New York: Free Press.

Jorm, A. F. & Jacomb, P. A. (1989). The informant questionnaire on cognitive decline in the elderly (IQCODE): Socio-demographic correlates, reliability, validity and some norms. *Psychological Medicine, 19*, 1015-1022.

Kahn, R. L., Goldfarb, A. I., Pollack, M., & Peck, A. (1960). Brief objective measure for the determination of mental status in the aged. *American Journal of Psychiatry, 117*, 326-328.

Karno, M., Burman, M. A., Escobar, J. I., & Eaton, W. W. (1993). Development of the Spanish-language version of the National Institute of Mental Health diagnostic interview. *Archives of General Psychiatry, 40*, 1183-1188.

Katzman R., Zhang, M., Orang-Ya-Qu, Wang, S., Liu, W. R., Wong, S., Salmon, D. P., & Grant, I. (1988). A Chinese version of the Mini-Mental State Examination: Impact of illiteracy in a Shanghai dementia survey. *Journal of Clinical Epidemiology, 41*, 971-978.

Kittner, S. J., White, L. R., Farmer, M. E., Wolz, M., Kaplan, E., Moes, E., Brody, J. A., & Feinlieb, M. (1986). Methodologic issues in screening for dementia: The problem of education adjustment. *Journal of Chronic Disease, 39*, 163-170.

LaRue, A. (1987). Methodological concerns: Longitudinal studies of dementia. *Alzheimer's Disease and Associated Disorders, 1* (3), 180-192.

Lowenstein, D. A., Arguelles, T., Arguelles, S., & Linn-Fuentes, P. (1994). Potential cultural bias in the neuropsychological assessment of the older adult. *Journal of Clinical and Experimental Neuropsychology, 16* (4), 623-629.

Matthews, C. G. (1992). Truth in labeling: Are we really an international society? *Journal of Clinical and Experimental Neuropsychology, 14*, 418-426.

Mungas, D. (1996). The process of development of valid and reliable neuropsychological assessment measures for English- and Spanish-speaking elderly persons. In G. Yeo & D. Gallagher-Thompson (Eds.), *Ethnicity and the dementias* (pp. 33-46). Washington, DC: Taylor and Francis.

Pfeiffer, E. (1975). A short portable mental status questionnaire for the assessment of organic brain deficit in elderly patients. *Journal of the American Geriatric Society*, 22 (10), 433-444.

Rosselli, M. & Ardila, A. (1993). Effects of age, gender and socioeconomic level on the Wisconsin Card Sorting Test. *The Clinical Neuropsychologist*, 7, 145-154.

Sue, S. (1996). Measurement, testing and ethnic bias: Can solutions be found? In G. R. Sodowsky & J. C. Impara (Eds.), *Multicultural assessment in counseling and clinical psychology* (pp. 7-36). Lincoln, NE: Buros Institute of Mental Measurements.

Tanaka, Y., Miyazaki, M., Sugimoto, K., Yamaguchi, T., & Wolfe, N. (1992). Preliminary validation study of the Mental Status Examination (MSE) [in Japanese with English abstract]. *Neurological Medicine*, 36 (1), 51-56.

Taussig, I. M., Dick, M., Teng, E., & Kempler, D. (1993). *The Taussig Cross-cultural Memory Test*. University of Southern California, Andrus Gerontology Center, Los Angeles, CA.

Taussig, I. M. & Ponton, M. (1996). Issues in neuropsychological assessment for Hispanic older adults: Cultural and linguistic factors. In G. Yeo & D. Gallagher-Thompson (Eds.), *Ethnicity and the dementias* (pp. 47-58). Washington, DC: Taylor and Francis.

Teng, E. L., Hasegawa, K., Homma, A., Imai, Y., Larson, E., Graves, A., Sugimoto, K., Yamaguchi, T., Sasaki, H., Shui, E., & White, L. R. (1994). The Cognitive Abilities Screening Instrument (CASI): A practical test for cross-cultural epidemiological studies of dementia. *International Psychogeriatrics*, 6, 45-58.

Teng, E. L. (1996). Cross-Cultural Testing and the Cognitive Abilities Screening Instrument. In G. Yeo & D. Gallagher-Thompson (Eds.), *Ethnicity and the dementias* (pp. 77-85). Washington, DC: Taylor and Francis.

Valle, R. (1994). Culture fair behavioral symptom differential assessment and intervention in dementing illness. *Alzheimer's Disease and Associated Disorders*, 8 (3), 21-45.

Vernon, P. E. (1969). *Intelligence and cultural environment*. London: Methuen.

White, L., Petrovitch, H., Ross, G. W., Masaki, K. H., Abbott, R. D., Wergowske, G., Chiu, D., Foley, D. J., Murdaugh, D., & Curb, J. D. (1996). Prevalence of dementia in older Japanese-American men in Hawaii: The Honolulu-Asia Aging Study. *Journal of the American Medical Association*, 276 (12), 993-5.

Wolfe, N., Imai, Y., Otani, C., Nagatani, H., Hasegawa, K., Sugimoto, K., Tanaka, Y., Kuroda, Y., Glosser, G., & Albert, M. L. (1992). Criterion validity of the Cross-Cultural Cognitive Examination (CCCE) in Japan. *Journal of Gerontology*, 47 (4), 289-291.

Wolfe, N. (1993, February). *Psychometric issues in cross-cultural neuropsychology. Cross-cultural Issues in Neuropsychological Assessment*. Symposium held during the Twenty First Annual Meeting of the International Neuropsychological Society, Galveston, Texas, USA.

Yeo, G. & Gallagher-Thompson, D. (Eds.). (1996). *Ethnicity and the dementias*. Washington, DC: Taylor and Francis.

VALIDATION OF THE NEUROBEHAVIORAL EVALUATION SYSTEM (NES) IN PATIENTS WITH FOCAL BRAIN DAMAGE

Rhea Diamond, Roberta F. White, Maxine Krengel,
Karen Lindem, Robert G. Feldman, Carole Palumbo,
Richard Letz, Ellen Eisen, and David Wegman

INTRODUCTION

Several computer-based test batteries based upon methods used in neuropsychological and neurobehavioral assessment have been developed for use in studies of occupational and environmental health and related fields (Kane & Kay, 1992). The advantages of computer-based batteries include standardized and precise presentation of test materials and efficient, objective, and accurate collection of response data. The *Neurobehavioral Evaluation System* (NES) (Letz & Baker, 1988) has been the most widely used of these computerized systems in the fields of occupational and environmental health (Letz, 1990).

The primary purpose for which the NES was developed was investigation of the effects of exposure to substances suspected to be neurotoxicants. Several studies have provided data supporting the instrument's adequate psychometric properties. Evidence that the NES shows an acceptable level of reliability comes from test-retest correlations in the range 0.6 to 0.9, obtained under both laboratory and field conditions (Arcia & Otto, 1992; Letz, 1990). Selected NES subtests have correlated, albeit to a moderate degree, with the standardized tests to which they are related (Baker et al., 1985; Hooisma et al., 1990; Krengel, White, & Diamond, 1996) and with demographic variables such as age, sex, and education.

Direct evidence that deficits on NES subtests are seen in subjects exposed to neurotoxicants (relative to unexposed controls) has been obtained in several laboratory studies using acute experimental exposure to toxicants (Echeverria, Fine, Langolf, Schork, & Sampaio, 1989; Echeverria, Fine, Langolf, Schork, & Sampaio, 1990; Greenberg, Moore, Letz, & Baker, 1985; Mahoney, Moore, Baker, & Letz, 1988). Epidemiologic studies using the NES have confirmed dose-effect relationships between impaired performance on particular subtests and exposure to a number of industrial agents (Anger, 1990; Letz, 1990).

Although findings from both the inter-test reliability and neurotoxicant studies suggest that NES subtests are valid measures of brain function, a more direct and informative method of exploring this issue is available: the relation between performance on the NES and well-documented evidence of brain damage. The initial question of interest is the ability of the NES subtests to detect such damage. Damage to any part of the brain is believed likely to yield impaired conceptual and abstract thinking, slowing of ideation, and reduced capacity for attention and immediate memory (Goodglass & Kaplan, 1979). To the extent that performance on a particular NES subtest is affected by one or more of these deficiencies, that subtest will detect neurologic abnormality. In addition to these general effects, patients with a variety of neurologic syndromes have been described as showing selective neuropsychological impairments that often permit a diagnostic impression in an individual case and that may also suggest a possible etiology (Grant & Adams, 1986; Lezak, 1995; Luria, 1962/1980; White, 1992).

Several different types of assessment methodologies have contributed to the descriptions of specific brain-behavior relationships provided in the neuropsychological literature. One type involves a detailed characterization of the patient's behavior during performance of a finely graded set of tasks. This method seeks to specify the nature of the deficits associated with damage to particular brain systems; qualitative contrasts between the performance of the same task by patients with brain damage at different loci are often utilized for that purpose (Luria, 1962/1980). Another assessment methodology employs batteries of standardized tests with known psychometric properties to identify particular areas in which an individual is impaired relative to appropriate norms. The pattern of scores across individual tests (and at times certain qualitative features of performance) are typically used to generate a description of the patient's functional capacities (Grant, 1986; Lezak, 1995; White, 1992).

Specific neuropsychological tests are often assigned to functional domains that include general intelligence, manual motor functions, attention and executive function, language and verbal skills, visuospatial abilities, learning and memory, and mood. The assignment of tests to domains does not comprise a well-defined theoretical structure but rather a grouping with considerable face validity that has served the clinical purposes to which it has been applied. Findings on a variety of tests that are believed to assess a common function have contributed to the literature associating particular neurologic syndromes with impairments in particular domains. Direct comparisons of performance on the same test by groups of patients with lesions at different sites are often unavailable. Moreover, it is well understood that single tests reflect functioning in more than one domain and that task variables (such as whether items used in tests of memory are verbal or visual) play an important part in determining the level of performance observed. All mental functions are currently understood to be subserved by systems comprised of widely dispersed networks of neural units and thus to be subject to disruption by lesions occurring at a variety of sites or by lesions that interrupt the pathways between relevant sites. In conformity with this model, investigations using the techniques of cognitive psychology have dissected some of these functions, identifying component processes to which specific areas of the brain make discrete contributions (McCarthy & Warrington, 1990).

Although many of the subtests of the NES derive from neuropsychological tests that have been used in clinical assessments and may be assigned to the domains to which those tests have most often been assigned, they differ from those tests in many respects. In particular, the NES subtests tend to be less complex than many neuropsychological tests. Moreover, the NES subtests differ even from the specific traditional tests they most closely resemble in features such as mode of stimulus presentation (visual rather than auditory) and mode of response (key press rather than spoken response or graphic production of a symbol). These differences in task variables may or may not alter the patterns of impairment seen in patients with well-defined neurologic syndromes. Instances in which findings in the neuropsychological literature generalize to NES subtests despite differences in task structure support the utility of the concept of functional domain. Instances in which NES results differ from those expected on the basis of the neuropsychological literature invite analysis of the basis for those differences.

This report describes a validation study of the current version of the NES, the NES2 (Letz, 1991), in a group of neurologic patients who had sustained focal damage to grey matter and/or subcortical white matter, most frequently as a result of stroke. In each case the damage was either confined to a specific quadrant of the brain or the extension of the lesion to an adjacent quadrant was considered minimal. The study was designed to answer three distinct questions. The first is whether the NES2 subtests are able to detect the fact that these patients are neurologically abnormal. The second is whether there is evidence that performance on particular NES2 subtests is differentially vulnerable to damage localized to specific quadrants of the brain. The third, given evidence of differential vulnerability to quadrant of brain damage, is the extent to which such patterns cohere with the associations between sites of brain damage and selective functional impairments that are described in the neuropsychological literature.

In the present investigation each group of patients is compared separately with neurologically normal controls. To the extent that these patients are impaired relative to controls, the NES2 subtests are validated as detecting brain damage. To the extent that the patterns of impairments on NES2 subtests of patients with focal lesions localized to left, right, anterior, and posterior quadrants conform to expectations derived from the neuropsychological literature, the NES2 subtests are also validated as detecting brain damage related to those areas. (A validation study of performance on the NES2 by patients with two other types of neuropathology, the white matter lesions of multiple sclerosis and the basal ganglia, and dopaminergic system dysfunction of idiopathic Parkinson's disease, has been reported separately by White, Diamond, Krengel, Lindem, and Feldman, 1996.)

A broad description of patterns of deficits associated with focal damage to the brain can be extracted from the neuropsychological literature (Lezak, 1995; Luria, 1962/1980; Reitan, 1986). (Expectations derived from this literature for performance of specific NES2 subtests are deferred to the *Results* section.) General intelligence, a composite measure, usually includes subscales measuring verbal and nonverbal abilities. Damage to any part of the brain may result in a decline in abilities of both types but lesions localized to the left hemisphere have regularly been associated with deficits in language and verbal skills whereas lesions localized to the right hemisphere have been associated with deficits in nonverbal skills.

Impairments in the control of movements of the hands, including measures of strength, speed, dexterity, and coordination, have been associated with damage localized to the frontal lobes. Attentional functions have been reported to be compromised by damage to any quadrant of the brain but to be especially sensitive to damage to areas of the frontal lobe; there is also evidence that attentional impairments such as unilateral neglect are found more frequently after damage to the right hemisphere rather than to the left (Bisiach & Vallar, 1988). Executive functions, which involve the planning and organization of all types of action, have also been shown to be especially vulnerable to lesions of the frontal lobe. Visuospatial functions have generally been reported to be impaired by lesions localized to parietal and parieto-occipital areas of either hemisphere, although deficits associated with posterior lesions of the right hemisphere have frequently been reported to be especially severe. Both anterior and posterior brain structures have been implicated in learning and memory: Lesions of the temporal lobe of the left hemisphere have been found to be especially detrimental to learning, retention, and retrieval of verbal materials whereas parieto-occipital lesions of either hemisphere have been associated with defects in learning and memory of visuospatial materials. Mood disorders of several kinds have frequently been described in patients who have sustained focal brain damage. Anxiety and depressive reactions have often been observed in patients with left-hemisphere lesions and a range of affective responses, including jocularity, euphoria, and anger, have frequently been reported in patients with right-hemisphere lesions (Gainotti, 1989; Starkstein & Robinson, 1991).

METHODS

Participants

Patients were recruited from the in-patient and out-patient Neurology services at the Boston Department of Veterans Affairs Medical Center and the Boston University Medical Center. Spouses, other family members, and friends of neurologic patients seen on those services were enrolled to form a group to serve as age- and sex-matched controls. All procedures were approved by the Institutional Review Board of both institutions and all subjects signed informed consent forms before entering the study. The patients' medical charts were reviewed in order to exclude individuals with neurologic or psychiatric disorders predating or co-existing with the current disorder (e.g., seizure disorder, encephalitis, psychiatric diagnosis of affective or psychotic illness, current substance abuse). Questions relevant to these exclusion criteria were also incorporated into an initial interview with each potential subject. This interview was also used to obtain an educational history; subjects reporting a history suggestive of the presence of a learning disability or of an attention deficit disorder were excluded. Controls were screened during the initial interview for a history of any neurologic disorder and for the remaining exclusion criteria applied to patients. All subjects were also screened for dementia using three traditional neuropsychological tests (see below).

A total of 42 patients participated, of whom the majority ($n = 32$) had sustained a unilateral CVA. Time since stroke onset was between one month and three years in 20 cases and greater than three years for the remaining 12 cases. CT scans obtained within the year prior to testing were reviewed and CT slices labeled according to the method developed by Naeser and associates (Naeser & Hayward, 1978). Lesions were classified based on laterality (left or right cerebral hemisphere) and location within each hemisphere (anterior or posterior). Where available, current MRI scans of the head (within one year of testing) were reviewed to exclude patients with lacunar state or leukoariosis not evident on CT (Omerod et al., 1987). The non-stroke cases included in the study included focal lesion patients who had recently undergone resection of a tumor ($n = 5$), patients with closed head injury ($n = 3$), and patients who had recently undergone clipping of an aneurysm ($n = 2$). Severely aphasic patients were not included in the study group. Alexic subjects were included, provided they could decipher single numbers or letters. There were four such patients, all of whom had sustained left-hemisphere damage. For these participants and for two other patients who appeared to have some difficulty reading, the on-screen instructions for the computer-assisted tests were read to them by the examiner. Hemiparetic subjects ($n = 13$) were not excluded. There were eight hemiparetic patients in the left anterior group, two in the left posterior group, one in the right anterior group, and one in the right posterior group.

PROCEDURE

The subjects were first interviewed briefly to obtain demographic information, educational history, and medical and psychiatric history. Three traditional neuropsychological tests were administered and were used as screening instruments: the *Mini-Mental State Examination* (MMSE) (Folstein, Folstein, & McHugh, 1975) and the information and picture completion subtests of the WAIS-R (Wechsler, 1981). To qualify for inclusion in the study subjects were required either to attain a score of 23/30 on the MMSE or to attain an age-scaled score of 7 (1 *SD* below the mean for age) on at least one of the WAIS-R subtests. Subjects retained in the study after completion of these procedures were administered the computer-assisted tests.

MATERIALS

The NES2 is an individually-administered battery consisting of subtests of motor and cognitive functions and affect. It is computer-assisted in that the examiner uses a script designed for testing neurologic patients, clarifying on-screen instructions as required and facilitating the subject's performance by such means as repeating practice trials and assisting the subject to adopt an optimal position for using the computer keyboard where this assistance is needed. All test parameters remain constant. The NES2 provides 17 subtests, intended for selection according to the purposes of particular investigations. To span the entire range of cognitive functions available while reducing the time required for testing, 14 tests were selected for the present study. The NES2 software automatically records data to raw data files in ASCII format and additional software permits computation of summary scores for each test. Summary scores for each subject were input into SAS. When a subject was unable to complete a test, the score representing the worst performance of a subject completing that test was assigned for purposes of analysis. Subtests used are described briefly below, in the order in which they were administered. A more complete description of each test is given in the test manual (Letz, 1991).

Finger Tapping

A test of manual motor speed requiring key tapping with the index finger of the preferred hand, the non-preferred hand, and, using two keys, the preferred and non-preferred hands in alternation. Each response produces a visual marker on screen. The measure is number of taps in 30 seconds.

Continuous Performance

A task measuring reaction time and accuracy in responding to a target letter randomly embedded in a series of large letters presented successively in the center of the screen. The test continues for five minutes. The measures are *latency*, *variability*, *number of false positives*, and *number of omissions*.

Hand-eye Coordination

A test of ability to control, with the dominant hand (using a joystick), the vertical location of a cursor, the horizontal movement of which is constant, and to keep it coincident with a sine wave pattern displayed on the screen. The measure is *distance from the target*.

Paired-associate Learning

A verbal learning task in which seven names and occupations are presented successively in statement form for encoding. Three learning trials are given with feedback after each response. The measure is *total number of correct pairings*.

Digit Span

An attention task in which digits are presented successively on screen for subsequent reproduction of the sequence guided by a display of dashes representing the number of digits required. Separate spans are determined for forward and backward production. The measure is *span length*.

Grammatical Reasoning

A verbal reasoning task in which the subject must verify whether an instance (*AB* or *BA*) is concordant with a statement (e.g., *A follows B*). The statements vary in grammatical form (active vs. passive), verb (*follows* vs. *precedes*), in whether the statement is positive or negative, in whether the first item mentioned is *A* or *B*, and in whether the statement is true or false. The measure is *number of errors*.

Symbol/Digit

A psychomotor coding task in which the subject must find and enter the digit associated with the appropriate symbol in an array that changes on each trial. The measure is *latency*.

Pattern Recognition

A pattern comparison task in which three matrices of 10 x 10 blocks are presented. Blocks are either light or dark. Two of the matrices are identical; the third contains blocks that differ in value. The subject is asked to choose the pattern that differs from the other two. The measure is *latency*.

Pattern Memory

A matrix similar to those in the pattern recognition task is presented alone. After an unfilled interval, a matching pattern and two other patterns, each of which differs from the target, are presented. The subject is asked to choose the matching pattern. Measures are *number correct* and *latency*.

Serial Digit Learning

Eight digits are presented successively on screen for reproduction of the sequence in the same format used for *Digit Span*. The measure reflects errors to the criterion of two correct trials in succession (or a maximum of eight trials).

Horizontal Addition

The subject is asked to enter a two-digit sum of three one-digit numerals presented horizontally. Measures are *latency* and *number of errors*.

Vocabulary

A multiple-choice test of word meanings. The measure is *number correct*.

Delayed Recall

A single trial of the names and occupations previously presented for paired-associate learning is given once, without feedback. The measure is *number correct*.

Mood Scales

A 25-item inventory assessing self-report of degree of anger, confusion, depression, fatigue, and tension for the preceding week. It consists of descriptors for these moods similar to those used in the *Profile of Mood States* (POMS) (McNair, Lorr, & Droppleman, 1971). The measures reflect *number of items endorsed*, weighted for severity. Total scores range from 0 to 260.

DATA ANALYSIS

Linear regression was used to estimate the mean difference for each test result between each of the four patient groups (Left Anterior – LA; Left Posterior – LP; Right Anterior – RA; and Right Posterior – RP) and the controls. A separate model was fitted to the results for each test outcome and the regression coefficient of a dichotomous group variable was interpreted as the mean difference in performance. The difference in test performance was adjusted for potential confounding by including age, gender, and education as other independent variables in the model for each outcome. The adjustments reflect the fact that these variables affect performance on NES2 subtests; thus, they were applied even when the groups did not differ on the variable in question.

An adjusted mean performance was estimated for each test in each patient group by adding the appropriate regression coefficient (with the appropriate sign) to the mean in the control group. The ratio of the adjusted mean to the control mean was calculated for each measure. After multiplying by 100, the ratios can be interpreted as an adjusted percentage difference in performance between the patient groups and controls. For measures in which a smaller score indicates better performance, such as latency, the percentage in the patient groups would be expected to be greater than or equal to 100%. For measures in which a larger score indicates better performance, such as number correct, the percentage in the patient groups would be expected to be less than or equal to 100%.

RESULTS AND DISCUSSION

The results for each measure are compared with expectations that can be derived from the clinical neuropsychological literature. Where the literature includes the results of tests that closely resemble NES2 subtests, those findings are given. In other cases, extrapolations from findings from traditional tests in the same functional domain are provided. Instances in which changes in task structure between traditional tests and NES2 tests appear likely to have influenced differences in outcome are noted. Because the four quadrant groups were not sufficiently large to provide adequate statistical power for direct comparison, evidence of the relative vulnerability of each subtest to lesions localized to each quadrant of the brain is offered in terms of the robustness (p values) of differences between each group and controls. These values also reflect differences in the size of the four patient groups.

Demographic data for the controls and for each of the patient groups, along with their scores on the traditional neuropsychological tests (MMSE, WAIS-R information and picture completion subtests) are given in Table 1. Differences between patient groups and controls were statistically adjusted for group differences in age, gender, and education. With the exception of the RA group, all patient groups were impaired relative to controls on the MMSE, as would be expected for this global measure of cognitive functioning. These results suggest that the RA group may have an advantage in overall cognitive functioning over the other patient groups that might be expected to influence their pattern of performance in all domains.

Table 1. Demographic Data and Results of Traditional Neuropsychological Tests

	Controls	Left Anterior	Left Posterior	Right Anterior	Right Posterior
N	67	13	8	11	10
Age	56.5 (12.2)	57.8 (8.1)	61.3 (11.5)	46.2 (16.7)	47.3 (17.6)
Percentage male	42.4	92.3	75.0	90.9	70.0
Percentage left-handed	10.4	7.7	12.5	9.1	0.0
Education (years)[a]	14.5 (2.5)	14.6 (3.8)	13.1 (3.4)	12.7 (2.2)	13.5 (2.6)
Mini-Mental Status Exam[a]	28.8 (1.0)	24.0 (7.0)[4]	23.7 (5.5)[3]	28.8 (2.0)	26.8 (2.5)[4]
WAIS-R information[a, b, c]	12.0 (2.4)	9.7 (4.2)[4]	7.9 (2.4)[4]	11.4 (2.9)	9.6 (3.6)
WAIS-R picture completion[a, b, c]	11.1 (2.2)	11.9 (3.7)	9.6 (2.2)[1]	10.6 (3.7)[1]	7.2 (2.6)[4]

[a] mean (SD)
[b] significance levels are for differences from controls, after adjustment for age, gender, and education
[c] scaled scores

[1] $p \leq 0.05$ [2] $p \leq 0.01$ [3] $p \leq 0.001$ [4] $p \leq 0.0001$

Both WAIS-R information (O'Brien & Lezak, 1981) and WAIS-R picture completion (Crosson, Greene, Roth, Farr, & Adams, 1990; Hom & Reitan, 1984) are considered relatively resistant to the effects of focal brain damage. However, low scores on information have in some studies been selectively associated with left-hemisphere damage (Hom & Reitan, 1984; Smith, 1966; Spreen & Benton, 1965). Consistent with those reports, LA and LP patients were impaired on WAIS-R information, and RA and RP patients were not. Patients in the RA, RP, and LP groups were impaired on WAIS-R picture completion, consistent with deficits in visuospatial skills expected from the neuropsychological literature to be associated with posterior lesions of either hemisphere and with the known contribution of the right hemisphere to processing of visual materials (Lezak, 1995). In accord with these expectations, the most robust differences between controls and patients were seen in the RP group. These results suggest that the sample of patients examined in this study is similar to those who have been evaluated with these traditional neuropsychological instruments in the past.

The results for NES2 tests of motor function are given in Table 2. Patients with left-hemisphere lesions were slowed on Finger Tapping when using either hand but their difference from controls was more robust when using the dominant hand (for 19 of the 21 subjects, the right hand). Patients with right-hemisphere lesions were also impaired when using either hand; their difference from controls was more robust when using the non-dominant hand (for 20 of 21 cases, the left hand). Brain damage has tended to be associated with slowing of finger tapping rate (Haaland, Cleveland, & Carr, 1977; Lansdell & Donnelly, 1977; Stuss et al., 1985); and lateralized brain lesions have often been found to slow the tapping rate of the contralateral hand (Brown, Spicer, Robertson, Baird, & Malik, 1989; Finlayson & Reitan, 1980; Haaland & Delaney, 1981), a pattern with which the NES2 results are in conformity. Tapping with the two hands in alternation was impaired relative to the performance level seen in controls in the LA, LP, and RP groups, an effect that was especially robust for the latter group. The neuropsychological literature suggests that deficits in the temporal organization of motor sequences are found in association with left frontal and fronto-temporal lesions (Luria, 1962/1980), observations with which the findings for the left-hemisphere patients are consistent. The particular difficulty with alternation seen in the RP group may reflect the fact that intact right posterior structures are believed to play an essential role in spatially directed attention (Mesulam, 1981). On *Hand-eye Coordination*, a visual-motor tracking task carried out using the dominant (generally right) hand, all patient groups tended to be less accurate than controls, with the deficit reaching a conventional level of significance in the LA group. Precise movements of the right hand would be expected to be most affected by damage to premotor, motor, and sensory cortex areas of the left hemisphere (Luria, 1962/1980), expectations with which this result is in agreement.

The results for tests of attention and executive function are given in Table 3. These functions have most often been associated with the frontal lobes of the brain (Lezak, 1995; Luria, 1962/1980). The first task categorized in this domain, *Continuous Performance*, requires sustained focused attention. Patients with lesions in any of the four quadrants were impaired on this task in latency, variability, and in number of false positive responses. Deficits in vigilance tasks

Table 2. Performance on Tests of Motor Function

Task	Controls[a]	Left Anterior[b] Percentage	Left Posterior[b] Percentage	Right Anterior[b] Percentage	Right Posterior[b] Percentage
Finger tapping (number of taps):					
dominant hand	149.6 (27.2)	77.2[3]	64.5[4]	83.8[1]	85.9[1]
non-dominant hand	140.3 (23.9)	82.9[1]	84.7[1]	82.2[1]	76.1[2]
alternating hands	196.3 (51.6)	68.3[2]	78.3[1]	84.0[1]	50.0[4]
Hand-eye coordination (distance from target)	2.3 (0.4)	108.7	108.7	104.3	108.7

[a] mean (SD)
[b] percentage of control scores, after adjustment for age, gender, and education
[1] $p \leq 0.05$ [2] $p \leq 0.01$ [3] $p \leq 0.001$ [4] $p \leq 0.0001$ for differences from controls

Table 3. Performance on Tests of Attention and Executive function

Task	Controls[a]	Left Anterior[b] Percentage	Left Posterior[b] Percentage	Right Anterior[b] Percentage	Right Posterior[b] Percentage
Continuous Performance:					
latency	352.1 (37.6)	131.8[4]	127.5[4]	117.9[3]	137.7[4]
variability	53.8 (16.1)	160.2[4]	150.6[2]	173.4[4]	198.1[4]
false positives	0.0 (0.2)	5666.7[4]	3666.7[4]	2166.7[1]	16833.36[4]
omissions	0.6 (1.0)	133.3	133.3	200.0	483.3[4]
Digit Span (length):					
forward	7.0 (1.6)	71.4[2]	75.7[1]	82.8[1]	81.4[1]
backward	5.5 (1.7)	65.4[2]	65.4[1]	87.3	70.9[2]
Serial Digit Learning (log errors)	1.9 (1.5)	221.0[4]	157.9	131.6	115.8
Horizontal Addition:					
latency	3.4 (1.1)	300.0[4]	161.8[2]	182.4[4]	161.8[4]
errors	1.1 (1.3)	545.4[4]	400.0[4]	209.1[1]	172.7
Grammatical Reasoning (errors)	7.5 (5.7)	100.0	88.0	33.3	104.0

[a] mean (SD)
[b] percentage of control scores, after adjustment for age, gender, and education
[1] $p \leq 0.05$ [2] $p \leq 0.01$ [3] $p \leq 0.001$ [4] $p \leq 0.0001$ for differences from controls

have often been noted as a consequence of brain damage without specification of the role of locus of brain lesion in the extent or type of impairment (Franz, 1970; Strub & Black, 1985). Nevertheless, in some traditional neuropsychological tasks that also require sustained focused attention (searching for visual targets in an array containing many distractors), patients with brain damage at different sites have been noted to differ in discrete ways. Thus, a tendency to neglect the left half of the display has frequently been observed in patients with right-hemisphere lesions, and an overall slowing of performance has been described in patients with lesions of the left temporal lobe (Lezak, 1995). On some tasks of this type patients with anterior lesions of the right hemisphere were observed to perform more poorly than those with left anterior lesions whereas no laterality differences were seen in groups with posterior lesions (Ruff, Niemann, Allen, Farrow, & Wylie, 1992). On the NES2 vigilance task, only patients with RP lesions failed on a statistically significant number of occasions (relative to controls) to respond to the target, an effect that might reflect the particular difficulty in processing visuospatial stimuli previously noted to be expected in this group (Lezak, 1995).

Length of *forward Digit Span* was impaired in all four patient groups with the LA group showing the most robust effect. Digit span forward has been reported to be more vulnerable to lesions of the left hemisphere than to lesions of either the right hemisphere or to diffuse brain damage (Black, 1986; Hom & Reitan, 1984; Newcombe, 1969; Risse, Rubens, & Jordan, 1984; Weinberg, Diller, Gerstman, & Schulman, 1972). However, those observations were based upon tests using spoken digits (Wechsler, 1981; 1987). Because NES2 *Digit Span* presents digits visually (and presents a visual display of dashes for eliciting and monitoring the response sequence) neuroanatomic areas important in processing of visual stimuli, including right-hemisphere structures, might be expected to play a considerable role. The addition of this visual component may be related to the similarity of the four patient groups on this task – that is, for attenuation of an expected lateralized effect. Performance on *backward Digit Span* (a more complex attention task requiring holding of information in immediate memory along with simultaneous tracking of forward and backward sequences) was impaired in all but the RA group. The success of the RA group on this task may reflect their slightly better overall cognitive ability than the other patient groups, as noted previously in considering their performance on the MMSE. Reversed digit spans have been reported to be sensitive to many kinds of brain damage (Black, 1986; Hom & Reitan, 1984; Newcombe, 1969; Risse, Rubens, & Jordan, 1984; Weinberg, Diller, Gerstman, & Schulman, 1972), observations with which the NES2 results are in agreement.

Only LA patients were impaired to a statistically significant degree on *Serial Digit Learning*. However, the tendency for both left-hemisphere groups to show greater deficits on this task than did the right-hemisphere groups is consistent with the neuropsychological literature in which deficiencies in verbal learning (in a variety of tasks) have been associated with left-hemisphere damage (Lezak, 1995; Luria, 1962/1980). Recall of nonsense syllables has been shown to be more impaired by left- than by right-hemisphere damage (Newcombe, 1969). A direct comparison of serial digit learning in patients with unilateral temporal lobe seizures showed significantly more failures on this task in the left-hemisphere group (Loring, Lee, Martin, & Meador, 1988) and a much larger effect of left temporal lobectomy than of right temporal lobectomy on post-surgical performance of this task (Lee, Loring, & Thompson, 1989). Patients with lesions in either hemisphere were slow on *Horizontal Addition*, and both left-hemisphere groups also made many more errors than did controls. The results for the error measure are consistent with particular involvement of left- hemisphere substrate in the processing of visuospatial aspects of verbal stimuli such as numbers, as well as with the contribution of internal speech-like mediating processes to carrying out of arithmetic calculations (Luria, 1962/1980). On *Grammatical Reasoning*, patients performed similarly to controls, with the RA group actually making fewer errors than controls. All groups, including controls, showed high variability. The NES2 test manual (Letz, 1991) indicates that stable performance on *Grammatical Reasoning* requires considerable practice, a characteristic that suggests this test has limited usefulness as a neuropsychological measure of executive function.

The results for tests of verbal and visuospatial function are given in Table 4. Patients with left-hemisphere lesions were impaired on *Vocabulary* while those with right-hemisphere lesions were not. This result is consistent with the literature associating the left hemisphere preferentially with language functions (Lezak, 1995) and with findings on a similar multiple choice vocabulary test that has been used for neuropsychological assessment (Costa & Vaughan, 1962). All patient groups performed worse than controls on *Symbol/digit* with more robust differences in the LA, LP, and RP groups than in the RA group. *Symbol/digit* is a complex task: the subject must monitor the array in order to select the symbol to be responded to next, scan the code to find that symbol and its associated digit, and finally find and press the corresponding numeric key on the computer keyboard. The vulnerability of this task to lesions in all four quadrants may be taken to reflect the many components of the task; comparable traditional tests (paper-and-pencil versions similar in structure) are known to be extremely sensitive to brain damage but relatively non-specific to locus of injury (Butters & Cermak, 1976; Glosser, Butters, & Kaplan, 1977). On the remaining visuospatial task, *Pattern Recognition*, patients with lesions in all four quadrants were also slower than controls. Findings with traditional tests of visuospatial abilities would lead to an expectation of greater impairment in patients with posterior lesions, especially in the RP group (Lezak, 1995; Luria, 1962/1980), effects that were not clearly shown. It is likely that, in addition to visuospatial skills, *NES2 Pattern Recognition* makes demands on attention and executive function (to carry out a thorough comparison of all three patterns) to a greater extent than do many traditional visuospatial tests. The addition of these attentional and strategic components, thought to be largely mediated by anterior structures, might account for the similarity of all four patient groups on the NES2 task.

The results for tests of learning and memory are given in Table 5. Both Left-hemisphere groups tended to be impaired in learning paired associates, as was expected on the basis of selective deficits in patients with left-hemisphere lesions on several traditional verbal learning tasks (Lezak, 1995), including paired-associate learning on Wechsler Memory Scales (Chelune & Bornstein, 1988; Vakil, Hoofien, & Blachstein, 1988). No patient group in the current study differed from controls at a statistically significant level in accuracy of recall of the paired associates after a delay (*Delayed Recall*). Deficits in recall of newly learned verbal material have frequently been reported in patients with left-hemisphere lesions, especially in

Table 4. Performance on Tests of Verbal and Visuospatial Function

Functions and Task	Controls[a]	Left Anterior[b] Percentage	Left Posterior[b] Percentage	Right Anterior[b] Percentage	Right Posterior[b] Percentage
Verbal Ability:					
Vocabulary (correct)	20.9 (3.9)	71.3[4]	67.0[4]	95.2	85.2[1]
Visuospatial Functions:					
Symbol/digit (latency)	2.7 (0.8)	174.1[4]	144.4[4]	118.5[1]	155.6[3]
Pattern Recognition (latency)	5.0 (1.1)	148.0[4]	128.0[3]	158.0[4]	174.0[4]

[a]mean (SD)
[b]percentage of control scores, after adjustment for age, gender, and education
[1] $p \leq 0.05$ [2] $p \leq 0.01$ [3] $p \leq 0.001$ [4] $p \leq 0.0001$ for differences from controls

Table 5. Performance on Tests of Memory

Functions and Task	Controls[a]	Left Anterior[b] Percentage	Left Posterior[b] Percentage	Right Anterior[b] Percentage	Right Posterior[b] Percentage
Verbal Learning and Memory:					
Paired-associate Learning (correct)	11.5 (5.1)	69.6[1]	69.6	107.8	98.3
Delayed Recall (correct)	4.4 (2.2)	75.0	79.5	95.4	90.9
Visual Learning and Memory:					
Pattern Memory (correct)	12.5 (1.6)	84.8[2]	81.6[2]	92.0	77.6[4]
Pattern Memory (latency)	6.1 (1.4)	126.2[3]	104.9	116.4	145.9[4]

[a] mean (SD)
[b] percentage of control scores, after adjustment for age, gender, and education
[1] $p \leq 0.05$ [2] $p \leq 0.01$ [3] $p \leq 0.001$ [4] $p \leq 0.0001$ for differences from controls

Table 6. Assessment of Mood

Mood	Controls[a]	Left Anterior[b] Percentage	Left Posterior[b] Percentage	Right Anterior[b] Percentage	Right Posterior[b] Percentage
Anger	1.7 (0.6)	105.9	111.8	129.4[1]	117.6
Confusion	2.2 (0.6)	113.6	118.2	122.7	100.0
Depression	2.2 (0.5)	120.0	120.0	120.0	100.0
Fatigue	2.7 (0.7)	96.3	103.7	129.6[2]	92.6
Tension	2.7 (0.8)	88.9	100.0	107.4	85.2
Summary Score	2.2 (0.5)	104.5	109.1	122.7[1]	95.4

[a]mean (SD)
[b]percentage of control scores, after adjustment for age, gender, and education
[1] $p \leq 0.05$ [2] $p \leq 0.01$ for differences from controls

association with damage to medial temporal structures (Lezak, 1995). The absence of more robust effects of left-hemisphere damage on the verbal learning and memory measures may reflect the fact that the NES2 task is much more difficult than are traditional paired-associate tasks (controls produced only 11.5 correct responses out of 21 opportunities, or 55%; on the traditional tests controls of this age produce approximately 19 correct responses out of 24, or 79%) (Wechsler, 1987).

Performance of the visuospatial memory task, *Pattern Memory*, was impaired (in either speed or accuracy) in all but the RA group. In the neuropsychological literature, several visual memory tasks have shown selective vulnerability to right-sided lesions (Lezak, 1995). For example, in one study recognition memory for line drawings of natural objects (*flora* and *fauna*) was impaired in stroke patients with lesions lateralized to either the left or right hemisphere, but right-sided lesions had a more detrimental effect on both immediate and delayed memory (Trahan, Larrabee, & Quintana, 1990). In a multiple choice recognition task using matrices similar to those in the NES2 *Pattern Memory* subtest (Warrington & James, 1967) patients with either left or right parietal lesions were inferior to controls but those with right-hemisphere damage made many more errors than did those with left-hemisphere damage (Campbell & Oxbury, 1976; Oxbury, Campbell, & Oxbury, 1974).

The results for the NES2 *Mood Scales* are given in Table 6. Only RA patients acknowledged higher overall levels of dysphoric mood than did controls (*Summary Score*). RA patients reported elevated Anger, Tension and Fatigue to a statistically significant degree and their endorsement of feelings of Confusion approached that level. It is of interest that the RA group showed fewer cognitive deficits than any other patient group while indicating greater impairment of mood. On the other hand, the RP group, whose cognitive deficits often seemed the most severe, reported less dysphoria than did controls. A failure of patients with right-hemisphere lesions to acknowledge their physical or cognitive disabilities or to complain of dysphoric mood has often been observed. However, the absence of acknowledgement of impaired mood by LA and LP groups is at variance with previous findings (Gainotti, 1989).

GENERAL DISCUSSION

On 20 of the 22 NES2 measures of cognitive functioning examined, one or more groups of patients with focal lesions showed deficits relative to controls. Thus, the majority of the NES2 subtests appear to meet the gold standard criterion for neuropsychological tests – that is, the ability to detect the fact that these patients are neurologically abnormal. This result suggests that the majority of NES2 subtests can be considered to detect CNS dysfunction, validating their use in studies of the effects of exposure to suspected neurotoxicants. The subtests that did not meet this standard were *Grammatical Reasoning* and *Paired-associate Delayed Recall*, both of which failed to differentiate patients from controls at a statistically significant level. In addition, the NES2 *Mood Scales* revealed dysphoric symptoms only for the RA group, whereas expectations based upon the neuropsychological literature were for disturbances of mood in other groups as well.

Performance on the majority of NES2 tests was affected by lesions in all four quadrants of the brain. This result accords with the observation that brain damage of any kind affects most cognitive functions, including speed of cognitive processing. Nevertheless, differences between patients with lesions of the left and right hemisphere were seen on several NES2 measures, in agreement with expectations based upon the neuropsychological literature. Among these findings were the demonstration of more pronounced manual motor slowing when using the hand contralateral to the lesion, deficits in verbal processing and in learning of verbal materials preferentially associated with left-hemisphere lesions, and deficits in visuospatial skills preferentially associated with right-hemisphere lesions, with the RP group showing the most pronounced effect.

These results suggest that the NES2 may be useful in the evaluation of patients who have sustained focal brain damage. However, validation of the NES2 for clinical purposes also requires that performance on the battery be evaluated with respect to its implications for daily living. In addition, several limitations of the present battery are evident that prevent it being considered a substitute for a full neuropsychological assessment using traditional tests. Formal language processing tasks (such as naming) are not represented in the NES2 and such measures are essential for the evaluation of functioning in this domain. The visual memory tasks included in the NES2 appear to make heavy demands on attention and executive function, making those measures less able to discriminate impairments specific to visuospatial processing. Finally, verbal learning and memory might be more precisely delineated by a task (such as list learning) in which several component processes involved in these functions may be assessed. These and other refinements have been developed and incorporated in a new version of the NES, the NES3. Studies are now underway in which the new instrument is being given to groups of neurologic and other clinical patients who are also being evaluated with traditional neuropsychological tests. This work is an important step toward validation of the NES for both clinical and epidemiological use.

ACKNOWLEDGMENTS

This project was supported by grant R01-OH02767 from the National Institute of Occupational Safety and Health and by the Department of Veterans Affairs Boston Environmental Hazards Center grant.

REFERENCES

Anger, K. (1990). Worksite behavioral research: Results, sensitive methods, test batteries and the transition from laboratory data to human health. *Neurotoxicology*, *11*, 629-720.

Arcia, E. & Otto, D. A. (1992). Reliability of selected tests from the Neurobehavioral Evaluation System. *Neurotoxicology and Teratology*, *14*, 103-110.

Baker, E., Letz, R., Fidler, A., Shalat, S., Plantamura, D., & Lyndon, M. (1985). Computer-based neurobehavioral testing for occupational and environmental epidemiology: Methodology and validation studies. *Neurotoxicology and Teratology*, *7*, 369-377.

Bisiach, E. & Vallar, G. (1988). Hemineglect in humans. In F. Boller & J. Grafman (Eds.), *Handbook of neuropsychology* (Vol. 1, pp. 195-222). Amsterdam: Elsevier.

Black, F. W. (1986). Digit repetition in brain-damaged adults: Clinical and theoretical implications. *Journal of Clinical Psychology*, *42*, 770-782.

Brown, G. G., Spicer, K. B., Robertson, W. M., Baird, A. D., & Malik, G. (1989). Neuropsychological signs of lateralized arteriovenous malformations: Comparisons with ischemic stroke. *The Clinical Neuropsychologist, 3*, 340-352.
Butters, N. & Cermak, L. S. (1976). Neuropsychological studies of alcoholic Korsakoff patients. In G. Goldstein & C. Neuringer (Eds.), *Empirical studies of alcoholism* (pp. 153-193). Cambridge, MA: Ballinger.
Campbell, D. C. & Oxbury, J. M. (1976). Recovery from unilateral spatial neglect. *Cortex, 12*, 303-312.
Chelune, G. J. & Bornstein, R. A. (1988). WMS-R patterns among patients with unilateral brain lesions. *The Clinical Neuropsychologist, 2*, 121-132.
Costa, L. D. & Vaughan, H. G. Jr. (1962). Performance of patients with lateralized cerebral lesions. *Journal of Nervous and Mental Disease, 134*, 162-168.
Crosson, B., Greene, R. L., Roth, D. L., Farr, S. P., & Adams, R. L. (1990). WAIS-R pattern clusters after blunt head injury. *The Clinical Neuropsychologist, 4*, 253-262.
Echeverria, D., Fine, L., Langolf, G., Schork, A., & Sampaio, C. (1989). Acute neurobehavioral effects of toluene. *British Journal of Occupational Medicine, 46*, 483-495.
Echeverria, D., Fine, L., Langolf, G, Schork, A., & Sampaio, C. (1990). Acute neurobehavioral effects from social consumption of alcohol. In B. Das (Ed.), *Advances in industrial ergonomics and safety II* (pp. 865-872). London: Taylor & Francis.
Finlayson, M. A. J. & Reitan, R. M. (1980). Effects of lateralized lesions on ipsilateral and contralateral motor functioning. *Journal of Clinical Neuropsychology, 2*, 237-243.
Folstein, M. F., Folstein, S., & McHugh, P. R. (1975). Mini-mental state: A practical method for grading the cognitive state of patients for the clinician. *Journal of Psychiatric Research, 12*, 189-198.
Franz, S. I. (1970). *Handbook of mental examination methods*. New York: Johnson Reprint.
Gainotti, G. (1989). Disorders of emotion and affect in patients with unilateral brain damage. In F. Boller & J. Grafman (Eds.), *Handbook of neuropsychology* (Vol. 3, pp. 345-361). Amsterdam: Elsevier.
Glosser, G., Butters, N., & Kaplan, E. (1977). Visuoperceptual processes in brain damaged patients on the Digit Symbol Substitution Test. *International Journal of Neuroscience, 7*, 59-66.
Goodglass, H. & Kaplan, E. (1979). Assessment of cognitive deficits in the brain-injured patient. In M. S. Gazzaniga (Ed.), *Handbook of behavioral neurobiology: Neuropsychology* (Vol. 2, pp. 3-22). New York: Plenum Press.
Grant, I. & Adams, K. M. (Eds.). (1986). *Neuropsychological assessment of neuropsychiatric disorders*. New York: Oxford University Press.
Greenberg, B. D., Moore, P. A., Letz, R., & Baker, E. L. (1985). Computerized assessment of human neurotoxicity: Sensitivity to nitrous oxide exposure. *Clinical Pharmacology and Therapeutics, 38*, 656-660.
Haaland, K. Y., Cleveland, C. S., & Carr, D. (1977). Motor performance after unilateral hemisphere damage in patients with tumor. *Archives of Neurology, 34*, 556-559.
Haaland, K. Y. & Delaney, H. D. (1981). Motor deficits after left or right hemisphere damage due to stroke or tumor. *Neuropsychologia, 19*, 17-27.
Hom, J. & Reitan, R. M. (1984). Effects of lateralized cerebral damage upon contralateral and ipsilateral sensorimotor performances. *Journal of Clinical and Experimental Neuropsychology, 12*, 644-654.
Hooisma, J., Emmen, H. H., Kulig, B. M., Muijser, H., Poortvliet, D., & Letz, R. (1990). Factor analysis of tests from the neurobehavioral evaluation system and the WHO neurobehavioral core test battery. In B. Johnson (Ed.), *Advances in behavioral toxicology* (pp. 248-256). Chelsea, MI: Lewis.
Kane, R. L. & Kay, K. G. (1992). Computerized assessment in neuropsychology. *Neuropsychology Review, 3*, 1-117.
Krengel, M., White, R. F., & Diamond, R. (1996). A comparison of NES2 and traditional neuropsychological tests in a neurologic patient sample. *Neurotoxicology and Teratology, 18*, 435-439.
Lansdell, H. & Donnelly, E. F. (1977). Factor analysis of the Wechsler Adult Intelligence Scale subtests and the Halstead-Reitan Category and Tapping tests. *Journal of Consulting and Clinical Psychology, 45*, 412-416.
Lee, G. P., Loring, D. W., & Thompson, J. L. (1989). Construct validity of material-specific memory measures following unilateral temporal lobe ablations. *Psychological Assessment, 1*, 192-197.
Letz, R. (1990). The neurobehavioral evaluation system: An international effort. In B. Johnson (Ed.), *Advances in behavioral toxicology* (pp. 189-210). Chelsea, MI: Lewis.
Letz, R. (1991). *NES2 user's manual* (Version 4.4). Winchester, MA: Neurobehavioral Systems.

Letz, R. & Baker, E. L. (1988). *Neurobehavioral evaluation system NES user's manual.* Winchester, MA: Neurobehavioral Systems.

Lezak, M. D. (1995). *Neuropsychological assessment* (3rd ed.). New York: Oxford University Press.

Loring, D. W., Lee, G. P., Martin, R. C., & Meador, K. J. (1988). Material-specific learning in patients with partial complex seizures of temporal lobe origin: Convergent validation of memory constructs. *Journal of Epilepsy, 1,* 53-59.

Luria, A. R. (1980). *Higher cortical functions in man* (2nd ed., B. Haigh, Trans.). New York: Plenum Press. (Original work published 1962)

Mahoney, F. C., Moore, P. A., Baker, E. L., & Letz, R. (1988). Experimental nitrous oxide exposure as a model system for evaluating neurobehavioral tests. *Toxicology, 49,* 449-453.

McCarthy, R. A. & Warrington, E. K. (1990). *Cognitive neuropsychology: A clinical introduction.* San Diego, CA: Academic Press.

McNair, D. M., Lorr, M., & Droppleman, L. F. (1971). *Profile of mood states.* San Diego, CA: Educational and Industrial Testing Service.

Mesulam, M. M. (1981). A cortical network for directed attention and unilateral neglect. *Annals of Neurology, 10,* 309-325.

Naeser, M. A. & Hayward, R. W. (1978). Lesion localization in aphasia with cranial computed tomography and the Boston Diagnostic Aphasia Exam. *Neurology, 28,* 545-551.

Newcombe, F. (1969). *Missile wounds of the brain.* London: Oxford University Press.

O'Brien, K. & Lezak, M. D. (1981, July). *Long-term improvements in intellectual function following brain injury.* Paper presented at the meeting of the International Neuropsychological Society, Bergen, Norway.

Omerod, I., Miller, D., McDonal, W., duBoulay, E., Rudge, P., Kendall, B., Moseley, I., Johnson, G., Tofts, P., Halliday, A., Bronstein, A., Scaravilli, F., Harding, A., Barnes, D., & Zilka, K. (1987). The role of NMR imaging in the assessment of multiple sclerosis and isolated neurological lesions. *Brain, 110,* 1579-1616.

Oxbury, J. M., Campbell, D. C., & Oxbury, S. M. (1974). Unilateral spatial neglect and impairments of spatial analysis and visual perception. *Brain, 97,* 551-564.

Reitan, R. M. (1986). Theoretical and methodological bases of the Halstead-Reitan Neuropsychological Test Battery. In I. Grant & K. M. Adams (Eds.), *Neuropsychological assessment of neuropsychiatric disorders* (pp. 3-30). New York: Oxford University Press.

Risse, G. L., Rubens, A. B., & Jordan, L. S. (1984). Disturbances of long-term memory in aphasic patients. *Brain, 107,* 605-617.

Ruff, R. M., Niemann, H., Allen, C. C., Farrow, C. E., & Wylie, T. (1992). The Ruff 2 and 7 Selective Attention Test: A neuropsychological application. *Perceptual and Motor Skills, 75,* 1311-1319.

Smith, A. (1966). Intellectual functions in patients with lateralized frontal tumors. *Journal of Neurology, Neurosurgery, and Psychiatry, 29,* 52-59.

Spreen, O. & Benton, A. L. (1965). Comparative studies of some psychological tests for cerebral damage. *Journal of Nervous and Mental Disease, 140,* 323-333.

Starkstein, S. E. & Robinson, R. G. (1991). The role of the frontal lobes in affective disorder following stroke. In H. S. Levin, H. M. Eisenberg, & A. L. Benton (Eds.), *Frontal lobe function and dysfunction* (pp. 288-303). New York: Oxford University Press.

Strub, R. L. & Black, F. W. (1985). *Mental status examination in neurology* (2nd ed.). Philadelphia: F. A. Davis.

Stuss, D. T., Ely, P., Hugenholtz, H., Richard, M. T., LaRochelle, S., Poirier, C. A., & Bell, I. (1985). Subtle neuropsychological deficits in patients with good recovery after closed head injury. *Neurosurgery, 17,* 41-47.

Trahan, D. E., Larrabee, G. J., & Quintana, J. W. (1990). Visual recognition memory in normal adults and patients with unilateral vascular lesions. *Journal of Clinical and Experimental Neuropsychology, 12,* 857-872.

Vakil, E., Hoofien, D., & Blachstein, H. (1992). Total amount learned versus learning rate of verbal and nonverbal information, in differentiating left- from right-brain injured patients. *Archives of Clinical Neuropsychology, 7,* 111-120.

Warrington, E. K. & James, M. (1967). Disorders of visual perception in patients with localized cerebral lesions. *Neuropsychologia, 5,* 353-266.

Wechsler, D. (1987). *Wechsler memory scale* (Rev. ed.). San Antonio, TX: The Psychological Corporation.

Wechsler, D. (1981). *Wechsler adult intelligence scale-Revised (WAIS-R) manual.* New York: Psychological Corporation.

Weinberg, J., Diller, L., Gerstman, L., & Schulman, P. (1972). Digit span in right and left hemiplegics. *Journal of Clinical Psychology, 28,* 361.

White, R. F. (Ed.). (1992). *Clinical syndromes in adult neuropsychology: The practitioner's handbook.* Amsterdam: Elsevier.

White, R. F., Diamond, R., Krengel, M., Lindem, K., & Feldman, R. G. (1996). Validation of the NES2 in patients with neurologic disorders. *Neurotoxicology and Teratology, 18,* 441-448.

NEUROLOGY OF AGING

Janice E. Knoefel and John C. Adair

INTRODUCTION

The neurology of old age is not a newcomer to the stage of neuroscience. MacDonald Critchley's series of essays in the 1930s (Critchley, 1932) explored the phenomenology of geriatric neurology. In this series of three articles he pointed out the importance of neurological dysfunction in the elderly, categorized a number of conditions, and is generally given credit for focusing early attention on the impact of aging upon society. In the past two or three decades the issues of aging and disease have aroused the renewed interest of clinicians and neuroscientists. For the most part, this has to do with the increased recognition among both scientists and society that the rapid aging of Western society has produced and will produce many more millions of aged individuals. For neuroscientists and neurologists, this translates to a markedly increased prevalence of neurodegenerative conditions with the widespread accompanying societal implications. As the century closes, the astute observations of Dr. Critchley 70 years ago are coming to have even more pertinence.

In the United States in 1900 there were three million people over the age of 65 and 72 thousand people over the age of 85. By 1996 those numbers had increased to 33.3 million and 2.2 million (Katzman, 1997). This is a projected rate of annual growth of 3.14 percent in men and 4.94 percent in women (Riggs, 1996). This projection of rapid aging of the United States population is not expected to level off for approximately 50 years. Hence, the impact of markedly increased numbers of aged individuals and the functional dependence caused by neurodegenerative conditions is of serious concern. The emphasis has long been on the neurological conditions in this age group due to the fact that the neurological illnesses of Alzheimer's disease, other dementias, Parkinson's disease, malignant brain tumors, amyotrophic lateral sclerosis, and other neurological conditions contribute inordinately to high disease prevalence and disability rates in the elderly.

What does the increased rate of aging represent? The increased survival due to declining mortality at all ages in society, especially in the old, results in the markedly increased prevalence of the old (those between 65 and 85) and old-old (greater than 85 years of age) (Olshanski et al., 1993). This will inevitably result in increased frequency of neurological disease and disability from it in the elderly population. The recognition of the uncertain, differential, and sometimes conflictual relationships between aging and disease has furthermore stimulated interest in studying and understanding the biomechanisms of aging. As improved understanding of the pathology of disease processes occurs, our understanding of underlying aging processes will also undoubtedly benefit. The reverse, the unraveling and understanding of the various mechanisms of the aging process, will undoubtedly aid our understanding of a number of disease processes as well.

COGNITION

Decline in cognitive abilities is so frequently observed in elderly people that the term *old age* (senescence) and dementia (disease) are perceived as being virtually synonymous (Keefover, 1998). It has been known for millennia that aged individuals are at greater risk for intellectual decline. What is less obvious, however, is the contribution of either systemic or neurologic disease processes, however well controlled and treated, to the decline. The presence of presumed Alzheimer's disease in the aged population had, for many centuries, been accepted as part of the aging process. It was only when this process appeared in a much younger individual, mid 50s in the first patient described by Alzheimer, that it became clear that this was a pathological, and not a normal aging, process (Alzheimer, 1907). Neuroscientists, neuropsychologists, and neurologists have been trying ever since to unravel this mysterious question: What is aging and what is disease?

One of the most challenging aspects of the study of aging is to identify a disease-free elderly population for the study of cognitive decline, that is, decline related to aging alone. Although this may be quite easy to achieve by elimination of diagnosed or screened-for systemic illnesses, the diagnosis of neurological impairment of insidious onset may only be made in retrospect; thereby such individuals contaminate normal aging studies while in the early throes of a diagnosable dementing illness (LaRue et al., 1995).

Perhaps even more difficult than identifying disease-free elderly individuals for study participation is the task of following such a selected group in a longitudinally designed study. Most studies looking at age-associated cognitive decline have employed cross-sectional designs out of practical considerations. Unfortunately, well-described *cohort-effects*, such as educational history, nutritional history, previous medical care, vocation, avocation, social activities, medication use, etc., are well known to engender substantive differences among age cohorts.

In addition to the uncertain relationship of cognitive changes to aging, there are other examples of physiological changes with an unknown relationship to normal or abnormal aging; these include progressive cerebral atrophy (Coffey et al., 1992), decreased cerebral glucose and oxygen metabolism in PET (positron emission tomography scanning) (De Santi et al., 1995), visual, auditory, and somatosensory age-related increase in latencies or decrease in amplitude (Gilmore, 1995), and patterns of temporal EEG activity (Rice et al., 1995). The conclusion from this summary of years of study of physiological parameters of aging is that these differences, common in groups of older individuals compared to younger groups of subjects, cannot be presumed to be normal due simply to their prevalence (Keefover, 1998).

Within the context of the above-described limitations in study design, there are a number of changes in cognition affecting the intellectual functions of attention, memory, language, and higher cortical functions that indeed do appear to change with age. Performance speed, as measured by reaction time, has long been recognized to be age dependent (Birren & Fisher, 1991). This concept has also been encapsulated in the well described and well-known age-related declines observed in the performance subtests as compared to the verbal subtests of the Wechsler Adult Intelligence Scale (WAIS) (Wechsler, 1981). This decline in performance on the performance subtests has been attributed to the fact that they are timed tasks, whereas the verbal subtests are not timed. However, even when time is removed from the equation, there is a decline in scores of the older as compared to a younger group of subjects (Storandt, 1977). Decrements in motor performance speed have been noted in such simple tasks as finger tapping (Shimoyama et al., 1990) as well as in complex motor tasks such as ambulation (Bohannon, 1997).

Though the concept of crystallized intelligence (i.e., an accumulated knowledge base repeatedly accessed and expanded throughout an individual's life span) versus fluid intelligence (i.e., the ability to dynamically assess and respond to novel situations arising in the environment) has been investigated for decades (Horn & Cattell, 1967), this distinction is still driving new research (Baltes, 1993). Although such a comparison may be difficult to quantify, nonetheless it is a useful construct to describe qualitatively differences in performance in younger compared to aged subjects (Kaufman & Horn, 1996). It may well be, however, that executive cognitive function generally classified as solely influenced by fluid intelligence may be substantially confounded with slowed processing speed, thereby rendering it less susceptible to unitary cognitive deficit than formerly appreciated (Salthouse, 1996).

The study of memory and memory deficits amongst the aging has been prompted by clinical and colloquial observations that such memory complaints and impairments are very common (Schofield et al., 1997) and, as importantly, also valid (Jonker et al., 1996). The above-mentioned critical potential failings of aging studies with regard to study design and cohort effects, as well as confounding effects of processing and cognitive speed, also apply to the study of memory impairment in aging. Notwithstanding these caveats, however, it does appear that disturbances in memory functions can accompany otherwise normal aging. The debate regarding normal/usual aging compared to optimal/successful aging can also be waged in regard to memory impairment. In fact, there is at least one study demonstrating that effects of age on memory functions can be ameliorated somewhat by both education and training (Shimamura et al., 1995). Table 1 describes the various types of memory functions and the effects seen with aging (Keefover, 1998).

To summarize, although effects of aging upon memory include relatively preserved registration of new information as well as retrieval of old information, new information recently learned appears to be forgotten more rapidly in the aged compared to a younger age population. There are a number of testing conditions that can be found to affect this pattern of memory strengths and weaknesses. Short-term memory is better for cued recall and recognition memory than for free recall memory (Wahlin et al., 1995). Other conditions that magnify apparent memory

Table 1. Effects of Aging on Memory Functions

Memory Function	Description	Change With Age
Registration (immediate)	Retention for seconds	No
Short-term, delayed recall (secondary or intermediate)	Retention for minutes to hours	Yes
Free recall	Items recalled without benefit of cues or associated stimuli	Yes
Cued recall	Item-associated stimuli or other cues provided	Minimal
Recognition	Items presented mixed with non-target distracter items	Minimal
Episodic	Recollection of context-specific information (e.g., word lists recall after a delay)	Yes
Semantic	Retrieval of vocabulary or general knowledge	Minimal
Explicit	Conscious recall of specified information	Yes
Implicit	Unconscious recollection of facts/skills acquired during earlier exposures	No
Working	Retention of information for transformation or manipulation	Yes
Primary	Simple recall of non-transformed data	Minimal
Long-term permanent	Retention for months to years	Minimal

failings with advanced age include manipulation, or transformation, of the information to be remembered. These conditions are contrasted with primary memory, which allows for storage but not processing of information. Primary memory function is unaffected by aging but any task requiring manipulation or processing of information shows a prompt reduction in efficiency with aged subjects (Brebion et al., 1995).

Recent investigations utilizing electrophysiological studies (Chao & Knight, 1997) and PET scanning (Furey et al., 1997) demonstrate activation of frontal and prefrontal cortical areas, which may be preferentially affected during aging. Impairment in these systems may affect working memory tasks to a greater degree than primary or long-term memory tasks. Whether disruption of these prefrontal systems leading to executive dysfunction and further amplification in the memory function is a condition of aging or of pathology also remains to be seen.

Communication, written and spoken, verbal and nonverbal, is a crucial cognitive function in everyday life. In the absence of disease, the elderly perform as well as younger groups on formal testing of language functions. The initial 1955 standardization of the WAIS showed a drop of less than one standard deviation in the score of the verbal subtests across the ages of 25 to 74 (Weschler, 1955). The cross-sectional standardization was hypothesized to reflect major cohort differences in education rather than indicate a true age effect. Longitudinal studies have shown that the major language functions of vocabulary, information and comprehension do not change (but see Obler et al., 1991) until well past age 70 (Eisdorfer & Wilker, 1973). Qualitative differences are seen with active naming, suggesting that the elderly have difficulty retrieving precise target words from an intact lexicon (Sandson et al., 1987). This helps to explain a common complaint of older individuals, that of not easily finding the intended word or name, as well as the oft-observed tendency towards loquaciousness in the elderly (Knoefel & Albert, 1990).

MOTOR CHANGES IN AGING

A motor act is required for all behaviors to be produced. From the simplest reflex to the most complex cognitive problem-solving tasks, a motor performance ultimately forms the basis upon which other cognitive and perceptual processes are judged. Change in any aspect of motor performance can be expected to have broad implications and wide-ranging effects for function. Of all the aspects of aging in humans, motor performance is the most significantly affected. As mentioned above, there are a number of neuropsychological tests which sample motor performance. In general, these are timed tasks such as the performance scale subtests of the WAIS. Speed of response can be tested by reaction time tests, both simple and choice. Tests designed to assess manual dexterity include finger tapping tests (Goldstein et al., 1973) and the Perdue Pegboard tests (Perdue Research Foundation, 1948). Normative scores need to be adjusted with increasing age in these timed tasks of motor performance.

Data primarily from cross-sectional studies have shown a moderate decrement of muscular strength (from 40 to 60 percent) and a decrement of 30 to 40 percent in upper-extremity- and manual-dexterity (Potvin et al., 1998; Faulkner et al., 1990). Changes in muscular tone are also noted to be mildly increased in the very aged, but this may be due more to changes in the musculoskeletal system than to changes in the peripheral or central nervous system (Jenkyn, 1985). However, evidence of rigidity or spasticity on neurological neuromuscular exam suggests an underlying pathological process.

Physical conditioning and practice appear to delay age-related decay in strength (Gersten, 1991). In fact, in a study of optimal aging, physical exercise was determined to be the number one key factor for successful healthy aging (Rowe & Kahn, 1998). Although optimal nutrition is required to maintain strength and muscle bulk, nutritional status alone does not seem to alter muscle composition or strength (McCarter & McGee, 1987). Although the sum total of changes described above is a slowing of activities, nonetheless, elderly individuals remain able to improve performance with practice to a degree equivalent to that of a younger comparison group. This principle, the so-called practice effect, is the theoretical basis for geriatric exercise groups and rehabilitation aimed at improving neuromuscular condition. This practice effect refers not only to strength and muscular conditioning but also to speed and accuracy of motor acts.

A number of pathological changes in the basal ganglia have been reported with advanced age (McGeer et al., 1997). As a function of aging there is an apparent reduction in the number of neurons in the substantia nigra. There is also a relative decrease in the amount of dopamine and in dopamine-synthesizing enzyme systems found in the basal ganglia (Cote & Kremzner, 1983). These described changes, added to changes in speed, muscular strength and endurance, and sensory decrements described in the next section, impair gait in a quite characteristic pattern in advanced age. These changes include slightly flexed posture in the upright position, slower forward progress with ambulation, shortened length of stride, decreases in clearance of the foot and heel from the ground, increased extra steps in turning, and increase in side-to-side sway. Ambulation remains quite functional and falling or extreme slowness are again indicative of a pathological condition, not normal aging.

Neurophysiological studies have shown slowing in both peripheral and central components associated with motor activity. It has been shown that nerve conduction velocities slow in motor and sensory nerves, but only to a mild degree (LaFratta & Canestrari, 1966). In an elegant neurophysiological study, Birren and Botwinick (1955) found a greater degree of decrease in the speed of central motor processing than in the speed of the peripheral component.

In summary, age-related slowing in all aspects of motor performance has been demonstrated. Performance deteriorates additively when simple motor skills are combined with other skills known to be vulnerable to the aging process. Hence, complex integrated motor tasks of ambulation are affected to a greater degree than simple reflex reaction time. Tasks which utilize greater cognitive processing and interpretation show a greater decline in the elderly than simple perceptual or motor tasks. Of note, however, is a positive practice effect for motor tasks, which is equal in both elderly and younger age groups. Thus, if one's definition of being old is "when he can't stand on one leg and pull on his pants" (Cowley, 1976) then one can postpone that by practicing putting on one's pants a leg at a time while standing.

SENSORY CHANGES

Somatosensory function is sensation coming from the skin and viscera; *kinesthesis* is information of movement coming from the muscles and joints. These senses are important for all tasks of mobility, ambulation, for internal homeostasis, and for overall well-being and function.

In the elderly there is a loss of receptors in the skin, of heavily myelinated nerve fibers, and of neurons in the spinal cord and parietal cortex. The largest and longest nerve fibers of the posterior columns, subserving vibration and position in the distal lower extremities, seem to be the most affected (Dorfman & Bosley, 1979). There is estimated to be a 30 to 50 percent loss of motor units in persons over the age of 60 years as determined by electrophysiological techniques (Brown et al., 1988). Latencies of sensory nerve conduction of the remaining motor units are also prolonged with age (Kimura, 1993), demonstrated by a loss of vibratory sensation of up to 60 percent in the lower extremities and up to 40 percent in the upper extremities (Potvin et al., 1980). Little change is found in touch sensation in the elderly. Diminished deep tendon reflex response, especially in the lower extremities and particularly at the ankle, is also seen clinically and is considered to be within the acceptable range of normal for the elderly.

The somatosensory system as described in the aged displays slight but real reductions in sensory function. These decrements in sensation, when compounded with complex motor actions, do interfere with some activities and occupational skills. The sensory functions, as opposed to the motor functions described above, have not been demonstrated to be responsive to repeated practice and exercise.

SUCCESSFUL AGING

As more studies are undertaken of aging, it is clear that such factors as disease, lifestyle choices, social factors, and social activities play a much larger role in healthy aging than previously appreciated. In a recently published study looking at the Swedish twin registry, McClearn et al. (1997), showed that there was a substantial genetic influence on the cognitive abilities of twins in old age; however, this genetic influence accounted for only 50 percent of the variance that was found. This leaves 50 percent of cognitive function attributable to things such as disease states, injuries, lifestyle choices, and other psychological and social factors. An earlier study by the same group estimated that genetic make-up accounted for only about 30 percent of the variance in physical functioning seen with aging (McClearn et al., 1994). As noted above, there is a real practice effect for motor abilities, an improvement in physical functioning that can be made with repeated exercise and activity. As also noted by the study of successful aging by Rowe and Kahn (1998), the absence of disease is also a major determinant of physical functioning.

What is becoming clearer is that cognitive functions also may well be responsive to a *practice effect*. One of the major findings of the recently published McArthur foundation study of successful aging notes that optimal cognitive functioning and otherwise successful aging were seen most often in those individuals who had a high degree of social connectedness and were actively engaged in productive activities (Rowe & Kahn, 1998). With what is being discovered about brain plasticity in health and in disease (Cohen et al., 1998), it appears that the brain is far more plastic, regenerative, and responsive to activities and experience than previously appreciated. Thus it would seem that successful aging is less an issue of choosing the right parents, with the optimal genetic make-up, than of committing to a healthy lifestyle of active physical and cognitive functioning.

REFERENCES

Alzheimer, A. (1907). Über eine eigenartige Erkrankung der Hirnrinde (Regarding an unusual disease of the cerebral cortex). *Allgemeine Zeitschrift für Psychiatrie, 64*, 146-148.
Baltes, P. B. (1993). The aging mind: Potential and limits. *Gerontologist, 33*, 580-594.
Birren, J. E. & Botwinich, J. (1955). Age differences in finger, jaw and foot reaction time to auditory stimuli. *Journal of Gerontology, 10*, 429-432.
Birren, J. E & Fisher, L. M. (1991). Aging and slowing of behavior: Consequences for cognition and survival. *Nebraska Symposium of Motivation, 39*, 1-37.
Bohannon, R. W. (1997). Comfortable and maximum walking of adults aged 20-79 years: Reference values and determinants. *Age and Aging, 26*, 15-19.
Boyle, P., Maisonneuve, P., Saracci, R., & Muir, C. S. (1990). Is the increased incidence of primary malignant brain tumors in the elderly real? *Journal of the National Cancer Institute, 82*, 1594-1596.

Brebion, G., Ehrlich, M. F., & Tardieu, H. (1995). Working memory in older subjects: Dealing with ongoing and stored information in language comprehension. *Psychological Research, 58*, 225-232.

Brown, W. F., Strong, M. J., & Snow, R. S. (1988). Methods for estimating numbers of motor units in biceps-brachialis muscles and loss of motor units with aging. *Muscle and Nerve, 11*, 423-432.

CDC: Center for Disease Control (1991). Mortality from Alzheimer's Disease-United States 1979-1987. *Journal of American Medical Association, 265*, 313-317.

Chancellor, A. M. & Warlow, C. P. (1992). Adult onset motor neuron disease: Worldwide mortality, incidence, and distribution since 1950. *Journal of Neurology, Neurosurgery and Psychiatry, 55*, 1106-1115.

Chao, L. L. & Knight R. T. (1997). Age-related prefrontal alterations during auditory memory. *Neurobiology of Aging, 18*, 87-95.

Clarke, C. E. (1993). Mortality from Parkinson's Disease in England and Wales 1921-1989. *Journal of Neurology, Neurosurgery and Psychiatry, 56*, 690-693.

Cohen, L. G., Ziemann, U., Chen, R., Claussen, J., Hallett, M., Gerloff, C., & Butefisch, C. (1998). Studies of neuroplasticity with transcranial magnetic stimulation. *Journal of Clinical Neurophysiology, 15*, 305-324.

Coffey, C. E., Wilkinson, W. E., Parashos, I. A., Soady, S. A. R., Sullivan, R. I., Patterson, L. J., Figiel, G. S., Webb, M. C., Spritzer, C. E., & Djang, W. T. (1992). Quantitative cerebral anatomy of the aging human brain: A cross-sectional study using magnetic resonance imaging, *Neurology, 42*, 527-536.

Cote, L. J. & Kremsner, L. T. (1983). Biochemical changes in normal aging in human brain. In R. Mayeux & W. G. Rosen (Eds.), *The dementias. Advances in neurology* (Vol. 38, pp. 19-30). New York: Raven.

Cowley, M. L. (1976). *The view from 80*. New York: Viking Press.

Critchley, M. (1932). The neurology of old age. *Lancet, 1*, 1119-1127, 1221-1230, 1331-1337.

DeSanti, S., deLeon, M. J., Convit, A., & Tarshish, C. (1995). Age-related changes in brain: II. Positron emission tomography of frontal and temporal lobe glucose metabolism in normal subjects. *Psychiatric Quarterly, 66*, 357-370.

Dorfman, L. J. & Bosley, T. M. (1979). Age-related changes on peripheral and central nerve conduction in man. *Neurology, 29*, 38-44.

Eisdorfer, C. & Wilker, F. (1973). Intellectual changes with advancing age. In L. F. Jarvik, C. Eisdorfer, & J. E. Blum (Eds.), *Intellectual functioning in adults* (pp. 21-29). New York: Springer Publishing.

Faulkner, J. A., Brooks, S. V., & Zerba, E. (1990). Skeletal muscle weakness and fatigue in old age: Underlying mechanisms. *Annual Review of Gerontology and Geriatrics, 10*, 147-166.

Furey, M. L., Pietrini, P., Haxby, J. V., Alexander, G. E., Lee, H. C., Van Meter, J., Grady, C. L, Sketty, U., Rappaport, S. I., Schapiro, M. B., & Freo, U. (1997). Cholinergic stimulation alters performance task-specific regional blood flow during working memory. *Proceedings of the National Academy of Science, 94*, 6512-6516.

Gerstein, J. W. (1991). Effect of exercise on muscle function decline with aging. *Western Journal of Medicine, 154*, 579-582.

Gilmore, R. (1995). Evoked potentials in the elderly. *Journal of Clinical Neurophysiology, 12*, 132-138.

Goldstein, S. G., Deysach, R. E., & Kleinknecht, R. A. (1973). Effect of experience and amount of information on identification of cerebral impairment. *Journal of Consulting and Clinical Psychology, 41*, 30-34.

Horn, J. L. & Cattell, R. B. (1967). Age differences in fluid and crystallized intelligence. *Acta Psychobiologica, 26*, 107-129.

Jenkyn, L. R., Reeves, A. G., Warren, T., Whiting, R. K., Clayton, R. J., Moore, W. W., Rizzo, A., Tuzan, I. M., Bonnett, J. C., & Culpepper, B. W. (1985). Neurologic signs in senescence. *Archives of Neurology, 42*, 1154-1157.

Jonker, C., Launer, L. J., Hooijer, C., & Lindeboom, J. (1996). Memory complaints and memory impairments in older individuals. *Journal of American Geriatric Society, 44*, 44-49.

Katzman, R. (1997). The aging brain, limitations on our knowledge and future approaches. *Archives of Neurology, 54*, 1201-1205.

Kaufman, A. S. & Horn, J. L. (1996). Age changes on tests of fluid and crystallized ability for women and men on the Kaufman Adolescent and Adult Intelligence Test (KAIT) at ages 17-94 years. *Archives of Clinical Neuropsychology, 11*, 97-121.

Keefover, R. W. (1998). Aging and cognition. In J. E. Riggs (Ed.), The neurology of aging. *Neurologic Clinics, 16*, 635-648.

Kimura, J. (1993). Nerve conduction studies and electromyography. In P. J. Dyck, P. K. Thomas, J. W. Griffin, P. A. Low, & J. F. Poduslo (Eds.), Peripheral neuropathies (3rd ed., pp. 598-644). Philadelphia: W. B. Saunders.

Knoefel, J. E. & Albert, M. L. (1990). Neurologic changes. In M. R. Katlic (Ed.), *Geriatric surgery* (pp. 153-172). Baltimore: Urban & Schwarzenberg.

LaRue, A., O'Hara, R., Matsuyama, S. S., & Jarvik, L. F. (1995). Cognitive changes in young-old adults: Effect of family history of dementia. *Journal of Clinical and Experimental Neuropsychology, 17*, 65-70.

McCarter, R. & McGee, J. (1987). Influence of nutrition and aging on the composition and function of rat skeletal muscle. *Journal of Gerontology, 42*, 432-441.

McClearn, G. E., Svartengren, M., Pedersen, N. L., Heller, D. A., & Plomin, R. (1994). Genetic and environmental influences on pulmonary function in aging Swedish twins. *Journal of Gerontology, 49*, M264-M268

McClearn, G. E., Johansson, B., Berg, S., Pedersen, N. L., Ahern, F., Petrill, S. A., & Plomin, R. (1997). Substantial genetic influence on cognitive abilities in twins 80 or more years old. *Science, 276*, 1522-1523.

McGeer, P. L., McGeer, E. G., & Suzuki, J. S. (1977). Aging and extrapyramidal function. *Archives of Neurology, 34*, 33-35.

Obler, L. K., Fein, D., Nicholas, M., & Albert, M. L. (1991). Auditory comprehension and aging: Decline in syntactic processing. *Journal of Applied Psycholinguistics, 12* (4), 433-452.

Olshansky, S. J., Carnes, B. A., & Cassel, C. K. (1993). The aging of the human species. *Scientific American, 268*, 6-52.

Potvin, A. R., Syndulko, K., Tourellotte, W. W., Lemmon, J. A., & Potvin, J. H. (1980). Human neurologic function and the aging process. *Journal of the American Geriatrics Society, 28*, 1-9.

Purdue Research Foundation (1948). Examiner's Manual for the Purdue Pegboard. Chicago: Science Research Associates.

Rice, D. M., Buchsbaum, M. S., Hardy, D., & Burgwald, L. (1991). Focal left temporal slow EEG activity is related to a verbal recent memory deficit in a non-demented elderly population. *Journal of Gerontology, 46*, P144-P151.

Riggs, J. E. (1996). Changing demographics and neurologic disease in the elderly. *Neurologic Clinics, 14*, 477-486

Rowe, J. W. & Kahn, R. L. (1998). *Successful aging*. New York: Pantheon Books.

Salthouse, T. A. (1996). The processing-speed theory of adult age differences in cognition. *Psychological Reviews, 103*, 403-428.

Sandson, J., Obler, L. K., & Albert, M. L. (1987). Language changes in healthy aging and dementia. In S. Rosenberg (Ed.), *Advances in applied psycholinguistics* (pp. 264-292). New York: Cambridge University Press.

Schofield, P. W., Marder, K., Dooneief, G., Jacobs, D. M., Sano, M., & Stern, Y. (1997). Association of subjective memory complaints with subsequent cognitive decline in community-dwelling elderly individuals with baseline cognitive impairment. *American Journal of Psychiatry, 154*, 609-615.

Shimoyama, I., Ninchoji, T., & Uemura, K. (1990). The finger tapping test: A quantitative analysis. *Archives of Neurology, 47*, 681-684.

Storandt, M. (1977). Age, ability level and method of administering and scoring the WAIS. *Journal of Gerontology, 32*, 175-186.

Index

A

abstract reasoning, 353
affect, 78, 233, 247, 252, 255, 362-363. *See also* emotion
age, 4, 7-9, 13, 15, 18, 56, 63, 77, 82, 126, 213, 215-217, 219-220, 224-226, 246, 327, 347-348, 352, 354, 381-387. *See also* aging, elderly
aggression, 153, 328, 337
aging, 204, 213-218, 220, 223, 225-226, 228-234, 347-348, 355, 381-387. *See also* age, elderly
agitation, 328, 331, 333-335
agraphia, 77-83, 85-88, 152, 270
alcoholism, 48, 213-221, 223-226, 228-234
alexia, 96, 105, 152, 269-270, 272, 274-275, 294, 299, 302, 363
Alois Alzheimer, 77
Alzheimer's disease (AD), 5, 11, 45-50, 54-57, 61-63, 72, 75, 77-79, 81-88, 149-151, 155, 166-168, 173, 259, 299-300, 327-341, 381-382
amnesia, 259, 261, 319, 321
amphetamine, 161
amyotrophic lateral sclerosis, 254, 381
aneurysm, 363
angular gyrus, 125, 223
anomia, 100, 150-151, 154, 160, 165-166, 170, 299, 302
anosognosia, 259-267, 271
anterior brain regions, 78, 118, 123, 135-136, 144-146, 154, 159-160, 162, 166, 194, 207-208, 216, 223, 227, 361-363, 371-372
antidepressants, 102, 337
antipsychotics, 336
anxiety, 102, 233, 328, 330-332, 336-337, 339, 340
aphasia, 86, 96, 100, 101, 103, 105, 110, 112, 116, 146, 149, 159, 160, 161, 162, 163, 167, 168, 170, 171, 173, 271, 299
    Broca's, 78, 87-88, 141-142, 149-152, 294
    fluent, 87-88
    primary progressive (PPA), 149-151, 153, 155
    semantic, 167
    severity, 99-104, 111, 120, 161, 167, 335, 365
    transcortical motor aphasia, 96, 102, 162-163, 207-208
    transcortical sensory aphasia, 151
    Wernicke's, 78, 87-88, 137, 141, 144-146, 149-152, 165, 171, 259
apraxia, 150-151, 153, 259
assessment, 347-349, 351, 353-355, 359-361, 372, 377
atrophy, 153-155, 214-215, 217-218, 226, 254, 299-300, 302-304, 382
attention, 9, 28, 78, 85, 87, 100-101, 161, 165-166, 170, 179-180, 193-196, 203-208, 214, 221-222, 224-225, 227-228, 230, 233, 252, 266-267, 302, 304, 316, 318, 320, 350, 360, 362, 364, 368, 371-372, 377, 383. *See also* concentration
attitude, 23-24, 27-28, 30, 32-33, 36, 38-40, 354

automaticity, 299

B

Babinski, 259-260
basal ganglia, 97, 152, 154, 159, 165, 254, 361, 385
behavioral rating scales, 332, 335
bifemelane, 167-168
bilingualism, 352
Block design, 220, 222, 226-227, 300
Boston Assessment of Severe Aphasia exam (BASA), 118-120, 127, 134-137
Boston Diagnostic Aphasia Examination (BDAE), 86, 99, 103-104, 301
Boston Naming Test (BNT), 99, 301
brain imaging. *See* imaging
Broca, 150-151
Broca's aphasia, 78, 141-145, 150-151, 203, 294
Broca's area, 121, 124-125, 135, 141, 146, 160, 165
bromocriptine, 96, 102, 159, 161-163, 165, 173, 194-196, 207
buffer, 46, 57
    graphemic, 80, 85

C

caffeine, 161
canonical forms, 65, 203, 205, 243
caudate, 124, 135, 159
cerebellum, 216
cholinergic system
    agents, 167-168, 170, 336, 339
cholinergic system, 166, 168-169, 171
    agents, 166
    therapy, 338
cingulate gyrus, 217, 252
circumlocution, 100
closed head injury, 363
closed-class words, 202, 269-272, 274, 276-277, 279-282, 285-288, 292, 294
cloze procedure, 11-13, 23
cognition, 4-5, 7-10, 17, 26-27, 32-33, 38-40, 46, 56, 62, 78, 87, 97-102, 105-106, 150, 161, 165-166, 168, 170, 173, 179-180, 182-185, 188, 191, 193-197, 201-202, 204-205, 208, 213-221, 223-225, 227-234, 247, 251, 255-256, 302, 304, 316, 320, 328-331, 334-338, 340-341, 348-351, 354, 360, 363, 366, 371, 376-377, 382-387
Cognitive Abilities Screening Instrument (CASI), 349-350
cognitive flexibility, 25-27, 33, 39
communication, 23-24, 61, 101, 111, 114, 118, 122, 125, 134-135, 137, 162-163, 214, 217, 259

Community Screening Instrument for Dementia (CSI'D), 350-351
comprehension, 3-4, 7, 10, 17, 23-25, 27-30, 40, 48-49, 52, 54, 56, 61, 63-64, 67, 72, 77, 79, 150-151, 153, 242, 245, 249-250, 255, 304
concentration, 101, 194, 349. *See also* attention
confabulation, 264
confrontation naming, 104, 206
confusional states, 78, 261
connectionism, 79
construction abilities, 328
content, 13, 15, 61-62, 67, 75, 77, 86, 244-245, 248-249, 255, 318, 320, 322, 353
content words, 78. *See* substantives
continuous performance, 364, 368, 370
converging evidence, 182-183, 196-197
corpus callosum, 217, 226, 228
cortex, 47, 77-78, 152, 154, 247, 251-252, 254-256, 299-300, 302
corticobasal degeneration (CBD), 153, 155
Creutzfeldt-Jakob disease, 154, 299
cross-cultural issues, 347, 349, 351, 355
cross-sectional study, 335, 382, 384-385
cued recall, 384
cueing, 96, 104-105, 138

D

d-amphetamine, 162
deblocking, 105
deep dyslexia, 270, 272, 274, 285-289, 291-294
delayed recall, 365, 372, 374, 376
dementia. *See* Alzheimer's disease, Lewy body dementia, Parkinson's disease
denial, 260-261
dependency relations, 143
depression, 153, 252, 327-329, 333-334, 336-337, 339
diaschisis, 96, 98, 196
digit span, 6, 8, 49, 53-54, 56-57, 87, 167-168, 300, 353, 364-365, 370-371
digit symbol task, 218, 220
disconnection, 264
discourse, 4, 78, 85, 87
disinhibition, 96, 98, 101, 106, 150, 252-254, 330-331, 337, 339-340
dopamine, 4, 159, 161, 164, 194-196, 201, 204-208
Down's syndrome, 328
dual route model, 46, 57
dual-task studies, 10
Ducarne Aphasia Battery, 271

E

education, 24, 348, 350, 352-354
EEG, 159, 167, 341, 382
elderly, 3-5, 7-13, 15-18, 57, 64, 82-83, 86, 348-351. *See also* age, aging
emotion, 153, 213, 230, 232-233, 246-247, 251-252, 259
encoding, 3, 4, 11, 318
ephedrine, 161-162
epidemiology, 349
episodic memory, 77, 150, 315, 320-322
estimation, 62, 315-322
event-related brain potentials (ERP), 227, 229-231
exception words, 80-82. *See also* irregular words
executive function, 9, 100-101, 179-180, 182-183, 194, 196-197, 204, 206, 218, 301-302, 327, 360, 362, 368, 372, 377, 383-384
extrapyramidal symptoms, 153

F

face processing, 231-233
finger tapping, 364, 368
fluency, 45, 47, 151, 202, 204, 206-208, 349
fluent aphasia, 87-88, 149-150, 154
fMRI. *See* functional MRI. *See also* imaging.
free recall, 384
frequency, 6, 45, 47, 56, 63, 81-82, 86, 152, 276
frontal lobes, 150-151, 153-154, 163, 165, 179, 201, 207, 214-215, 217-218, 221, 223, 226-228, 231, 233, 247, 250, 253, 255, 304, 315-316, 321-322, 338-339, 362, 368
frontal operculum, 125
frontotemporal dementia (FTD), 150-151, 155
function words, 87, 273, 275. *See also* closed-class words
functional MRI (fMRI), 180, 182, 184-185, 187-188, 191, 193, 196, 227

G

gait, 201, 386
galanthamine, 166
gap (syntactic), 143-145
gating paradigm, 10
gender, 48, 215
genetic factors, 154
Geschwind-Galaburda Questionnaire, 28, 35
global-local tasks, 225
grammatical reasoning, 364, 370, 372, 376

H

haloperiodol, 207
hand-eye coordination, 364, 368
Hasegawa Dementia Screening Scale, 349
head trauma, 328, 335
hearing loss, 5
hemianopia, 299-300, 302
hemiplegia, 259-262, 264-267
hippocampus, 3-4, 166, 170, 201, 216, 218, 252
horizontal addition, 365, 370, 372
Hughlings Jackson, 103, 165
humor, 241-253, 255-256

I

imaging, 83, 153-154, 300, 304. *See also* functional MRI, MRI
imipramine, 102, 161, 338
Informant Questionnaire on Cognitive Decline in the Elderly (IQCODE), 351
initiation
    limbic, 135
    of speech, 96, 124, 159-163, 165-166, 170-171, 206, 208
intelligence, 95, 100, 179, 361, 383
intonation, 105
irregular words, 81-82, 152, 291, 293. *See also* exception words

J

jargon aphasia, 171

K

Korsakoff's syndrome, 215, 259, 315-316, 319-322

L

language, 4, 7, 10, 17-18, 23-30, 32-33, 35-40, 45-47, 49, 56, 61, 63, 75, 77-79, 84-87, 100, 103, 141, 145, 149-151, 153, 155, 161, 163, 167-168, 171-172, 204-205, 264, 301-302, 348-350, 352-354
laterality, 219, 228, 233, 363, 371
L-dopa, 161-162
learning, 300, 328, 360, 362, 364-365, 372, 377
left hand, 219
left hemisphere, 214, 217, 220, 222-225, 227-228, 230, 233-234, 249, 251, 254-255, 260-262, 264-267, 304, 361, 363, 368, 371-372, 376-377
    left-hemisphere damage (LHD), 246, 249-250, 252, 266

left-hemisphere, 78, 88
length effect, 275
lesion size, 125, 129, 134
Lewy bodies, 337
Lewy body dementia, 341
lexicon, 11, 47, 80, 84. *See also* naming
limbic system, 77, 247, 252, 255, 338
literal alexia, 269
longitudinal study, 62, 81, 332, 335, 382

M

matched-guise procedure, 23
maze learning, 230
Melodic Intonation Therapy, 97, 105
memory, 3-6, 8, 13, 56, 61-62, 64, 67, 77, 79-80, 100-102, 104, 150, 152-153,
    154-155, 159, 165-166, 168, 170-171, 184-185, 203, 216, 219, 227, 229-230,
    292-293, 299-300, 302, 315-323, 327-328, 350, 360, 362, 371-372, 376-377, 383
    episodic, 77, 150, 315, 320-322, 384
    explicit, 218, 230, 232, 384
    immediate, 360, 371
    implicit, 230, 384
    long-term, 213, 219, 231-232, 234, 349, 384
    pattern, 365, 374, 376, 383
    primary, 384
    procedural, 230
    recognition, 10-11, 13, 25, 46, 105, 112-113, 218, 232-233, 263, 265, 376, 381,
        383-384
    remote, 222
    semantic, 47, 56, 61, 384
    short-term, 7, 45, 48-49, 54, 56-57, 231, 349, 383-384
    spatial, 180
    verbal, 180
    working, 4-5, 7-10, 72, 75, 80, 85, 170, 182-185, 188, 190-197, 204, 206, 208,
        221, 231, 318, 384
mental imagery, 223
mental rotation, 223
mesencephalon, 167
mesocortical system, 159-160, 163, 165, 201, 205-206
mesolimbic system, 159-160
Mini-Mental State Examination (MMSE), 48, 51, 56, 330-331, 348-349, 352, 363,
    366, 371
modularity, 79
mood disorders, 362

motor processes, 78, 80, 96, 102, 104-105, 118, 124, 129, 150-153, 155, 159-160, 162-163, 165-166, 171, 179, 183-186, 193-196, 201-202, 205, 207-208, 219-221, 234, 247, 254, 256, 265-266, 328, 331, 336, 339-340, 360, 363-364, 368, 377, 383, 385-387
MRI, 217-218. *See* also fMRI
multiple sclerosis, 254, 361
music, 220, 231
mutism, 149, 151

N

naming, 45, 47, 57, 63, 77, 79, 81, 84, 86, 88, 97-98, 100, 102-104, 125, 137, 161-162, 166-168, 170, 206, 269, 271, 289, 302, 305-312, 328, 353, 377, 385. *See also* lexicon
    colors, 305-312
narrative, 62, 84, 86-88, 248-249
neglect, 262
neologisms, 86, 100
neurofibrillary tangles, 328
neuroimaging. *See* imaging
neuropathology, 154
neuropsychological tests, 197, 352, 354
neurotransmitters, 4, 159, 165-166, 170-173, 194, 201, 215
    acetylcholine, 101, 165-168, 170, 215, 328, 338
    dopamine, 102, 159-161, 163, 165, 170-171, 194, 215, 386
    gamma-aminobutyric acid, 328
    glutamate, 328
    norepinephrine, 328, 338
    serotonin, 328, 338
    somatostatin, 328
neurovegetative disturbances, 331
nonverbal aphasic patients, 122, 137-138
nonverbal communication, 117, 134, 137

O

object assembly, 222
occipital lobe, 217, 223, 227-228, 300, 302
occupation, 352
open-class words, 269-270, 285. *See also* substantives
organization, 86
orientation, 45, 302, 319, 349
outcome, 117-118, 121, 124-125, 131-137

P

paired-associate learning, 221, 364, 374

paralexias
    formal paralexias, 277-279, 285-286, 288
    verbal paralexias, 269-270, 275, 278-281, 292-293
paralimbic structures, 339
parallel distributed processing, 79
paranoia, 328
paraphasias, 78, 102, 151, 170-171, 259, 271
parietal lobe, 78, 87, 129, 136, 153-154, 166, 170, 181, 188, 207, 214, 217, 222-224, 226-228, 252, 299, 328, 362, 376, 386
Parkinson's disease (PD), 96, 160, 182, 194, 201-208, 361, 381
parkinsonism, 336-337
pattern
    memory, 365, 374, 376
    perception, 225
    recognition, 365, 372-373
peripheral impairments, 88
perisylvian areas, 125
perseveration, 85-86, 99, 104, 138, 170, 301, 322
personality changes, 328, 330
PFC. *See* prefrontal cortex
phantom movements, 263
pharmacology. *See names of specific medications*
phonological dyslexia, 289
phonology, 27, 32, 38, 45-47, 57, 62, 72, 79-81, 83, 88, 97, 100, 151-152, 168, 289, 293-294, 312
physostigmine, 166-167, 338-339
Pick complex, 150
Pick's disease (PiD), 149-151, 153, 155
picturability, 276
picture description, 62, 86-87
Pierre-Marie's three-papers test, 272
piracetam, 102, 167
plaques, 328
pontine region, 254
Porch Index of Communicative Ability (PICA), 121, 162
Positron Emission Tomography (PET), 137, 153, 168, 217, 227, 382, 384
posterior areas, 217, 223, 227-228, 231-232
posterior lesion, 362, 368, 371-372
praxis, 78, 87
predictability, 14-16, 81, 255
prefrontal cortex, 4, 179, 181-182, 185, 188-189, 191-192, 194-197, 206, 247, 250, 253, 255, 316, 322

presbycusis, 5
process approach, 98-99, 106, 221
processing modes, 214-215, 219, 221-222, 224-234
propositional content, 61-63, 67, 75, 103
pseudowords, 46-47, 49, 54-57, 79-81, 83
psychosis, 329
putamen, 159

Q

quality of life, 341

R

rate
    heart, 241
    presentation, 13
    processing, 10, 319
    speech, 7, 15, 17
    time passing, 316
rating, 244
reaction time, 194, 266, 364, 383, 385-386
reading, 45, 47, 77, 102, 105, 109, 111, 114, 161, 166, 168, 269, 270-274, 276, 282-283, 285-289, 291-294, 299-301, 304-312, 317-318, 363
recall, 5, 8, 10, 13, 15-17, 300, 353
registration, 384
regularization, 80, 82
rehabilitation, 95-96, 98, 101, 103, 105-106, 109, 138, 259, 385
rehearsal, 72, 188
repetition, 45-50, 54-57, 77, 86, 102, 125, 138, 144-145, 151, 161, 168, 271, 353.
    See also perseveration
restitution, 97, 105
retrieval, 15, 84, 188, 301, 311, 318, 320, 362
right hemisphere, 97, 105, 125, 136-137, 214, 217, 219-220, 222-228, 231, 233-234, 248, 250-252, 255, 260-264, 266-267, 271, 361, 368, 371-372, 376-377
    right-hemisphere damage (RHD), 248-249, 250-253

S

scanning, 221
scopolamine, 166, 168
semantics, 45-47, 56, 61-63, 75, 77, 79-80, 83-84, 86, 87, 97, 99-100, 104-105, 135, 137-138, 141-146, 149-152, 159, 165-167, 170, 232, 243-244, 270, 272-273, 277-289, 291-293, 300, 316
sensory processing, 196, 219-220, 229-230, 234, 386
sentence completion, 84

sentence construction tasks, 62
serial digit learning, 365, 370-371
set-shifting, 206
severity, 47-48, 51, 54, 56, 62-63, 82, 86-88, 117-118, 120-122, 129, 137, 302
short-term memory, 7, 45, 48-49, 54, 56-57, 231, 349, 383-384
Single Photon Emission Computerized Tomography (SPECT), 154, 300, 302, 304
sleep, 328, 331
socioeconomic status, 352
sodium amytal, 102, 161
Spanish and English Neuropsychology Assessment Scale (SENAS), 351, 353
spatial phenomena, 5, 9, 45, 78, 153-154, 180-181, 183, 185, 188, 190-194, 214, 217-225, 227-231, 233-234, 252, 262, 266-267, 302, 350. *See also* visual processing
speed, 105, 195, 221-222, 299, 305, 307-308, 311-312, 350, 353, 362, 364, 376-377, 383, 385-386
spelling, 79-86, 88, 301. *See also* exception words, irregular words
stereotypic
    behaviors, 150, 331
    expressions, 103
striatonigral region, 159-160
striatum, 160, 165, 195, 201, 207
stroke, 102-103, 109-110, 112, 114, 117-120, 125-127, 132-133, 137, 149, 151-152, 161-162, 168, 220, 248-249, 252, 254, 259-362, 376
Stroop effect, 304-305, 307-308, 311-312
subcortical areas, 3, 97, 118, 123-124, 130, 155, 171, 201, 216, 233, 251-252, 254-255, 299, 361
substantia nigra, 159, 165, 201, 385
subtraction, 184-185, 191, 193, 196
supplementary motor area (SMA), 118, 124, 129-133, 135, 159-160, 163, 165, 171, 208
supramarginal gyrus, 125
surface dyslexia, 291
syntax, 45, 61-64, 67, 75, 77, 86-87, 141-142, 150-151

T

tacrine, 167-168, 335, 338-339
Taussig Cross-Cultural Memory Test, 351
tegmental region, 165
temporal lobe, 3-4, 15, 87, 97, 118, 123-124, 126, 130-133, 135, 144-145, 153-154, 160, 165-166, 168, 170-171, 181, 188, 217, 223, 227, 273, 317, 319, 328, 330, 338-339, 341, 362, 368, 371-372, 376, 382
thalamus, 97, 160
The Cross-Cultural Cognitive Examination (CCCE), 350
theory of mind, 250

therapy, 95-98, 100-106, 112-113, 134, 137, 160, 162, 206, 273-274, 340. *See also* treatment
time, 64, 67, 72, 84, 152, 266, 305-308, 310-312, 315-322
toxicants, 213, 216, 359, 376
traces, 142
traumatic brain injury (TBI), 182, 196, 254
treatment, 117, 119-120. *See also* therapy
Treatment of Aphasic Perseveration (TAP), 104-105
tumors, 254, 363, 381

V

vigilance, 368, 371
visual fields, 224-225
visuoperceptual error, 100
visuospatial processing, 45, 78, 100-101, 153-154, 168, 195, 214, 217-220, 222, 224, 227-231, 233-234, 327, 360, 362, 368, 371-372, 376-377. *See also* spatial phenomena
vocabulary, 8, 15, 86, 300, 365, 372-373
Voluntary Control of Involuntary Utterances (VCIU), 103-104

W

Wada test, 261
Wechsler Adult Intelligence Scale
    WAIS, 214, 218, 220, 222, 226, 300, 363, 366-368, 383-385
    WAIS-R, 218, 220, 222, 226, 300, 363, 366-368
Wechsler Memory Scale (WMS), 218
Wechsler Memory Scale-Revised (WMS-R), 101, 300-301
Wernicke's area, 121, 123, 126, 130, 135, 143-145, 160, 165, 168, 171
Western Aphasia Battery, 149
Wisconsin Card Sorting Test (WCST), 26, 32, 34, 101, 168, 322, 348
word
    class effect, 275
    discrimination, 99
word-finding, 95, 102, 163, 165-166, 168, 170, 202, 271, 300, 302
working memory, 4-5, 7-10, 72, 75, 80, 85, 170, 182-185, 188, 190-197, 204, 206, 208, 221, 231, 318, 384
writing, 45-47, 62, 77-88, 95, 102-103, 109, 111, 114, 117, 120, 151, 161, 168, 272, 281, 294, 301-302, 318